BRADY

BASIC FIRST RESPONSE

GRANT B. GOOLD, MPA/HSA, EMT-P
SCOTT VAHRADIAN, EMT-P

Contributors:
Lisa Dubnoff, EMT-P
David Zenker, EMT-P

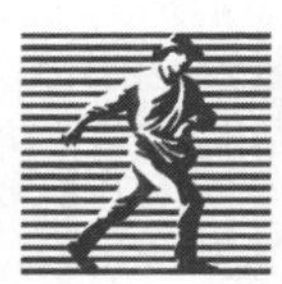

BRADY
PRENTICE HALL
UPPER SADDLE RIVER, NEW JERSEY 07458

Library of Congress Cataloging-in-Publication Data
Goold, Grant B.
Basic first response / Grant B. Goold, Scott Vahradian; contributors, Lisa Dubnoff, David Zenker.
P. cm.
Includes index.
ISBN 0-8359-4914-1
1. Medical emergencies. 2. Emergency medical technicians. I. Vahradian, Scott. II. Dubnoff, Lisa. III. Zenker, David. IV. Title.
RC86.7.G665 1997 96-22141
616.02'5—dc20 CIP

Publisher: Susan Katz
Editorial Assistant: Carol Sobel
Managing Development Editor: Lois Berlowitz
Project Editor: Josephine Cepeda
Editorial/Production Supervision: Janet McGillicuddy
Managing Production Editor: Patrick Walsh
Director of Production/Manufacturing: Bruce Johnson
Page Make-up: KR Publishing Services
Creative Director: Marianne Frasco
Interior Design: Claudia Durell
Photography Consultant: Michael Heron
Cover Photo: Marc Longwood, Inc.
Cover Design: Bruce Kenselaar
Prepress/Manufacturing Buyer: Ilene Sanford

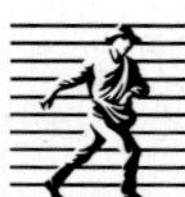

Printed in the United States of America

10 9 8 7 6 5 4 3 2 1

ISBN 0-8359-4914-1

Prentice-Hall International (UK) Limited, *London*
Prentice-Hall of Australia Pty. Limited, *Sydney*
Prentice-Hall Canada Inc., *Toronto*
Prentice-Hall Hispanoamericana, S.A., *Mexico*
Prentice-Hall of India Private Limited, *New Delhi*
Prentice-Hall of Japan, *Tokyo*
Simon & Schuster Asia Pte. Ltd., *Singapore*
Editora Prentice-Hall do Brasil, Ltda., *Rio de Janeiro*

Notice: The authors and the publisher of this book have taken care to make certain that the equipment and schedules of treatment are correct and compatible with the standards generally accepted at the time of publication. Nevertheless, as new information becomes available, changes in treatment and in the use of equipment and procedures become necessary. The reader is advised to carefully consult the instruction and information material included in each piece of equipment or device before administration. First Responders are warned that the use of any techniques must be authorized by their medical director, where appropriate, in accord with local laws and regulations. The publisher disclaims any liability, loss, injury, or damage incurred as a consequence, directly or indirectly, of the use and application of any of the contents of this book.

Photo Credits:
All photography by Marc Longwood except figure numbers as noted below:

Robert J. Bennett:	8-1a
Michael Gallitelli:	24-1, 29-4
Richard Logan:	A1-8b, A1-9b
Charles Stewart, M.D.:	28-3a, 28-3b, 28-3c, 29-2b, 29-2c, 29-10a, 29-10b, 29-10c

Photography Assistance: The authors also wish to express their appreciation to the following organizations and individuals for invaluable assistance in the photography program for this book:

Seth Johnson, Michael Goold, Sacramento County Sheriff's Department, John Arribit, California Highway Patrol, Gary Kilbourne—Butler's Uniforms, Adam Carlson—Pro Med, Shelley & Renee Goold—Shelley's Catering Service, Sacramento County Fire Protection District, Sacramento County Fire Communications, Mercy San Juan Hospital, American River College—Paramedic and EMT Students, '95 & '96.

CONTENTS

SECTION 3 FIRST RESPONDER EMERGENCY CARE PLANS

PREFACE

Welcome to *Basic First Response*. As a First Responder you'll represent the first critical link between a patient's injury or illness and the care provided by other EMS professionals. We've written this book to provide you with the skills you'll need to take care of sick and injured people on the streets of your home town, in your workplace, your schools, your restaurants, your parks.

When we conceived of *Basic First Response*, it was extremely important to us that we communicated "need to know" information in a form that you could actually use out in the field. We wanted to provide you with a road map to help you negotiate the EMS terrain out there in the real world with real patients. We realized that this meant we'd need to present material that outlined specific strategies for managing patients, not merely laundry lists of tasks to perform. We believe that we've accomplished this.

CONTENT AND ORGANIZATION

Your book is divided into three sections. All three comply with the 1995 U.S. Department of Transportation, National Highway Traffic Safety Administration, "First Responder: National Standard Curriculum."

- **Section 1: First Responder Preparation.** Section 1 sets the foundation for the rest of the book. The first three chapters provide an overview of the EMS system, the well being of the First Responder, and legal issues. By the time you complete these three chapters, you'll understand the structure and function of EMS systems. You'll have a good grasp of the legal rules of the road. You'll also understand how the stress of EMS can affect you, and you'll learn strategies to help you handle that stress. The second part of Section 1 sets the foundation for patient care by introducing the human anatomy, body substance isolation (BSI), and lifting and moving. The last chapter of Section 1, "Patient Management Strategies," is the heart of this section. It sets forth our strategies for communicating effectively with patients and introduces our five-step approach to patient management.

- **Section 2: First Responder Skills.** Section 2 takes the five-step approach to patient management and breaks it down into its component parts. This section contains all the basic skills you'll need to work as a First Responder. We present these skills sequentially, as you would use them when you run a call, from scene size-up to patient hand-off. You'll learn about assessing and treating threats to your patient's airway, breathing, and circulation. You'll learn how to perform patient histories and physical exams that will guide your treatment strategies. You'll also learn how to tie all of these "pieces of a call" into a unified whole.

- **Section 3: First Responder Emergency Care Plans.** Section 3 takes all of the skills you learned in Section 2 and applies them to common medical and trauma emergencies. Each chapter provides you with important background on an illness or injury, which is followed by a specific "Emergency Care Plan" that applies our five-step approach to patient management. By the time you complete Section 3, you'll have the tools necessary to manage a wide variety of patients using an organized, systematic approach.

We've also included an appendix to your text that will introduce you to defibrillation and automatic external defibrillators (AEDs). We've placed this topic at the back of the book since First Responder courses don't routinely teach it. We believe that all First Responders ought to be trained to use AEDs. We also understand that most First Responder courses have neither the time nor the resources to include this as a standard curriculum topic.

ICONS

In Chapter 7 and then throughout the rest of this book, you'll notice the use of five symbols or icons. These symbols are used exclusively to strengthen your ability to recall material during actual emergencies. While simple, these symbols will combine with written explanations to increase your recall by as much as 40%. Recent research using content similar to *Basic First Response* has demonstrated the effectiveness of this "dual-coding" theory. We encourage you to give this proven technique a try. We are confident that you'll be impressed with your results.

FIRST RESPONDER CERTIFICATION

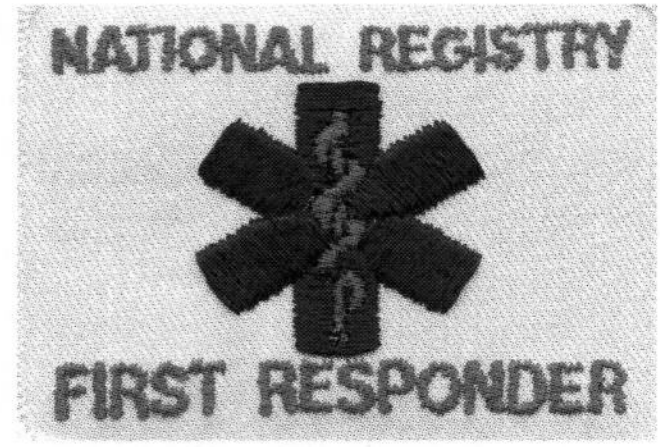

In 1970, the National Registry of Emergency Medical Technicians was formed to help promote and improve the delivery of emergency medical services across the nation. The National Registry has established a process to certify First Responders nationally. For information on entry requirements and registration procedures contact:

The National Registry of EMTs
6610 Busch Blvd.
Columbus, Ohio 43229
Phone 614-888-4484

A FINAL NOTE

You're beginning an educational process that will give you the tools to manage patients suffering all manner of medical and trauma emergencies. This increase in your training brings with it an increase in responsibility. Read each chapter of this textbook carefully. Actively participate in your First Responder course. Ask questions in class. Practice the steps in the "Emergency Care Plans."

As a First Responder you have the potential to become one of your local EMS system's greatest assets. Good luck!

Grant Goold
Scott Vahradian

Visit Brady's Web Site

http://www.bradybooks.com

ACKNOWLEDGMENTS

OUR CONTRIBUTORS

Our thanks to Lisa Dubnoff and David Zenker, who were an important part of the textbook development process. Lisa is a Firefighter-Paramedic at the Benicia Fire Department, Benicia, California. David is a Paramedic and Coordinator, Clinical and Education Services at American Medical Response West, San Jose, California.

REVIEWERS

Susan Barnes, RN, MEd., EMT-P
EMS Education Coordinator
State of Ohio
Columbus, Ohio

J. David Barrick, BS, NREMT-P
Chief-EMS
Newport News Fire Department
Newport News, Virginia

Brenda J. Beasley, RN, BS, EMT-P
Program Director, EMS Program
Southern Union State Community College
Opelika, Alabama

Michael D. Berg, NREMT-P
EMS Education Coordinator
Tidewater Emergency Medical Services Council, Inc.
Tidewater, Virginia

Liza K. Burrill
State of New Hampshire Training Coordinator
Northern NH EMS
Berlin, New Hampshire

Kerry Campbell, NREMT-P
Lakeshore Technical College
Cleveland, Wisconsin

Sandie Colbert, EMT-I, SEI
Yakima County Department of EMS
Yakima, Washington

Janet E. Crum, MA, EMT-A
Rescue Chief, Union Fire & Rescue
Titusville, New Jersey

Mike Helbock
Senior Firefighter, Paramedic
Bellevue, Washington
President, EMT-C

Sammy W. Hukkanen
Paramedic Captain
Kelseyville Fire Protection District
Kelseyville, California

Gerald W. Otto
EMS Coordinator
Willmar Technical College
Willmar, Minnesota

Jerry Reichel, EMT-P, EMSI/C
General Manager
Emergency Consultants, Inc.
West Columbia, Texas

Lisa Shelanskas, EMS-I, EMT-I/D
Suffield Volunteer Ambulance
Suffield, Connecticut

Carole Sloan, MEd., B-EMT, IC
Henry Ford Community College
Faculty, Health & Physical Education
Dearborn, Michigan

Craig Story, EMT-P
EMS Program Director
Polk Community College
Winter Haven, Florida

Richard Weigele, MPA, MICP
Coordinator, First Responder Program
John H. Stamler Police Academy
Scotch Plains, New Jersey

Joe Welsh, Medical Officer
Louisville Gas & Electric Co.
Emergency Response Team
Louisville, Kentucky

Brian J. Wilson, NREMT-P
Education Coordinator
Texas Technical University
El Paso, Texas

Chief Robert J. Wesche
Monroe Police Department
Monroe, Connecticut

PERSONAL ACKNOWLEDGMENTS

I would like to thank the following individuals for their efforts during this project:

Jo Cepeda, for your expertise, guidance, and unbelievable patience. I have come to better realize that behind many a successful author is a skilled editor. You are unconditionally the best.

To my wife, for her constant flexibility and understanding. As a partner, you provide the support and encouragement one hopes for. Thank you for raising our children wonderfully.

DEDICATION

I dedicate this work to my parents, Jay and Carol Goold. Their loving support is greatly treasured. My life is better because of your years of hard work and sacrifice. I am truly blessed.

—Grant Goold

DEDICATION

I dedicate this book to my family, as well as to all those EMS responders who daily take care of sick and injured people in the field.

—Scott Vahradian

First Responder: National Standard Curriculum Instructor's Lesson Plans

*CORRELATION OF 1995 U.S. DOT "FIRST RESPONDER: NATIONAL STANDARD CURRICULUM" WITH **BASIC FIRST RESPONSE***

National Standard Curriculum Instructor's Course Guide Modules	***BASIC FIRST RESPONSE*** Chapters	
MODULE 1: PREPARATORY	1	The EMS System and the First Responder
	2	The Well Being of the First Responder
	3	Legal and Ethical Issues for the First Responder
	4	The Human Body
	5	Body Substance Isolation (BSI)
	6	Lifting and Moving
	7	Patient Managemetn Strategies
	8	Scene Size-up
MODULE 2: AIRWAY	10	Airway and Breathing Management
MODULE 3; PATIENT ASSESSMENT	8	Scene Size-up
	9	Overview of Initial Assessment
	13	The Physical Exam
	14	Ongoing Assessment
	15	Patient Hand-off
MODULE 4: CIRCULATION	11	Circulation and CPR
	12	Shock and Bleeding Control
MODULE 5: ILLNESS AND INJURE	12	Shock and Bleeding Control
	16	Overview of Managing Medical Patients
	17	Chest Pain
	18	Shortness of Breath
	19	Altered Mental Status
	20	Abdominal Pain
	21	Poisoning and Overdose
	22	Allergic Reactions
	23	Environmental Emergencies
	25	Behavioral Emergencies
	26	Overview to Managing Trauma Patients
	27	Injuries to the Head and Spine
	28	Muscle and Bone Injuries
	29	Soft-Tissue Injuries
MODULE 6: CHILDBIRTH AND CHILDREN	24	Childbirth
	30	Infants and Children
MODULE 7: EMS OPERATIONS	7	Patient Management Strategies
	8	Scene Size-up

SECTION 1 FIRST RESPONDER PREPARATION

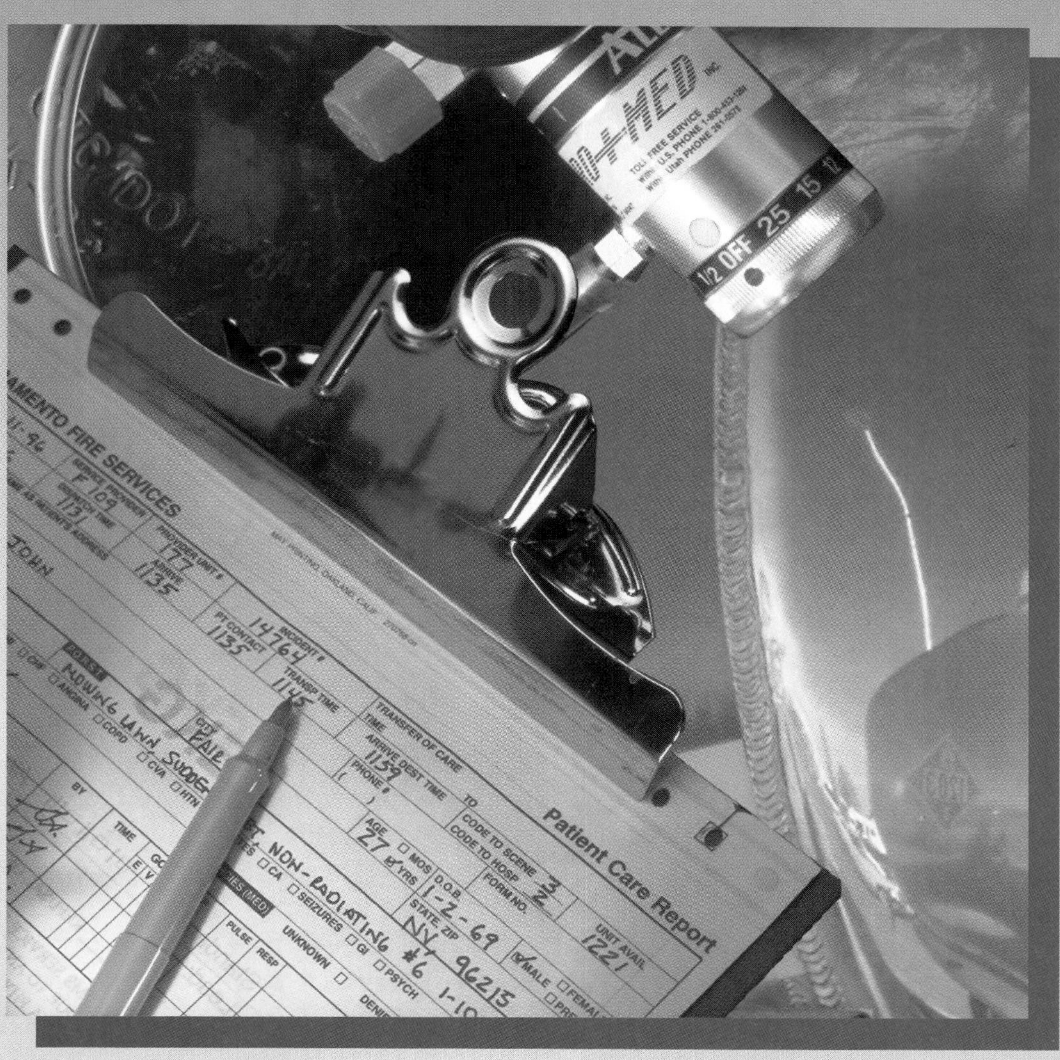

What is EMS? Do I have what it takes to be a good First Responder? What must I learn to be able to do a good job? Section 1 is meant to help you find the answers to questions like these. You'll be introduced to the basic parts of the EMS system. You'll read about important legal issues that'll affect how you handle yourself in the field. You'll learn some basic anatomy and physiology, strategies for protecting yourself against contagious diseases, and methods of lifting and moving equipment and patients safely. The final chapter of this section will introduce a step-by-step plan for managing patients that will be used throughout this book.

CHAPTER 1

THE EMS SYSTEM AND THE FIRST RESPONDER

FIRST RESPONSE

Trish and Bob are First Responders, part of the emergency response team at a large industrial park. According to EMS dispatch, a male worker fell from a scaffold. A bystander is providing rescue breathing.

As Trish and Bob approach the scene, they put on latex gloves. Bob looks around for hazards and for other victims. Trish focuses her attention on the fallen worker. The moment they get to the patient, Trish moves to hold his head and neck. Bob performs an initial assessment that reveals a pulse but no breathing. He immediately takes over rescue breathing.

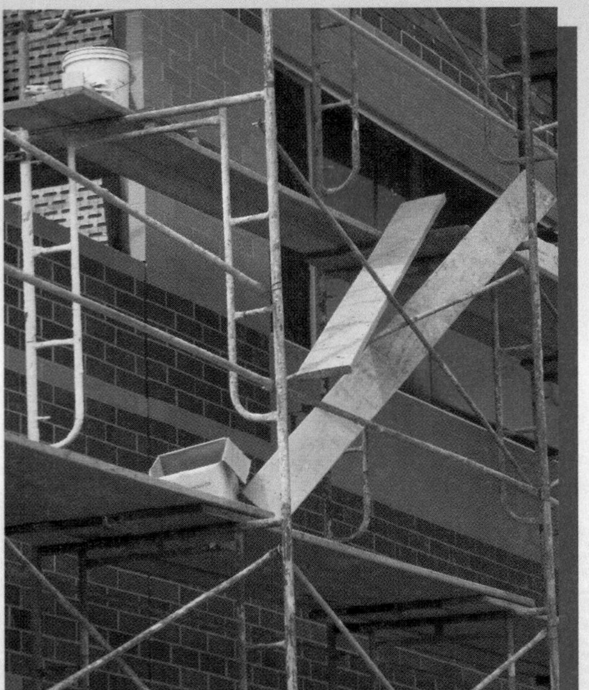

When two EMT-Basics from fire rescue arrive, Trish gives them a report. They take over. EMT-Paramedics are on the scene in an ambulance soon after. Trish and Bob fill them in on the accident and the condition of the patient.

The patient begins to vomit. The EMT-Paramedics suction his mouth and place a breathing tube into the windpipe. Minutes later the patient is completely immobilized, and rescuers work together to put him in the ambulance.

"He may have a head injury," an EMT-Paramedic says. "Can one of you give us a hand? Someone could ride in the back with us in case he vomits again." Trish volunteers to go to the trauma center with them.

Inside the ambulance she watches as the EMT-Paramedic prepares an IV. The rest of the ride is a blur of sirens. Finally, the ambulance stops. The waiting hospital team descends on them with organized urgency. It isn't long before the patient is examined, stabilized, and taken to surgery.

Trish decides to stay to help the EMTs clean the unit. Afterward she reflects on the call. She realizes that whether or not the patient survives, he was given the best chance possible to make it.

LEARNING OBJECTIVES

The "First Response" scenario on the previous page is a true-to-life description of a typical EMS call. As you read through the chapter, revisit it. It will help you understand the context in which you'll be working.

***By the end of this chapter, you should be able to:*†**

- 1-1.1 Define the components of Emergency Medical Services (EMS) systems. (pp. 3-6)
- 1-1.2 Differentiate the roles and responsibilities of the First Responder from other out-of-hospital care providers. (pp. 6-7)
- 1-1.3 Define medical oversight and discuss the First Responder's role in the process. (p. 8)
- 1-1.4 Discuss the types of medical oversight that may affect the medical care of a First Responder. (p. 8)
- 1-1.5 State the specific statutes and regulations in your state regarding the EMS system. (p. 8)

THE EMS SYSTEM

AN OVERVIEW

The **Emergency Medical Services (EMS) system** is a network of resources. In it people, equipment, and communications are organized to provide care to victims of sudden illness or injury (Figure 1-1). To get a good idea of how the system works, go back to the scenario at the beginning of the chapter. When the worker fell, a bystander immediately called EMS. How did he do it? In most parts of the country, anyone can by dialing 9-1-1. Some areas have "enhanced" computerized systems that identify a caller's location instantly. In other areas, the EMS system is activated only through a regular phone number.

In the scenario, both First Responders and EMTs responded to the emergency. (EMT is short for *emergency medical technician.*) Actually, there are four levels of out-of-hospital EMS workers (Figure 1-2). They are:

†Numbered objectives are from the 1995 U.S. DOT "First Responder: National Standard Curriculum."

The EMS System

Figure 1-1a
The accident occurs, and a bystander calls 9-1-1.

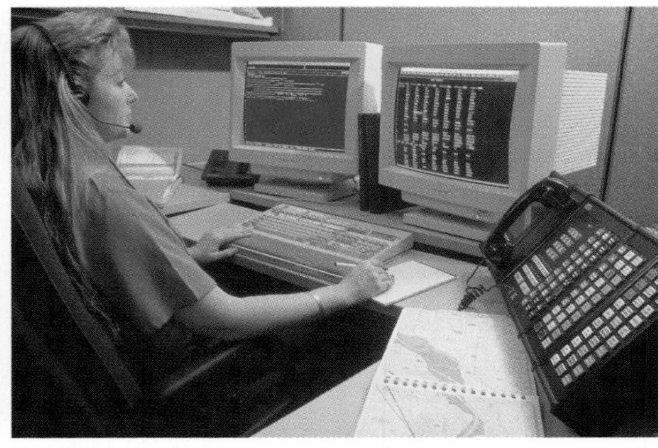

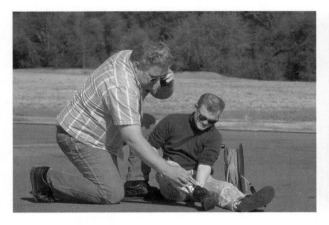

Figure 1-1b
The EMS dispatcher listens to the problem and alerts the appropriate EMS personnel.

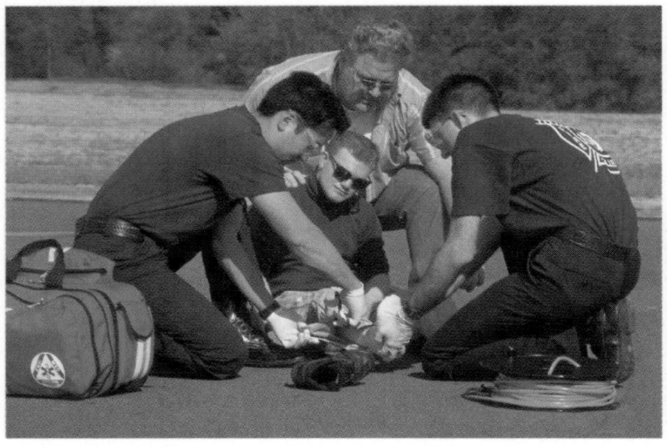

Figure 1-1c
First Responders arrive to assess the emergency and, if necessary, care for potential life threats.

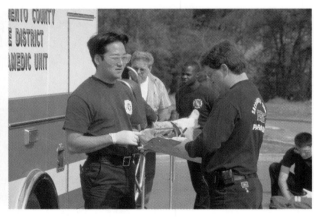

Figure 1-1d
When EMTs arrive, they take over to provide more advanced medical care.

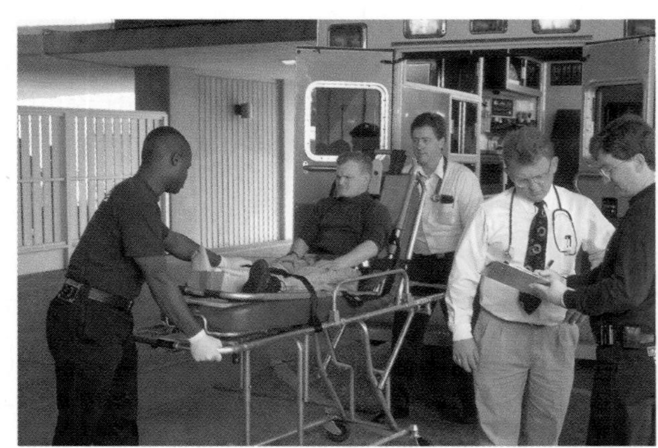

Figure 1-1e
EMTs finally hand-off the patient to the hospital emergency department physician.

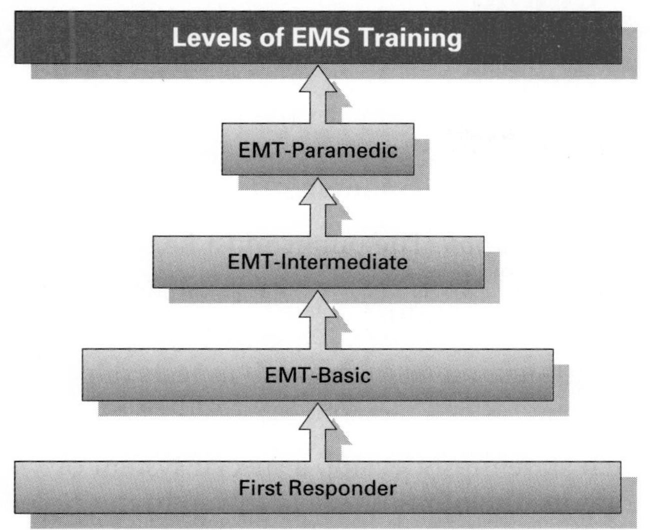

Figure 1-2

- *First Responder.* This EMS worker usually is the first trained rescuer at the scene of an emergency. He or she uses no or little equipment to assess and care for a patient.
- *EMT-Basic.* More highly skilled than a First Responder, the EMT-B may be certified as ambulance personnel.
- *EMT-Intermediate.* At this next highest level, the EMT-I performs advanced techniques and may administer some medications.
- *EMT-Paramedic.* More skills make this level of training the most advanced of the four.

Most patients who enter the EMS system are seen by doctors at a local hospital. In the scenario, the patient was taken to a **trauma center**, a hospital that specializes in caring for severe injuries. Other special hospitals focus on caring for burn patients, spine-injured patients, or infants and children.

Many EMS systems use helicopters. Some even have airplanes staffed by EMTs, nurses, and doctors. They work to cut transport time and to improve the quality of patient care en route to the hospital.

CLASSIC COMPONENTS

Each state in the U.S. controls its own EMS system. However, the federal government helps to set high standards. One example is provided by the National Highway Traffic Safety Administration. It recommends that every EMS system include 10 basic components. In summary, they are:

- *Regulation and policy.* Each state must have laws that govern its EMS system.
- *Resource management.* Each state must be sure that all patients have equal access to proper emergency care.
- *Human resources and training.* All workers in the EMS system are to be trained to a defined minimum standard.
- *Transportation.* All patients must be transported in a safe and reliable way.

- *Facilities.* All patients must be delivered to the closest, most appropriate medical facility.
- *Communications.* There must be a way for the public to access the EMS system. There also must be a way for dispatcher, ambulance, and medical control to communicate.
- *Public information and education.* The public must be told how to access the EMS system. EMS workers also may help the public learn to prevent illness and injury.
- *Medical oversight.* A physician must oversee all aspects of patient care.
- *Trauma systems.* Each state must develop a special system of care for trauma patients, including those involved in multiple-casualty incidents.
- *Evaluation.* Each state must have a program that helps to review and improve the quality of its EMS system.

ROLE OF THE FIRST RESPONDER

First Responders are the first medically trained rescuers on the scene. Because minutes, even seconds, matter to a patient's survival, First Responders are a critical part of the EMS system. The patient in the scenario at the beginning of the chapter, for example, may not have survived long enough to reach the hospital without First Responder help.

First Responders come from all walks of life (Figure 1-3). They may work for the fire department or law enforcement. They may be school teachers, park rangers, bus drivers, or community volunteers. All First Responders must perform the same basic tasks in an emergency. Those tasks are:

- *Assure scene safety.* This is always your first priority. If you can't assure scene safety, notify EMS dispatch immediately to ask for help. Don't enter the scene until it's safe.
- *Gain access to the patient.* Sometimes this can be difficult. A patient may be pinned in an overturned vehicle or trapped in a fire. In such cases, organize the scene so that specialized rescuers can enter and do their jobs.
- *Assess and treat the patient for life-threatening problems.* This is your most important task. If a patient has a problem with the ABCs—airway, breathing, or circulation, he or she can die unless treated quickly.

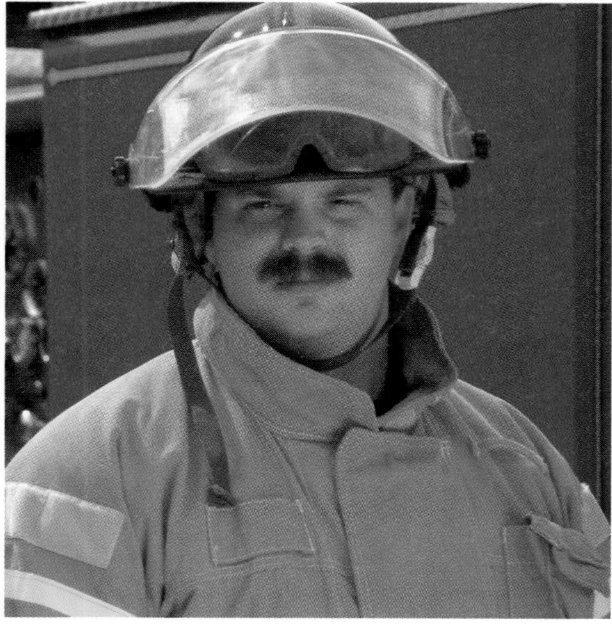

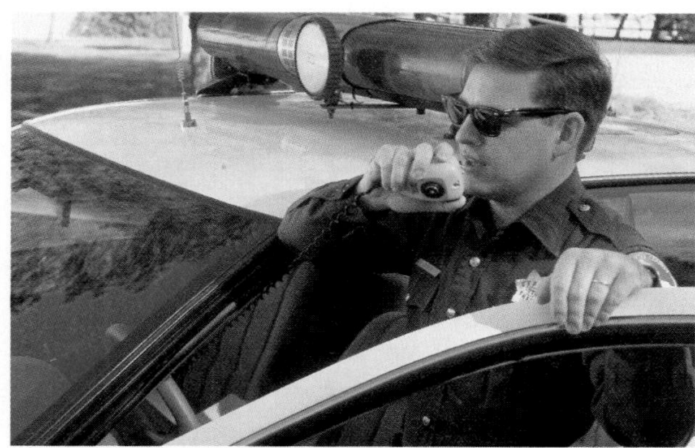

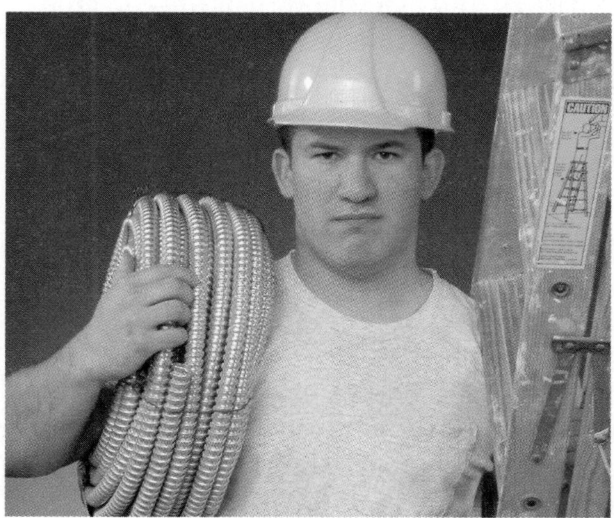

Figure 1-3
First Responders are people from many areas of the community.

- *Assist more highly trained EMS workers with patient care.* When the EMTs arrive, report your findings and transfer the patient to their care. If your help is needed, work under their direction.
- *Participate in record keeping and data collection.* Your instructor will tell you what's required by your state and locality.
- *Liaison with other public safety workers.* You'll work with a variety of specialized personnel. That includes local, state, or federal law enforcement, firefighters, and public utility workers, as well as other EMS personnel.

Once you master the nuts and bolts of running calls, there's more to do. You also must keep up your skills. So plan to take refresher courses, continue your education, and keep yourself in good physical condition.

Finally, in your role as a First Responder, you need to have certain attitudes and behaviors (Table 1-1). Because people will depend on your good judgment, you must maintain your composure, always be sure your attitude is a caring one, and always present yourself as a professional.

TABLE 1-1 RESPONSIBILITIES OF THE FIRST RESPONDER

1. Ensure personal health and safety.
2. Maintain a caring attitude.
3. Maintain composure.
4. Maintain a neat, clean, professional appearance.
5. Maintain up-to-date knowledge and skills.
6. Make patient's needs a priority without endangering self.
7. Maintain current knowledge of local, state, and national issues affecting EMS.

Information in this table is from the 1995 U.S. DOT "First Responder: National Standard Curriculum."

MEDICAL OVERSIGHT

Imagine what EMS would be like if rescuers practiced whatever brand of medicine they wished. The result would be chaos. So every EMS system is headed by a physician called the *medical director*. He or she is responsible for the medical care provided to every patient.

The physician oversees patient care in two ways—directly and indirectly. *Direct medical control* occurs when a rescuer speaks to the medical director or a surrogate on the radio, telephone, or on the scene. *Indirect medical control* includes system design, **protocols** (guidelines for field treatment), education, and quality improvement.

When caring for a patient, the First Responder is the designated agent of the medical director. The First Responder is considered to be an extension of the medical director's authority. Be sure to ask your instructor about your own state laws and regulations.

CONCLUSION

One EMS veteran explains what it means to be a First Responder: "Some calls use all of my skills. At others, I'm a social worker or even a mechanic. I've unstuck hands from drain pipes and helped to stabilize a patient who nearly drowned. While my primary job is to treat life threats, I figure I'm foremost a problem solver."

Remember, the EMS system is a network of resources, and you're an important part of it. When you're called to care for a victim of sudden illness or injury, first assure the safety of the scene. Then get to the patient and assess and treat life-threatening problems. Continue emergency care until medical personnel with more training take over.

KEY TERMS

You may wish to use this list to review your understanding of key terms introduced in the chapter.

Emergency Medical Services (EMS) system a network of resources–equipment, people, and communications—organized to provide emergency care to victims of sudden illness or injury.

EMT-Basic emergency medical technician trained to the minimum level of certification for ambulance personnel. *Also* EMT-B.

EMT-Intermediate emergency medical technician trained to perform essential advanced medical techniques and administer a limited number of medications. *Also* EMT-I.

EMT-Paramedic emergency medical technician who has the most advanced level of medical training among out-of-hospital EMS personnel. *Also* EMT-P.

First Responder usually the first medically trained personnel at the scene of an emergency. He or she uses a limited amount of equipment to perform patient assessment and care, and is trained to assist other EMS providers.

medical oversight refers to the formal relationship between EMS providers and the physician responsible for the out-of-hospital emergency medical care provided in a community.

protocols description of steps to be taken; guidelines for field treatment.

trauma center a regional hospital that specializes in caring for critically injured patients.

APPLICATION QUESTIONS

You may wish to use these questions to review your understanding of the chapter. For answers with page references, see Appendix 2.

1. You are a First Responder approaching the scene of a car crash. You see from a distance that it hit a large tree head on. The front of the car is crushed, and the driver is slumped over the steering wheel. What's the first thing you should do?

2. You are at the scene of the car crash described above. What's the difference between the care you provide as a First Responder and the care an EMT-Paramedic provides?

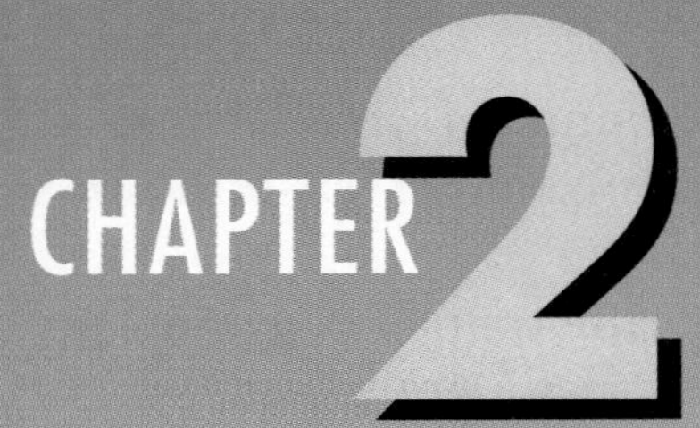

CHAPTER 2 THE WELL BEING OF THE FIRST RESPONDER

FIRST RESPONSE

Alan was glad that it was the end of his shift. A First Responder for a local fire agency, he had been up most of the night running medical calls. He was exhausted, and he didn't feel well. There was a hint of pressure in his chest, and he was having a problem catching his breath. He shook his head. He would have to stop smoking and soon. Everybody at work gave him grief about it. Alan, the pack-a-day king, they called him.

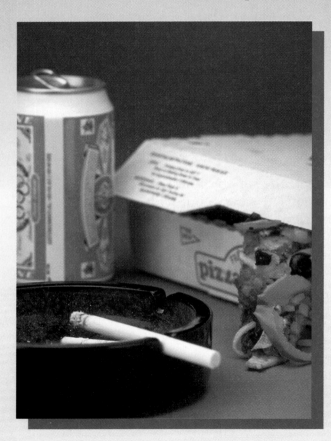

Alan was also the stress king. He worked too many shifts, got too little sleep, and too often indulged in hefty doses of fast food. Co-workers joked that he would be their next call, and that he ought to do TV testimonials for the American Heart Association. "Hi, my name is Alan. I'm 26 years old and headed for a heart attack...." Alan would laugh when people ribbed him. Hey, he was young. He could take it. He was tough.

A few nights later Alan woke with crushing chest pain. He felt as though he had a thousand pounds sitting on his chest, and he couldn't breathe. He managed to call 9-1-1 and saw the horrified faces of his friends.

An ambulance rushed Alan to the hospital. En route he went into cardiac arrest twice. Twice the EMTs successfully shocked his heart.

Alan arrived at the emergency room and doctors talked of rushing him into heart surgery, and of administering clot-busting drugs to unclog the offending artery in his heart. Alan was too exhausted to say anything. Hey, he wanted to say, this isn't necessary. I'm too young. All I need is to rest a bit....

Surgery corrected Alan's problem, and he managed to survive. In fact, Alan is back at work. Still smoking, still eating fatty foods, and still refusing to believe he needs help.

LEARNING OBJECTIVES

EMS work can be very stressful. In the scenario above Alan increased those stresses by managing his health poorly. However, the issue of First Responder wellness goes beyond physical health. You also must be able to keep yourself emotionally healthy. You have to. It's the only way you can be happy in your life outside of EMS.

By the end of this chapter, you should be able to:†

- 1-2.1 List possible emotional reactions that the First Responder may experience when faced with trauma, illness, death, and dying. (pp. 11-13)
- 1-2.4 State the possible reactions that the family of the First Responder may exhibit. (p. 13)
- 1-2.5 Recognize the signs and symptoms of critical incident stress. (pp. 12-13)
- 1-2.6 State possible steps that the First Responder may take to help reduce/alleviate stress. (pp. 13-15)

STRESS IN THE FIELD

Stress may be defined as the result produced when a person is acted upon by forces that disrupt equilibrium or produce strain. Think of situations in the field that might be especially stressful. For example:

- You're at the scene of a drowning. A child has been found in a backyard pool. Her parents are screaming at you to help. You perform CPR, but suspect that it won't be successful.
- As you approach the scene of a high-speed car crash, you see that there are three or more patients who may need immediate life-saving care.
- You're on vacation when you hear that your partner has been fatally injured on the job.

Most people associate stress with calls such as these. They're correct. However, stress and its accompanying feelings of fear, anger, and sadness don't have to be the result of one incident.

†Numbered objectives are from the 1995 U.S. DOT "First Responder: National Standard Curriculum."

Stress can build up over months, even years. This build-up of emotion may be even more difficult to handle, because you can't pinpoint an exact cause.

EMS work carries with it many kinds of stress (Figure 2-1). For example, First Responders who respond to a large number of calls may experience the stress of no sleep, missed meals, and too many patients. In other EMS systems, rescuers get stressed because they don't run enough calls to feel comfortable about their skills. As one First Responder describes it, "I remember my first few years in EMS as days and days of boredom broken by a few moments of sheer terror."

Every rescuer handles stress differently. The amount of stress a person can handle also varies. Even though your response to stress will be unique, look for the common warning signs. They'll help you recognize your emotional response to EMS work. Warning signs of stress include (Figure 2-2):

- Irritability to coworkers, family, friends.
- Inability to concentrate.
- Difficulty sleeping, nightmares.

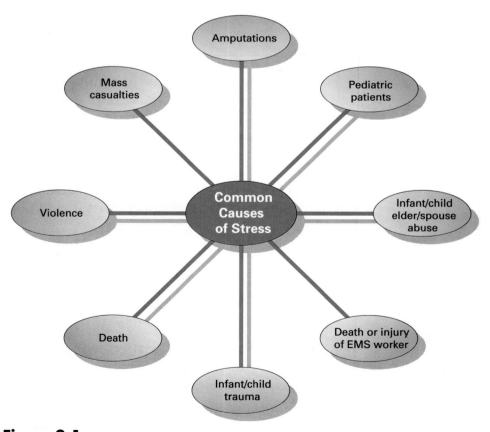

Figure 2-1
Common causes of stress.

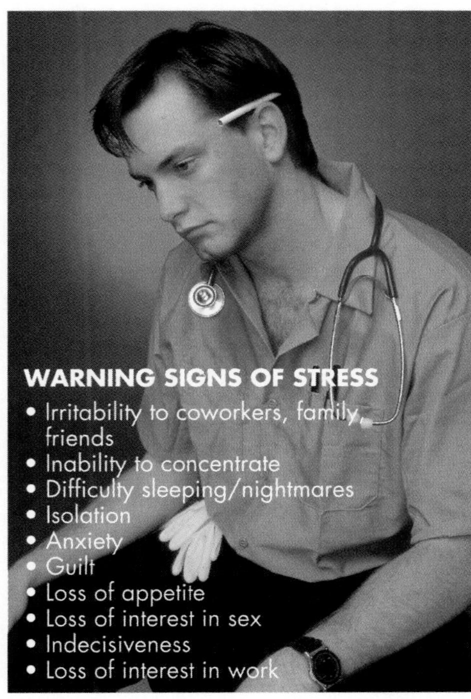
WARNING SIGNS OF STRESS
• Irritability to coworkers, family, friends
• Inability to concentrate
• Difficulty sleeping/nightmares
• Isolation
• Anxiety
• Guilt
• Loss of appetite
• Loss of interest in sex
• Indecisiveness
• Loss of interest in work

Figure 2-2
Watch for the warning signs of stress.

- Anxiety.
- Indecisiveness.
- Guilt.
- Loss of appetite.
- Loss of interest in sex.
- Isolation.
- Loss of interest in work.

MANAGING STRESS

There are many proven ways to help manage stress. Reducing your intake of sugar, fat, and caffeine will help. Regular exercise helps. So will reducing or avoiding alcohol. Many people also manage stress with relaxation techniques, meditation, and visual imagery.

All EMS workers take on the challenge of balancing work with their personal lives. Family conflicts are common. Family members may not understand a First Responder's job. They may feel as if they're being ignored, or they may have fears of separation. Frustration is also common; they want to share in the experience and obviously can't.

Good communication can help to resolve many of these problems. Don't carry the EMS pager to the family cookout when you're not on call. Turn it off when you've reserved time with your spouse and children. Prioritize your life. It's critical that family members feel valued and special, not second fiddle to a pager or scanner.

Another method to reduce your stress is to change your shift. Look for more flexible hours, for example, or request a rotation of duty assignment.

If these changes don't work, seek out counseling. A professional mental health worker, social worker, or the clergy may help you understand the causes of your stress, as well as to help you develop strategies to manage it effectively.

DEALING WITH CRITICAL INCIDENT STRESS

Critical incident stress is a normal stress response to abnormal circumstances. Before this type of stress was identified, rescuers were expected to "get over it." If you were tough enough for EMS, they thought, you could run a difficult call and walk away without showing any ill effects. We now know ignoring stress leads to "burnout."

Every EMS worker needs help in coping with critical incident stress. To address that need, EMS has developed services that are run by teams of peer counselors and mental health professionals. In general, those services include:

- Pre-incident stress education.
- On-scene peer support.
- One-on-one support.
- Disaster support services.
- Critical incident stress debriefing (CISD).
- Follow-up services.
- Spouse and family support.
- Community outreach programs.
- Other health and welfare programs such as wellness programs.

The **critical incident stress debriefing (CISD)** is key (Table 2-1). It provides a safe place for rescuers to review the call. Usually held within 24 to 72 hours after the incident, all rescuers associated with a major call are brought together. In a formalized way, they openly discuss their feelings, fears, and reactions. Note that CISD isn't an interrogation. Nothing said in the meeting may be used to investigate the incident. It's completely confidential.

Another technique for helping rescuers manage critical incident stress is called **defusing**. Less formal and less structured than a CISD, it's held a few hours after the event. It allows rescuers closest to the incident to "ventilate" their feelings. It also

TABLE 2-1	*WHEN TO ACCESS CISD*
• Multiple-casualty incidents. • Suicide of an EMS worker. • Line-of-duty death or serious injury. • Serious injury or death of infants and children. • Events with excessive media interest. • Victims known to the EMS workers. • Any event that has unusual impact on rescuers. • Any disaster.	

gives CISD leaders a chance to decide if a full CISD meeting might be needed.

Ask your instructor for information about CISD and related services offered in your EMS system.

CONCLUSION

Unmanaged stress will negatively affect your life, both on and off the job. Changes in lifestyle and work environment, and specific programs such as CISD, will help you to maintain both your emotional and physical health. Only by doing so, will you be able to effectively respond to the next EMS call for help.

KEY TERMS

You may wish to use this list to review your understanding of key terms introduced in the chapter.

critical incident stress debriefing (CISD) a formalized, peer-driven group counseling session in which rescuers have an open but confidential discussion of their feelings, fears, and reactions to the incident.

defusing shorter, less structured version of a CISD meeting, held for the rescuers most closely involved in a major call event.

APPLICATION QUESTIONS

You may wish to use these questions to review your understanding of the chapter. For answers with page references, see Appendix 2.

1. You're talking with another rescuer who is experiencing critical incident stress after a call to a two-car crash involving the death and injury of several children. She doesn't want to attend a CISD meeting. What argument could you use to convince her to attend?

2. Few if any of us can eliminate stress from our lives. So, we need to find ways of keeping ourselves fit for handling it. How can you improve your ability to manage stress?

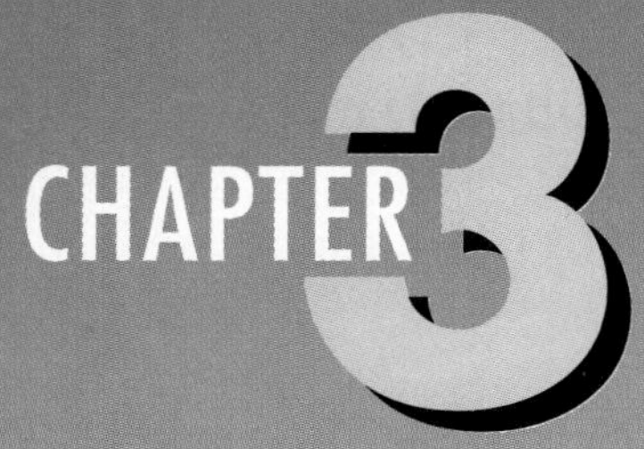

LEGAL AND ETHICAL ISSUES FOR THE FIRST RESPONDER

FIRST RESPONSE

It's 11 at night and Don and Phil are called to a "man down" in an alley behind Rau's Liquor Store. As they approach the scene, they see a heavily clothed figure stumble out from behind rows of garbage cans. The man shuffles down the alley, teetering slightly as he picks his way around obstacles. Don and Phil cautiously approach him. They observe that his forehead is bleeding from a two-inch long wound near the hairline. While Phil scans the scene and looks for others who may need help, Don asks the man, "Are you all right?"

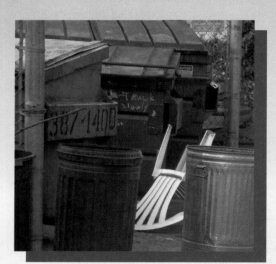

"I'm headin' home," is the hoarse reply. "That 'gainst the law?"

"Sir, we're not the law," Don says. "We're First Responders with the county hospital. We were told that someone in this alley may have fallen. Did you fall? May we take a look at that wound?"

"Naw," the man answers belligerently. "Leave me alone. I'm tryin' to find my hat." The man's words send the smell of alcohol and vomit into Don's face. He catches his breath.

"You could really be hurt," Don tells the man. "You have a head injury, and it may be serious. We should stop the bleeding and bandage it." Then clearly and firmly, Don asks, "May we help you?"

With a snarl, the man thrusts himself past them and out onto the street. As they watch him stumble away, Don wonders, "What are our legal obligations here? Should we force him to let us help? Does it matter that he's probably under the influence?" He decides it matters, and tells Phil to call for the police on the cellular.

A unit arrives almost immediately. "We were on the way here anyway," the police say. "Neighbors called to report someone knocking down garbage cans. What can we do for you?"

Don and Phil point out the man weaving up the street. The police woman's offer of "jail or the hospital" must convince him, because it isn't long before the EMTs arrive and put him in an ambulance. "He'll need stitches, and he may have a concussion," an EMT tells them. After they close the ambulance doors, Don and Phil head home.

LEARNING OBJECTIVES

Forgetting or disregarding the rules that govern EMS in the field can be downright dangerous. What would have happened to the patient—and to Don and Phil—if they had left the scene without calling for help? You'll find the answer to that question in the chapter. You'll also get a chance to become familiar with the most important legal concepts that affect First Responders.

By the end of the chapter, you should be able to:†

- 1-3.1 Define the First Responder scope of care. (p. 18)
- 1-3.2 Discuss the importance of Do Not Resuscitate [DNR] (advance directives) and local or state provisions regarding EMS application. (pp. 22-25)
- 1-3.3 Define consent and discuss the methods of obtaining consent. (pp. 20-21)
- 1-3.4 Differentiate between expressed and implied consent. (p. 20)
- 1-3.5 Explain the role of consent of minors in providing care. (pp. 20-21)
- 1-3.6 Discuss the implications for the First Responder in patient refusal of transport. (pp. 21-22)
- 1-3.7 Discuss the issues of abandonment, negligence, and battery and their implications to the First Responder. (pp. 20-22)
- 1-3.8 State the conditions necessary for the First Responder to have a duty to act. (p. 19)
- 1-3.9 Explain the importance, necessity and legality of patient confidentiality. (pp. 19-20)
- 1-3.10 List the actions that a First Responder should take to assist in the preservation of a crime scene. (pp. 25, 27)
- 1-3.11 State the conditions that require a First Responder to notify local law enforcement officials. (p. 25)
- 1-3.12 Discuss issues concerning the fundamental components of documentation. (p. 27)

†Numbered objectives are from the 1995 U.S. DOT "First Responder: National Standard Curriculum."

LEGAL AND ETHICAL RESPONSIBILITIES

THE SCOPE OF CARE

As a First Responder, you're only allowed to perform the skills defined by state law, local regulations, and EMS system medical direction. Together those skills are called your **scope of care**. Your instructor and this textbook will tell you what they are. Learn them. Practice until you master each one. Attend continuing education and refresher programs to keep them sharp. Participate in performance reviews, and always report patient findings honestly (Figure 3-1).

Warning *Never go beyond your scope of care. It's against the law!*

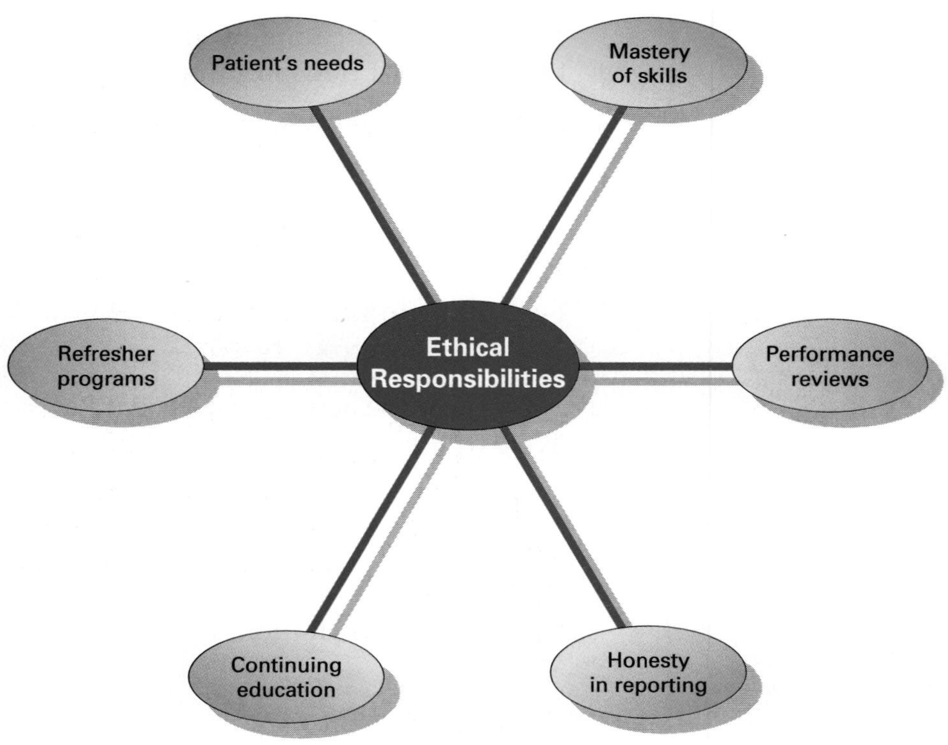

Patient's needs
Mastery of skills
Refresher programs
Ethical Responsibilities
Performance reviews
Continuing education
Honesty in reporting

Figure 3-1
A First Responder's ethical responsibilities.

DUTY TO ACT

In the scenario at the beginning of this chapter, Don and Phil had a **duty to act.** That is, they had a legal obligation to care for their patient. Ask your instructor to tell you how your state legally defines the term. In general, a First Responder has a duty to act when on call, when there's a contract between his or her employer and the community, and when patient care has been started.

You also have a duty to act appropriately. You must stay within your scope of care, and you must provide the best care possible. Appropriateness is determined by comparing the care you give a patient to a *standard of care,* or what another similiarly trained First Responder would do in the same situation.

NEGLIGENCE

Negligence is another legal term. When proper care is not given to a patient and an injury results, an EMS worker may be negligent. In order for negligence to be proven, four conditions must be present:

- There must have been a duty to act.
- There was an unexcused breach of duty or a failure to provide the standard of care.
- The patient was injured, either physically or psychologically.
- There is proof that the failure to meet the standard of care caused the injury.

For example, let's say you are at the scene of a car crash. A drunk driver is fighting all your attempts to protect him from further injury. If the driver injures himself anyway, are you negligent? Probably not, if you acted as any trained First Responder would have in the same situation.

Always attempt to meet the standard of care. If you are unable to do so, carefully document your reasons and follow up with your medical director as soon as possible. Remember, negligence most often occurs through errors of omission. That is, rescuers fail to act, fail to perform a needed procedure, or fail to take a patient's injuries seriously. Always do all you can to act in the patient's best interest.

CONFIDENTIALITY

Protecting your patient's privacy is part of top notch First Responder care. It's not always easy. Look at any supermarket tabloid. However, it's the ethical thing to do, and it's the law.

I authorize any holder of medical information about me to release to the Social Security Administration or its intermediaries or carriers any information needed for this or a related medical claim. I permit a copy of the authorization to be used in place of the original and request payment of medical insurance benefits to provider of ambulance service.

Signature	DL#	SS#

Figure 3-2
One type of information release form.

In general, confidential information includes the patient's medical history, assessment findings, and treatment. You may not share it with anyone other than the EMS workers who take over the patient's care. In order to give that information to anyone else, you must have a written release form signed by the patient (Figure 3-2). If the state wants patient information or if you're subpoenaed by the court, a signed release isn't needed.

Remember *Unless the EMS team, hospital staff, or the patient's immediate family is making the inquiry, maintain patient confidentiality. Politely decline to answer questions about the patient. Refer all such inquiries to your supervisor or scene commander.*

PATIENT CONSENT AND REFUSAL

CONSENT

Consent may be defined as a patient's acceptance of medical care. Before you can help any patient, you must have consent. If you don't, you could be charged with assault (touching without consent) or battery (causing bodily harm). In general, there are three types of consent:

- **Expressed consent** is given when a competent adult agrees to emergency medical care. Also called "informed consent," it's given after you describe treatment and the patient has considered the risks and benefits.
- **Implied consent** involves the patient who is unresponsive. In such a case you may assume he or she would agree to life-saving care. Implied consent also is used to treat a minor or a disabled adult when a parent or guardian cannot be found.
- **Substituted consent** occurs when someone consents for another person. Minors and mentally incompetent adults cannot legally give consent. A parent or guardian must do so. Emancipated teenagers are an exception. They are considered

adults by the courts. (Ask your instructor to explain your state's laws regarding the age of minors.)

Getting consent is part of your normal routine. For example, when you approach a patient, identify yourself and your level of training. Then ask, "May I help you?" or "May we check you out?" Be sure to explain what you want to do and why. Look again at the First Responders in the scenario at the beginning of the chapter. Notice that by asking questions, they also were able to get some idea of the patient's competence.

A patient is *competent* when he or she is able to understand your questions and the implications of accepting or refusing care. When you first approach a patient, be alert for signs of intoxication and drug use. Severe injury or a mental disability also can interfere with a patient's ability to understand the situation.

PATIENT REFUSAL

Competent patients have the right to make decisions about treatment. They also have the right to stop treatment at any time. So always let them know what you're going to do before you do it.

What happens when a competent patient refuses care? It's your job to make sure the patient understands the risks. For example, you might say to a patient who was in a car crash: "I understand you don't want me to treat you. You have the right to refuse care. But let me tell you what can happen if I don't immobilize your head and neck. You told me you're having pain there as a result of the crash. That means you could have a spinal-cord injury. If we don't immobilize the area, it's possible that you'll be risking further injury to your neck and back. That could result in permanent damage, even paralysis. Do you understand this?"

If the patient still refuses care, don't decide by yourself to walk away. Call for medical direction, if possible. (Follow your local protocols.) Other EMS workers will evaluate your patient. Also consider calling law enforcement (as Don did in the scenario at the beginning of the chapter). At the end of the call, be sure to report all your observations and document the sequence of events.

ABANDONMENT

Abandonment is one of the greatest legal risks for the First Responder. In general, it's defined as terminating care of a patient without making sure that care will continue at the same level or higher. For example, in the scenario at the beginning of the chapter, Don and Phil's patient was injured and probably drunk. He appeared to be less than competent, and probably needed an examination. If the First Responders had simply walked away when he refused care, they could have been guilty of abandonment.

Abandonment also includes termination of care or level of care without the informed consent of the patient. Do everything you can to make sure the patient who refuses care understands the risks. Then carefully weigh your reasons for terminating care. Always confirm with medical direction before leaving the patient.

> **Street Notes**
>
> If at any time you're in doubt about what to do, err in favor of providing care.

Ask your instructor to describe your state's laws concerning patient refusal. You may need to get the patient's signature on an official refusal form.

SPECIAL SITUATIONS

MEDICAL IDENTIFICATION INSIGNIA

Some patients wear pins, bracelets, or necklaces that alert rescuers to medical conditions such as allergies, diabetes, and epilepsy (Figure 3-3). Most also include a phone number that may be called for specific medical treatment. When you examine a patient, be sure to look for these insignia. If you find one, report it to the EMTs during patient hand-off.

WITHHOLDING EMERGENCY CARE

ADVANCE DIRECTIVES

You already know that patients have the right to refuse treatment. Many patients make that decision well in advance of an emergency situation. Usually prepared by a private physician, this type of refusal is called an *advance directive.*

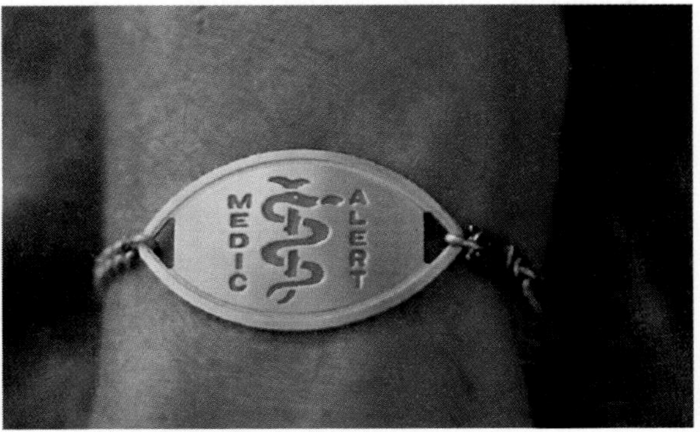

Figure 3-3
Medical identification insignia.

One type of advance directive is the organ donor card (Figure 3-4). It's found on the back of most driver licenses. Another type is the "Do Not Resuscitate" or DNR order (Figure 3-5). The DNR order is often used by terminally ill patients. It usually says that if the patient's heart or breathing stops, rescuers shouldn't start CPR or artificial ventilation.

When responding to a patient with a terminal illness, ask the caregiver if there is an advance directive. It may be a document, or it can be a medallion around the patient's neck or wrist. However, *you must have the actual document or medallion in your possession before you terminate emergency care.* You also may need to confirm the DNR order with medical direction. Remember, a family member's word is not enough. If you can't tell if an advance directive is valid, begin resuscitation efforts and contact medication direction for advice. Follow local protocols.

Check with your local EMS agency or medical society to find out what kinds of advance directives are used in your area.

General Guidelines

Did you know that under certain conditions a near-drowning victim may be resuscitated after as much as 30 minutes under water? Without special equipment and training, it's very difficult for a

Pursuant to the Uniform Anatomical Gift Act.
I hereby elect upon my death the following option(s):

A__To donate any organ or parts

B__To donate a pacemaker (date implanted__________)

C__To donate parts or organs listed________________

____

D__To not donate any organs, parts or pacemaker.

____

SIGNATURE DATE

DL 280 (REV 5/92)

- -

NOTICE

If you are at least 18, you may designate on your driver license or I.D. card a donation of any needed organs, tissues or pacemaker for medical transplantation. Under the Uniform Anatomical Gift Act (Sec. 7150, Health & Safety Code) donation takes effect upon your death.
NEXT OF KIN (OPTIONAL)

____

NAME

____

ADDRESS

____

TELEPHONE NO.

DETACH HERE

Figure 3-4
Example of organ donor card (front and back).

PREHOSPITAL DO NOT RESUSCITATE ORDERS

ATTENDING PHYSICIAN

In completing this prehospital DNR form, please check part A if no intervention by prehospital personnel is indicated. Please check Part A and options from Part B if specific interventions by prehospital personnel are indicated. To give a valid prehospital DNR order, this form must be completed by the patient's attending physician and must be provided to prehospital personnel.

A) ____________**Do Not Resuscitate (DNR)**:
No Cardiopulmonary Resuscitation or Advanced Cardiac Life Support be performed by prehospital personnel

B) ____________**Modified Support**:
Prehospital personnel administer the following checked options:

____________Oxygen administration
____________Full airway support: intubation, airways, bag/valve/mask
____________Venipuncture: IV crystalloids and/or blood draw
____________External cardiac pacing
____________Cardiopulmonary resuscitation
____________Cardiac defibrillator
____________Pneumatic anti-shock garment
____________Ventilator
____________ACLS meds
____________Other interventions/medications (physician specify)

____

Prehospital personnel are informed that (print patient name)________________________ should receive no resuscitation (DNR) or should receive Modified Support as indicated. This directive is medically appropriate and is further documented by a physician's order and a progress note on the patient's permanent medical record. Informed consent from the capacitated patient or the incapacitated patient's legitimate surrogate is documented on the patient's permanent medical record. The DNR order is in full force and effect as of the date indicated below.

______________________________ Attending Physician's Signature	______________________________ ______________________________
______________________________ Print Attending Physician's Name	______________________________ Print Patient's Name and Location (Home Address or Health Care Facility)
______________________________ Attending Physician's Telephone	
______________________________ Date	______________________________ Expiration Date (6 Mos from Signature)

Figure 3-5
Example of a Do Not Resuscitate (DNR) order.

First Responder to tell if a patient is beyond help. So, it's your duty to provide emergency care to any patient who needs it.

If the patient's heart has stopped beating, provide CPR. If the patient has stopped breathing, provide artificial ventilation. The only exceptions include finding the patient in a state of *rigor mortis* (the stiffness that follows death), decomposition, or with an obviously fatal injury such as decapitation or incineration.

SPECIAL REPORTING SITUATIONS

Once in a while you'll be expected to report an emergency to law enforcement or other appropriate authorities. Ask your instructor for your state, local, and EMS system requirements. In general, the emergencies you need to report include:

- Child abuse or neglect.
- Elder or dependent adult abuse or neglect.
- Domestic violence or partner abuse.
- Violent crimes such as sexual assault or shootings.
- Infectious disease exposure.

> **Remember** *Always report a suspected crime or abuse. A strong suspicion is all that is required. If you are unsure, ask your partner to evaluate the situation. Remember to trust your instincts. Let the authorities sort things out. Most states have legislation that will protect you from civil liability.*

CRIME SCENE RESPONSIBILITIES

Your first responsibility at any crime scene is your own safety. Never enter a crime scene before the police arrive to secure it. Once you enter, you have two responsibilities: patient care, which is the most important, and evidence preservation.

Here are some crime scene tips:

- Don't move anything unless it's necessary for patient care.
- Don't destroy evidence by cutting through stab marks or bullet holes.
- Keep the number of people at the scene down to a minimum. This will help reduce the chance of evidence being moved or destroyed.
- If you find a weapon, don't touch it. Immediately notify a police officer so that it can be handled properly.

COUNTY FIRE SERVICES — **Patient Care Report**

PATIENT

DATE | SERVICE PROVIDER | PROVIDER UNIT # | INCIDENT # | TRANSFER OF CARE TIME ___ TO ___

TIME OF INCIDENT | DISPATCH TIME | ARRIVE | PT CONTACT | TRANSP TIME | ARRIVE DEST TIME | CODE TO SCENE ___ CODE TO HOSP ___ | UNIT AVAIL

CALL LOCATION ☐ SAME AS PATIENT'S ADDRESS | PHONE # ( ) | FORM NO.

PATIENT NAME (LAST, FIRST) | AGE ☐ MOS ☐ YRS | D.O.B. | ☐ MALE ☐ FEMALE ☐ PREGNANT

PATIENT ADDRESS (STREET) | CITY | STATE, ZIP

PRIMARY

CHIEF COMPLAINT | P.Q.R.S.T

MEDICAL HISTORY ☐ UNKNOWN ☐ DENIED ☐ MI ☐ CHF ☐ ANGINA ☐ COPD ☐ CVA ☐ HTN ☐ DIABETES ☐ CA ☐ SIEZURES ☐ GI ☐ PSYCH

CURRENT MEDICATIONS UNKNOWN ☐ DENIED ☐ | ALLERGIES (MED) UNKNOWN ☐ DENIED ☐ | WT KG

VITALS

TIME	GCS E	GCS V	GCS M	BP	PULSE	RESP	EKG	BY	TIME	GCS E	GCS V	GCS M	BP	PULSE	RESP	EKG	BY

SECONDARY

HEAD ☐ ASSESSED & WNL | NECK ☐ ASSESSED & WNL | PUPILS ☐ PERL | CAP REFILL ☐ NORMAL ☐ DELAYED ☐ NONE

CHEST ☐ ASSESSED & WNL | LUNG SOUNDS ☐ ASSESSED & WNL | CRAMS ___ MECH ___ ANAT. ___

ABDOMEN ☐ ASSESSED & WNL | BACK ☐ ASSESSED & WNL | BLOOD SUGAR | TIME:

PELVIC ☐ ASSESSED & WNL | EXTREMITIES ☐ ASSESSED & WNL | CPR START TIME:

SKIN ☐ ASSESSED & WNL | NEURO ☐ ASSESSED & WNL | APGAR #1 TIME | APGAR #2 TIME

NARRATIVE

Document how Pt presented, treatments administered, response to treatments & transport condition.

AIRWAY

TIME: | OXYGEN ___ L/M | BY: ☐ MASK ☐ CANNULA ☐ BAG VALVE ☐ HHN | ☐ 02 SAT TIME % | ☐ 02 SAT TIME % | ☐ 02 SAT TIME % ☐

GAG YES ☐ NO ☐ | OPA ☐ TIME | NPA ☐ TIME | NTI ☐ TIME | OTI ☐ TIME | NEEDLE CRIC ☐ TIME | CHEST DECOMP ☐ L TIME R TIME

TIME: | ET SECURED AT ___ CM AT THE ___ (ANATOMY) USING ___ BY: ___ | TUBE SIZE: | NUMBER OF ATTEMPTS ___ NTI NUMBER OF ATTEMPTS ___ OTI

VERIFICATION OF TUBE PLACEMENT: ☐ = LUNG SOUNDS ☐ = CHEST RISE

IV

TIME	FLUIDS	SOLUTION	GAUGE	ATTEMPTS	LOCATION	RATE	TOT. VOL.	BY
	☐ IV ☐ IO					☐ TKO ☐ OPEN ☐ BOLUS		
	☐ IV ☐ IO					☐ TKO ☐ OPEN ☐ BOLUS		

TREATMENT

IMMOBILIZATION: ☐ NECK ☐ BACK ☐ LIMBS | TRANSP. POSITION: ☐ SUPINE ☐ LATERAL ☐ PRONE ☐ SITTING ☐ HEAD ELEV. ☐ FEET ELEV.

TIME	MEDICATION, TREATMENT AND RESPONSE	BY	TIME	MEDICATION, TREATMENT AND RESPONSE	BY

DESTINATION

TIME | MEDICAL CONTROL HOSPITAL CONTACTED ☐ MAR ☐ SGH ☐ MSJ ☐ MHS ☐ UCDMC ☐ NONE | ☐ PHONE ☐ RADIO | MICN # /NAME | M.D. | FORM LEFT W/PT? ☐ YES ☐ NO CONT. ATTACHED? ☐ YES ☐ NO

DESTINATION HOSPITAL | ☐ RAS ☐ AMA | RN ACCEPTING | ☐ PVT M.D. ☐ PT FAMILY REQUEST ☐ LAW ☐ TRAUMA CRITERIA ☐ CLOSEST ☐ BH ORDER ☐ DIVERSION ☐ SPECIALTY CENTER

☐ STANDING ORDERS ☐ COMMUNICATION FAILURE ORDERS | E.D. DIAGNOSIS/COMMENTS ☐ EXPIRED E.D. ☐ ADMIT ☐ HOME ☐ TRANSFER ☐ DEAD AFTER RESUS

EMT COMPLETING REPORT SIGNATURE # ___ | SECONDARY EMT SIGNATURE # ___ | PRECEPTOR SIGNATURE # ___

Figure 3-6
Example of a patient care report form.

- Always wear personal protective equipment, and try to control the amount of blood that is spread around the scene.

Don't underestimate the importance of trying to preserve evidence at the scene. You can make the difference between a violent criminal being convicted or set free.

DOCUMENTATION

Imagine the following scene: You are sitting on the witness stand in a brightly lit, crowded courtroom. You are holding a patient care report (PCR) that you filled out in haste one rainy night two years ago. Your patient that night is now accusing you of improper care. She's paralyzed from the neck down, and she says you did it. Unfortunately, you can't read your own handwriting. You feel a bead of sweat collect on your forehead....

The best way to avoid such a catastrophe is to accurately and legibly document your calls. Remember the adage, "If you don't write it down, it never happened."

A patient care report (PCR) is a legal document that can be used in a court of law (Figure 3-6). It's usually the only record you'll have from the host of calls you run in your career. Complete one every time you assess and treat a patient—for legal purposes as well as for other health care providers. Your PCR will provide them with the vital information they need to develop the best treatment plans possible for the patient.

CONCLUSION

Legal issues affect every area of your work as a First Responder. However, haggling over issues like consent, abandonment, or patient refusal is not how you'll want to spend your time. Learn the "rules of the road" now. Understanding them will free you up to make the best patient care decisions possible.

A final note: if you are ever in doubt about a particular legal issue when managing a patient, do what is best for the patient. This rule of thumb will see you through most difficult legal situations.

KEY TERMS

You may wish to use this list to review your understanding of key terms introduced in the chapter.

abandonment terminating care of the patient without ensuring that care will continue at the same level or higher. It also includes termination of care or level of care without the informed consent of the patient.

consent a patient's acceptance of medical care based on the information you provide.

duty to act a contractual, legal, and ethical obligation to render emergency medical care.

expressed consent a type of consent that is given when a competent adult agrees to emergency medical care. It's also called "informed consent" because it's given after you describe treatment and the patient has considered the risks and benefits.

implied consent a type of consent that assumes the unresponsive patient would agree to life-saving care. It also is used to treat a minor or a disabled adult when a parent or guardian cannot be found.

negligence a legal term referring to the unjustified departure from the accepted standard of care which results in injury to the patient.

scope of care all the emergency medical care skills First Responders are allowed to perform by state law, local regulations, and EMS system medical direction.

substituted consent a type of consent in which someone consents for another person. An example is a parent giving consent for a child.

APPLICATION QUESTIONS

You may wish to use these questions to review your understanding of the chapter. For answers with page references, see Appendix 2.

1. You have responded to an 89-year-old patient with terminal lung cancer. She is without a pulse and is not breathing. Her caregiver assures you that DNR orders exist, but she can't find them. How should you proceed?

2. You have responded to a chest-pain emergency. The patient is a well known politician. During assessment, he tells you that he has tested positive for HIV. This information is not public knowledge. With whom at the scene should you share this information?

3. You are approaching the scene of a patient who is very short of breath. When you ask if you may examine her, she says "Absolutely not." How should you proceed?

CHAPTER 4 THE HUMAN BODY

FIRST RESPONSE

As 17-year-old Nathan struggles on the roof with the air conditioning unit, he accidentally falls 20 feet down onto a concrete slab. Stunned coworkers call out for help. A second later George, Nathan's supervisor, sees someone running to him. "Nathan fell," Susan shouts. George grabs his jump kit and the cellular phone, and they both head to the scene of the accident. George puts on his gloves the second he can and pushes a pair at Susan. "Put them on. I think we'll need them."

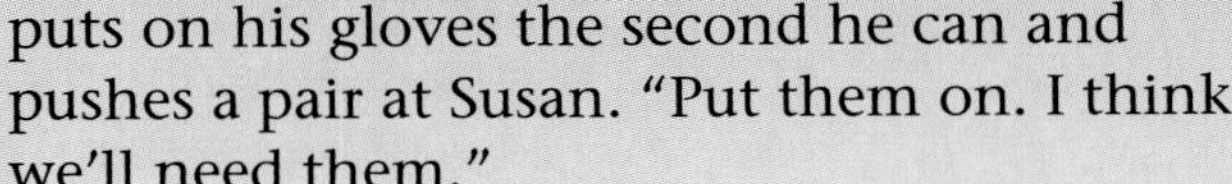

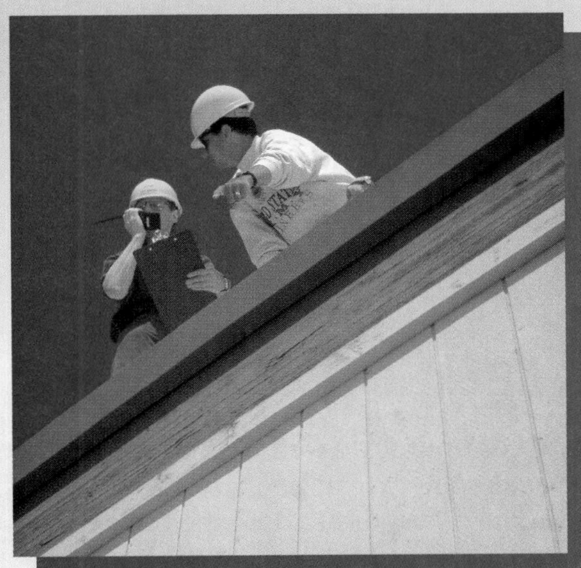

As George approaches the scene, he scans the roof. It appears to be safe. No falling debris. Then he looks at Nathan. His first impression is of blood streaming from the scalp and the right leg bent at an odd angle. He tells Susan, "Tell someone to get up there to secure the air conditioner. Come back right away to help me." He kneels beside Nathan and asks "How do you feel?"

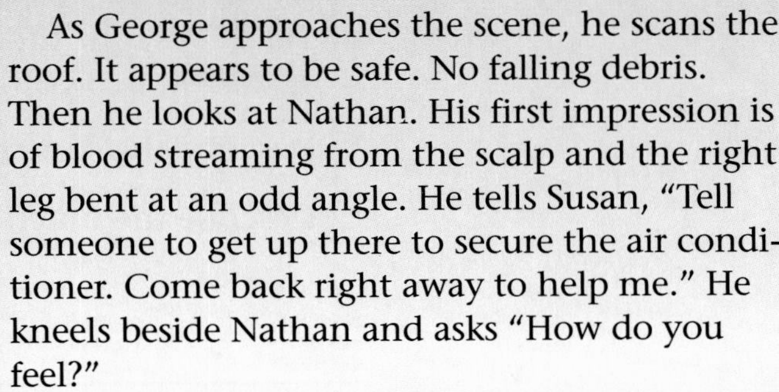

"What? Where am I?" Nathan responds, confused and in pain.

George tells him firmly, "Stay still, Nathan. I'm calling for help." He dials 9-1-1 on his cellular and relays Nathan's obvious injuries to the dispatcher. Then George begins the initial assessment. Nathan is awake and talking, so he knows the airway is open and that breathing is adequate. "Hold Nathan's head still like this." He quickly shows Susan how to hold the cervical spine. As she takes over, George tells Nathan, "You might have injured your back, son. So keep as still as you can. Don't move your head."

After George assesses circulation, he applies direct pressure to the scalp wound. He then looks down toward Nathan's leg injury. He sees that the deformity is in the thigh. No external bleeding, he notes, but a broken bone there can lead to life-threatening internal bleeding and shock. Quickly, he tells a bystander to get a blanket to keep Nathan warm. Just then he hears sirens. "Won't be long now," he reassures Nathan.

LEARNING OBJECTIVES

Do you know what led George to suspect serious internal bleeding? As a First Responder, he had been taught the necessary anatomy and physiology. He knew that a severe injury to the thigh could involve the femoral artery, one of the major arteries of the body. In this chapter you'll be introduced to important systems of the body. Learn them well. This knowledge will be the keystone to further learning.

By the end of the chapter, you should be able to:†

- 1-4.1 Describe the anatomy and function of the respiratory system. (pp. 32-34)
- 1-4.2 Describe the anatomy and function of the circulatory system. (pp. 34-37)
- 1-4.3 Describe the anatomy and function of the musculoskeletal system. (pp. 39, 40, 41)
- 1-4.4 Describe the components and function of the nervous system. (pp. 37-38)

* Describe the basic regions of the body. (p. 31)

* Describe the function of the skin. (p. 40)

DESCRIBING THE HUMAN BODY

One way you can be sure to communicate well with other EMS workers is to learn to speak the same language. Part of that language includes the terms EMS workers use to describe the external and internal parts of the body. Internal parts of the body are described throughout this chapter. The general surface areas of the body are described below (Figure 4-1).

- The area of the head includes:
  - skull
  - face
  - jaw
  - neck

†Numbered objectives are from the 1995 U.S. DOT "First Responder: National Standard Curriculum." Asterisks indicate supplemental material.

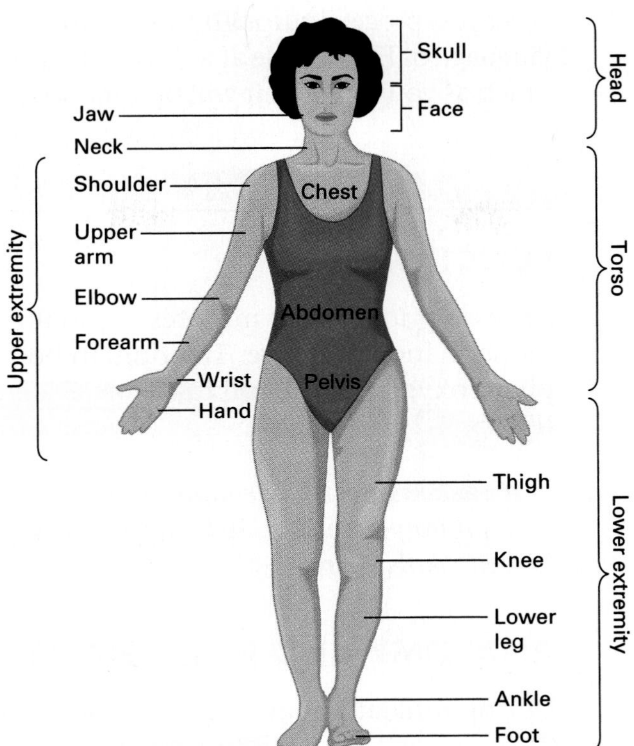

Figure 4-1
Regions of the body.

- The torso includes:
  - chest
  - abdomen
  - pelvis
- The upper extremity includes:
  - shoulder (collar bone and shoulder blade)
  - upper arm
  - elbow
  - forearm
  - wrist
  - hand
- The lower extremity includes:
  - thigh
  - knee
  - lower leg
  - ankle
  - foot

As you proceed through this course, you'll be introduced to the language of EMS a little at a time. Talk it. Write it. Think it. Use it as much as you can, and it will become second nature to you very soon.

THE RESPIRATORY SYSTEM

FUNCTION

After only four to six minutes without oxygen, the brain will suffer permanent damage. The human body requires a constant supply of oxygen. The basic function of the **respiratory system** (Figure 4-2) is to deliver that oxygen and remove carbon dioxide.

Remember *A large number of your critical patients will have respiratory problems. So keep your airway and breathing management skills sharp.*

ANATOMY AND PHYSIOLOGY

During inhalation, air enters the nose and mouth and passes through the throat, or **pharynx**. (The *oropharynx* is the area inside the mouth. The *nasopharynx* is the area above the roof of the mouth.) After passing through the **larynx** (voice box), air enters the **trachea** (windpipe). A leaf-shaped structure called the **epiglottis** prevents food and liquid from entering the trachea during swallowing.

Air then travels down to the right and left mainstream *bronchi.* Air travels through successively smaller *bronchioles* until it reaches the *alveoli*. The alveoli are air sacs which are surrounded by tiny blood vessels. This is where an exchange of oxygen and carbon dioxide occurs.

Another important part of the respiratory system is the **diaphragm**. Dividing the chest from the abdomen, this muscle is situated below the lungs. Movement of the diaphragm drives both inhalation and exhalation (Figure 4-3). During inhalation, the diaphragm moves down and the chest moves out. This causes air to rush into the lungs. During exhalation, the diaphragm moves up and the

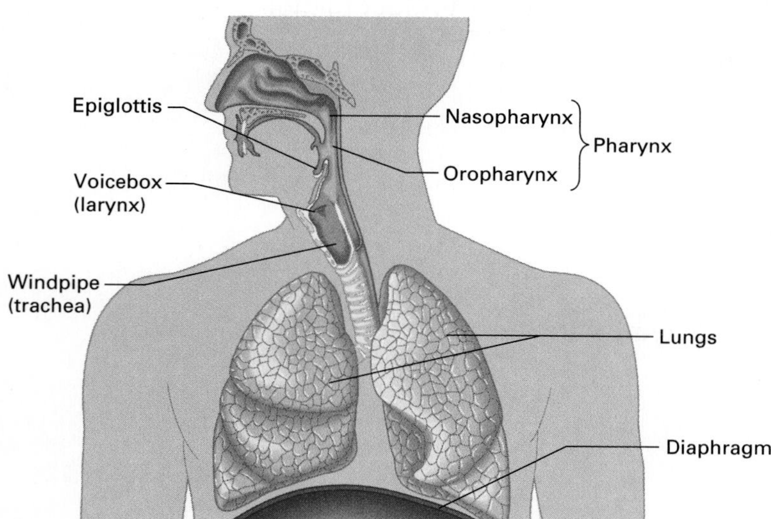

Figure 4-2
The respiratory system.

HOW RESPIRATION WORKS

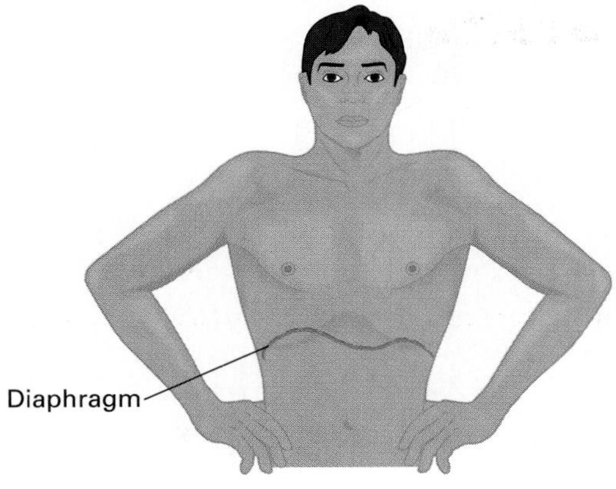
Inhalation:
Diaphragm moves down and chest moves out, drawing air into lungs.
Diaphragm

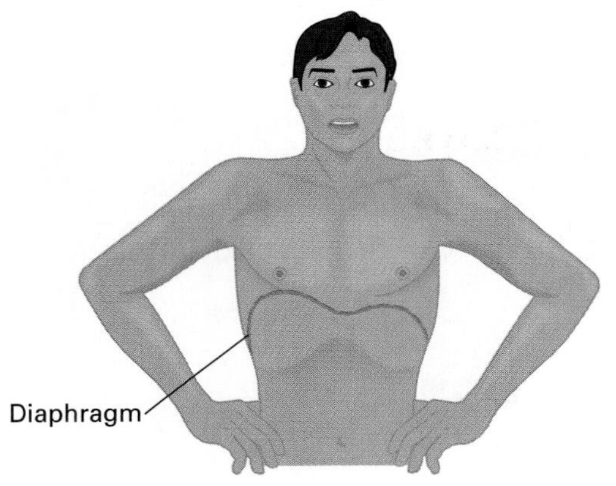
Exhalation:
Diaphragm moves up and chest wall moves in, causing air to exit the lungs.
Diaphragm

Figure 4-3
How respiration works.

TABLE 4-1	***BREATHING RATES FOR PATIENTS AT REST***
PATIENT'S AGE	BREATHS PER MINUTE
Infant	24-40
Child	20-30
Adult	12-20

chest wall moves in causing air to rush out of the lungs.

The human body can sense the levels of oxygen and carbon dioxide in the blood. Varying levels stimulate it to breathe. See Table 4-1 for normal breathing rates of patients at rest. Breathing rates are measured by counting a patient's respirations (an inhale plus an exhale equals one respiration). Notice that rates get slower as patients get older. Regardless of a patient's age, normal breathing should not be labored.

STREET NOTES

Labored breathing, or breathing with effort, is the number one sign of a respiratory problem.

The primary cause of the heart stopping in infants and children is a respiratory problem. It's critical that you always provide aggressive airway and breathing support to these patients. The respiratory systems of infants and children aren't the same as adults. The differences will affect the kind of care you give, so learn them well. The respiratory system of infants and children compare to an adult's in the following ways (Figure 4-4):

- Every part of the airway is smaller and more easily blocked.
- The most common cause of a blocked airway in an unresponsive patient—infant, child, or adult—is the tongue. In infants and children the tongue takes up proportionately more space. Therefore, it's even more likely to be the cause of a blocked airway for them.
- The trachea is more flexible and softer than an adult's. This makes it easier to kink or even close off when you perform airway maneuvers on an infant or child.
- An infant's or child's lungs may require more pressure and less air to inflate than an adult's.

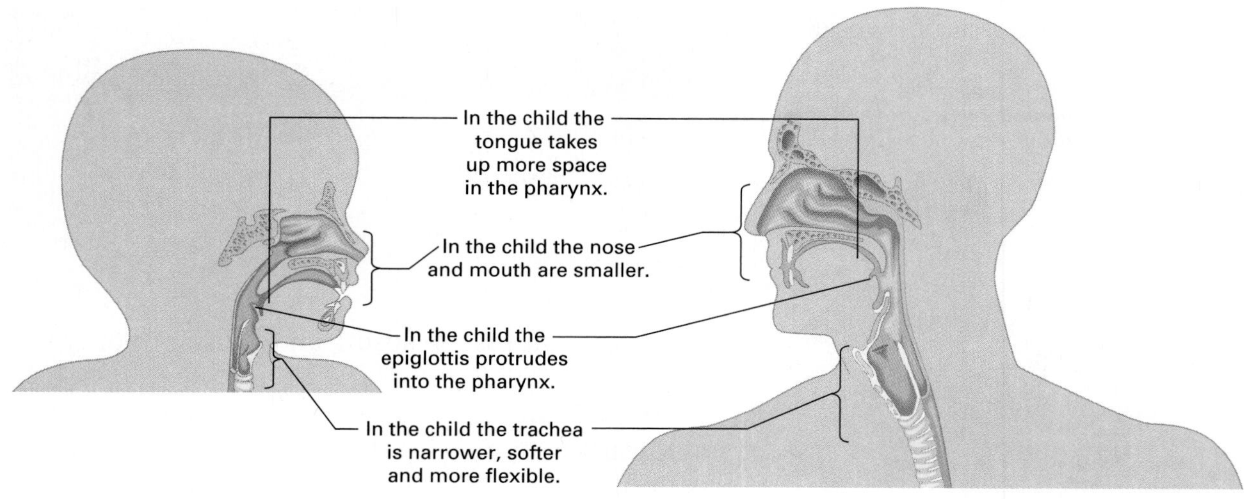
In the child the tongue takes up more space in the pharynx.
In the child the nose and mouth are smaller.
In the child the epiglottis protrudes into the pharynx.
In the child the trachea is narrower, softer and more flexible.

Figure 4-4
The respiratory systems of the adult and child are different.

THE CIRCULATORY SYSTEM

FUNCTION

Two major functions of the **circulatory system** are to deliver oxygen and nutrients to the body's tissues and to remove waste products. When the circulatory system doesn't deliver oxygen or remove wastes well enough, a life-threatening condition called **shock** may be the result.

ANATOMY AND PHYSIOLOGY

The basic components of the circulatory system are the heart, blood vessels, and blood (Figures 4-5 and 4-6).

THE HEART

The heart is a four-chambered pump. The top chambers are known as *atria*. The bottom chambers are called *ventricles*. The right atrium and ventricle together pump oxygen-poor blood into the lungs. The left atrium and ventricle together pump oxygen-rich blood from the lungs to the body. Valves between chambers prevent the blood from backing up.

The heart alternately contracts (pumps) and rests. Contraction of the heart is known as *systole*. The heart at rest between contractions is known as *diastole*. It's during diastole that the chambers of the heart fill up with blood. One way to measure how fast or how slow the heart's working is to feel for a pulse. Pulse rate refers to the number of contractions that occur each minute (Table 4-2).

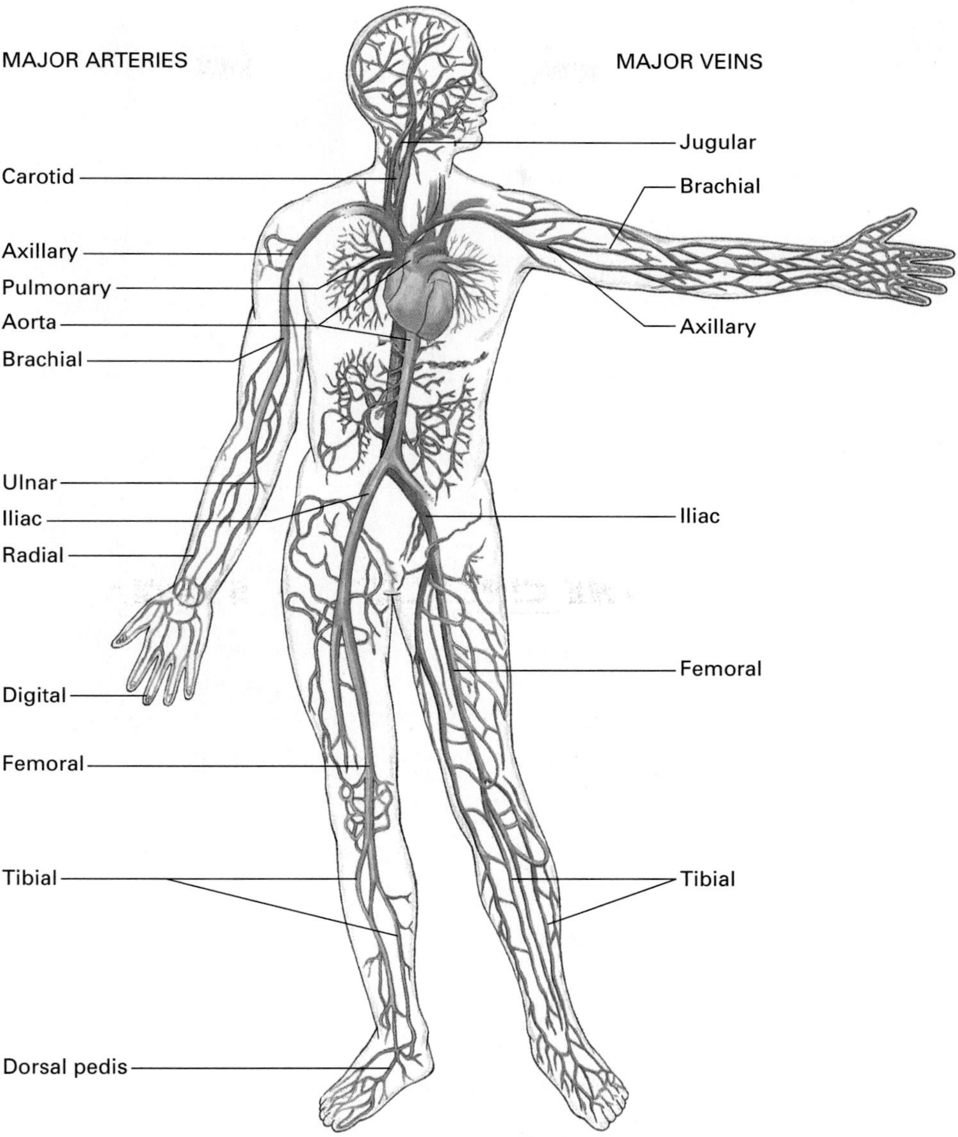

Figure 4-5
The circulatory system.

TABLE 4-2	***PULSE RATES FOR PATIENTS AT REST***
PATIENT'S AGE	CONTRACTIONS PER MINUTE
Infant	80-160
Child	80-120
Adult	60-100

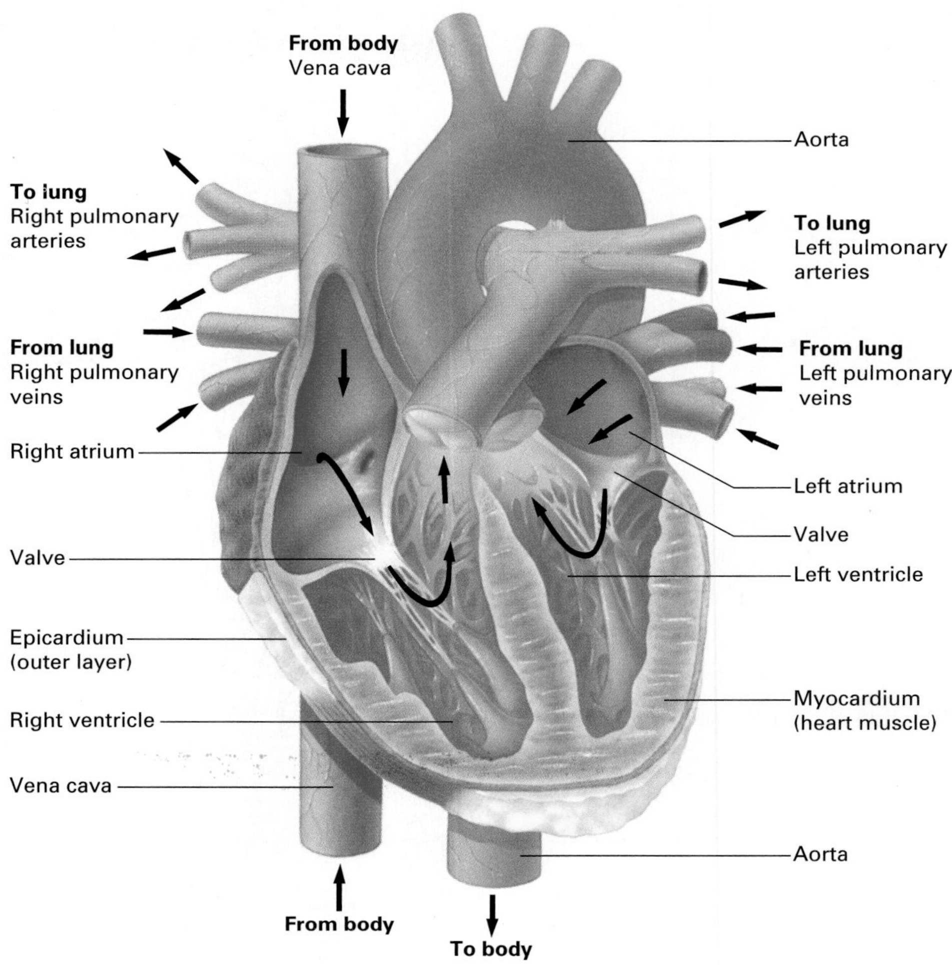

Figure 4-6
The heart.

Blood Vessels

The heart pumps blood to the body by way of a complex network of blood vessels. That network consists of **arteries, capillaries,** and **veins.**

The arteries carry blood under high pressure from the heart to the rest of the body. When an artery is located over a bone near the surface of the body, a **pulse point** is created (Table 4-3). There you can feel the body's pulse, or the wave generated by each contraction of the heart. As arteries network to all the organs and cells in the body, they become smaller and smaller. Finally, blood flows into the smallest vessels, the capillaries.

Capillaries deliver oxygen and nutrients directly to each cell of the body. They also take away carbon dioxide and waste products. Blood from the capillaries is then transported to the veins, which take it back to the heart.

TABLE 4-3 MAJOR ARTERIES		
ARTERY	LOCATION	PULSE POINT
Carotid	Neck	Side of neck
Radial	Lower arm	Inside wrist
Brachial	Upper arm	Inside upper arm
Femoral	Thigh	In groin
Dorsalis pedis	Foot	Top of foot

Blood

Blood is the fluid of the circulatory system. It's made up of many elements, including *red blood cells* and *plasma.* The red blood cells carry oxygen to the body. Plasma carries dissolved gases, nutrients, and a great variety of other substances. A newborn's total blood volume is about one cup. By the time the newborn is an adult, blood volume will have expanded to five or six liters.

THE NERVOUS SYSTEM

FUNCTION

The nervous system (Figure 4-7) controls the voluntary and involuntary activity of the body. It also provides for higher mental functions including thoughts and emotions.

ANATOMY

The **central nervous system** is the command center of the body. It includes the brain and the spinal cord. The brain is located in the *cranium* (skull). The spinal cord is located in the *spinal column* (backbone).

> **Remember** *The central nervous system, especially the brain, is very sensitive to changes in the body's oxygen supply. So constantly assess a patient's mental status. It can tell you when the patient's respiratory and circulatory systems aren't delivering enough oxygen.*

The central nervous system controls many of the body's activities through the **peripheral nervous system**. Made up of spinal and cranial nerves, this system connects organs in the body to the brain and spinal cord.

One set of peripheral nerves make up the **sympathetic nervous system**. This system controls the body's responses to

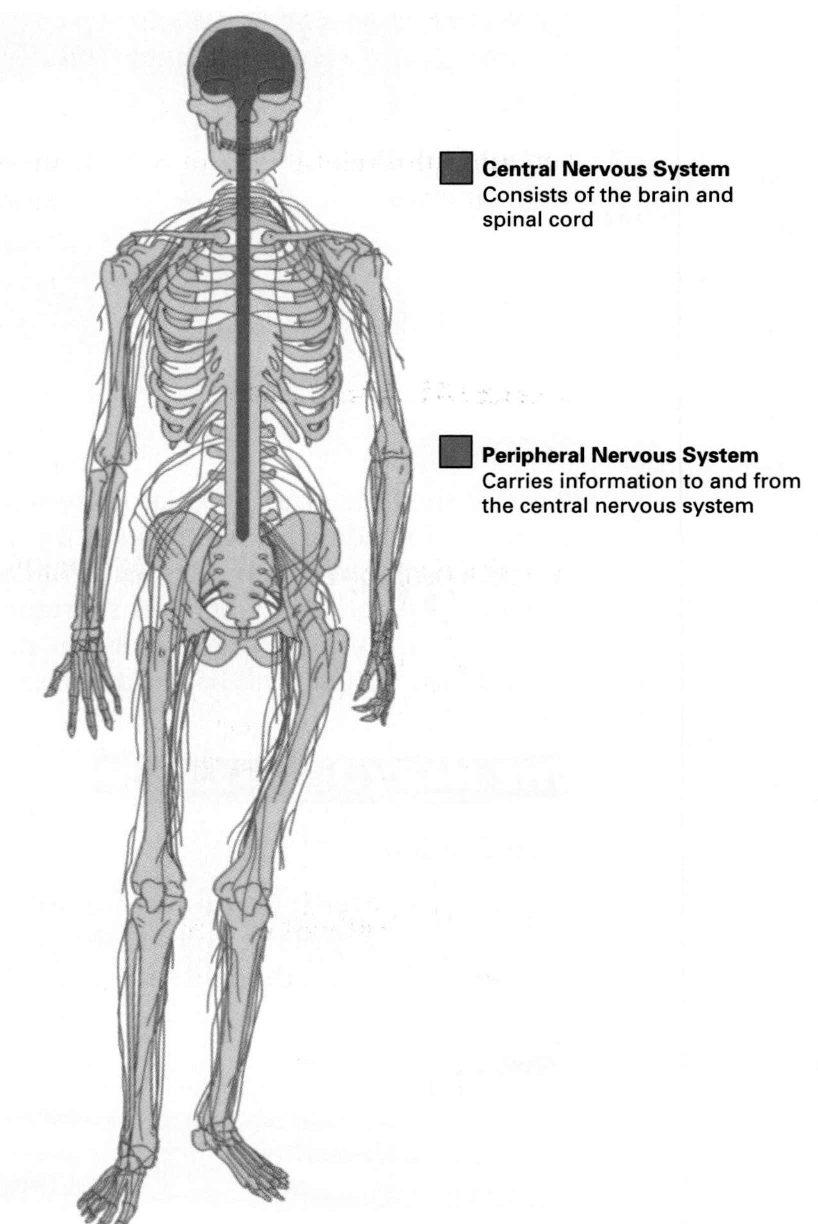
Central Nervous System
Consists of the brain and spinal cord
Peripheral Nervous System
Carries information to and from the central nervous system

Figure 4-7
The nervous system.

> **STREET NOTES**
>
> To help you find out if a patient is critically ill or injured, check mental status and look for a "sympathetic response."

stress. When the body is sick or injured, often it will have a "sympathetic response." This response includes a rapid pulse and pale, sweaty, cool skin. It's one of the best indicators that your patient has a serious problem.

THE MUSCULOSKELETAL SYSTEM

FUNCTION

The **musculoskeletal system** is made up of muscles, bones, and joints. It gives the body shape, protects its vital organs, and provides for movement. Certain bones also store calcium and produce red blood cells. The musculoskeletal system is the most commonly affected body system in trauma emergencies.

SKELETAL ANATOMY

See Figure 4-8 for a good description of the human skeleton. Here are a few specific comments on major bones of the body:

- The skull does a good job of protecting the brain. However, it also is a rigid container that doesn't expand when the brain is injured and swells. This can lead to further brain damage.
- The spinal column protects the spinal cord. However, notice that the neck, or the **cervical spine**, doesn't have the additional support provided by the ribs and pelvis. Add that to the fact that the neck has the job of supporting the heavy head. It's no wonder then that the cervical spine is the most often injured area of the spinal column.
- Notice the **xiphoid process**. It's the bony point that marks the lower border of the breastbone, or the **sternum**. It's also a "landmark" for positioning your hands when you perform CPR.
- Two of the biggest bones in the body are the pelvis and the **femur**. Injuries to these bones usually mean that the patient has sustained a tremendous blow. Such a blow can lead to massive bleeding and shock.

In general, infants and children have bones that are very flexible. Though less likely to break than adult bones, their bones provide less protection to the organs that lie beneath.

MUSCULAR ANATOMY

The three major types of muscles are *voluntary* (skeletal), *involuntary* (smooth), and *cardiac* muscle (Figure 4-9). Voluntary muscle is attached to bone and is responsible for movement. It's the only type of muscle that can contract and relax by will of the individual. Involuntary muscles line blood vessels, the walls of some organs, and so on. Cardiac muscle is found only in the heart.

THE SKELETAL SYSTEM

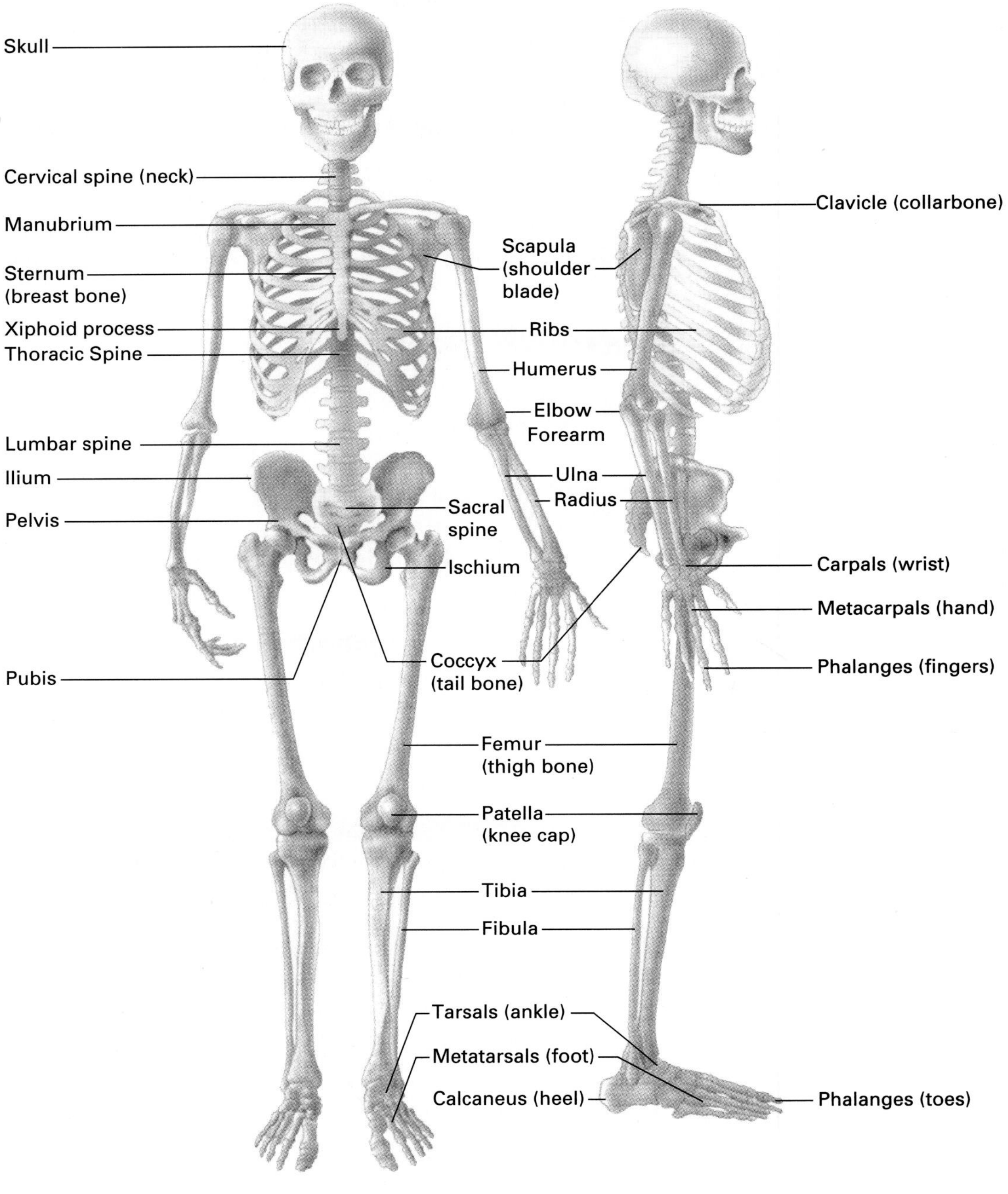

Skull
Cervical spine (neck)
Manubrium
Sternum (breast bone)
Xiphoid process
Thoracic Spine
Lumbar spine
Ilium
Pelvis
Pubis
Scapula (shoulder blade)
Ribs
Humerus
Elbow
Forearm
Ulna
Radius
Sacral spine
Ischium
Coccyx (tail bone)
Femur (thigh bone)
Patella (knee cap)
Tibia
Fibula
Tarsals (ankle)
Metatarsals (foot)
Calcaneus (heel)
Clavicle (collarbone)
Carpals (wrist)
Metacarpals (hand)
Phalanges (fingers)
Phalanges (toes)

Figure 4-8
The skeletal system.

THE SKIN

Skin protects the body from bacteria and other organisms. It helps to regulate body temperature and prevents dehydration. It senses heat, cold, touch, pressure, and pain. Skin also helps to ward off infection.

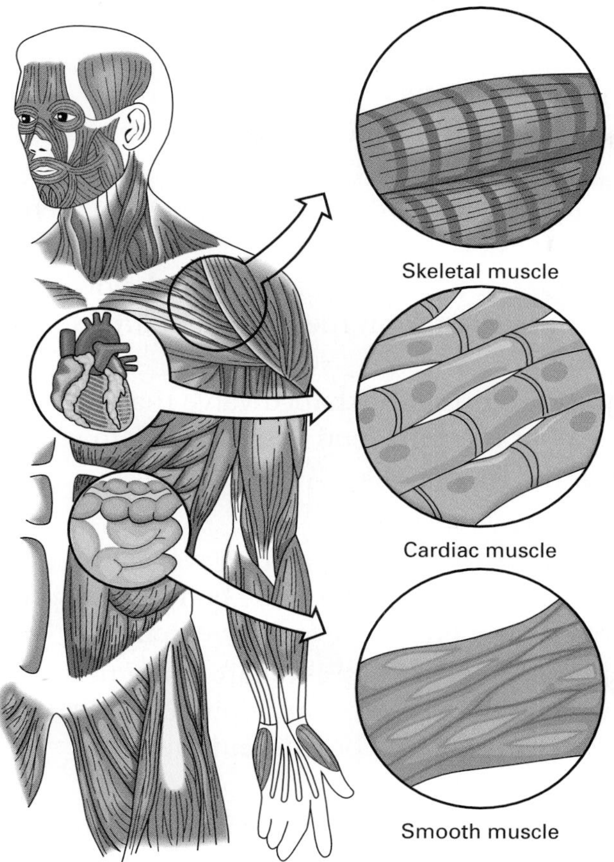

Figure 4-9
There are three types of muscle in the human body.

CONCLUSION

It's important for you to have a basic knowledge of the human body. That knowledge is the solid foundation on which to build your assessment skills. With it, you'll be better able to understand a patient's problems. You'll also be able to communicate those problems accurately to other health care professionals.

KEY TERMS

You may wish to use this list to review your understanding of key terms introduced in the chapter.

arteries blood vessels that carry blood away from the heart.

capillaries tiny blood vessels that connect the small arteries and veins and allow the exchange of oxygen and carbon dioxide at the cellular level.

central nervous system part of the nervous system that is made up of the brain and the spinal cord; acts as the master control for the entire nervous system.

cervical spine the first seven bones of the spinal column.

circulatory system a body system that delivers oxygen and nutrients and removes waste; major components are the heart, blood vessels, and blood.

diaphragm a muscle that is situated below the lungs and separates the chest from the abdomen; drives inhalation and exhalation.

epiglottis a thin, leaf-shaped valve that allows air into the trachea but prevents food and liquid from entering.

femur the thigh bone.

larynx the voice box.

musculoskeletal system a body system made up of muscles, bones, and joints, giving the body shape, protecting its vital organs, and providing for movement.

peripheral nervous system part of the nervous system that is made up of the cranial and spinal nerves; transmits nerve impulses between the organs and the brain.

pharynx the throat.

pulse point the point at which a pulse can be felt, usually where an artery lies over a bone close to the surface of the body.

respiratory system the body system that delivers oxygen and remove carbon dioxide; major components include the pharynx, epiglottis, larynx, trachea, lungs, and diaphragm.

shock the inability of the circulatory system to deliver oxygen to the body's tissues and cells.

sternum the breast bone.

sympathetic nervous system specialized spinal nerves that prepare the body to respond to stress.

trachea the windpipe.

veins blood vessels through which blood is transported from the body back to the heart.

xiphoid process the lowest part of the sternum.

APPLICATION QUESTIONS

You may wish to use these questions to review your understanding of the chapter. For answers with page references, see Appendix 2.

1. You are the first to arrive at the scene of a head-on car crash. One of the accident victims is a child. The other is an adult.

They aren't wearing seat belts. Both complain of chest pain from the impact. Based on what you know about adult and child musculoskeletal systems, how might their injuries be different?

2. You are a member of an emergency response team that is extricating a victim of a trench collapse. The patient is trapped about 10 feet down. He is complaining of a lack of feeling to his legs. When you finally reach him, which part of the spinal column will you immobilize first? Why?

3. You are evaluating a trauma patient. You have the choice of assessing only one of the following: mental status, pulse rate, or her physical injuries. Which single choice will give you the best information about how well her respiratory and circulatory systems are working? Why?

CHAPTER 5 BODY SUBSTANCE ISOLATION (BSI)

FIRST RESPONSE

Anna is a lifeguard. As she scans the beach, a man brings his ten-year-old son to the lifeguard tower. She observes that the boy has a small towel wrapped around his left foot. "Looks like someone has a flat tire," Anna says to them.

"Yes," says the father. "Are you trained in first aid? He knelt on a piece of glass. I took it out, but I think he needs a bandage."

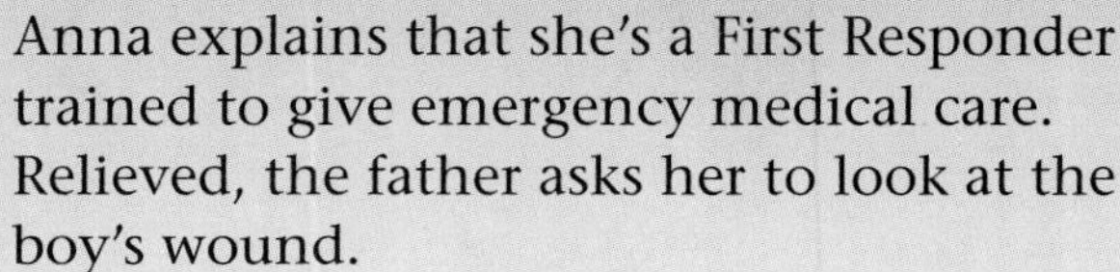

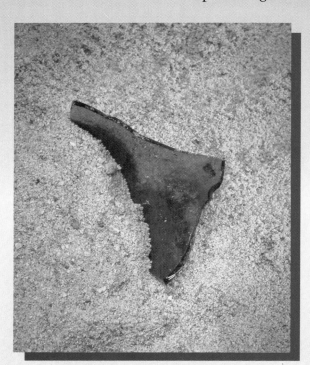

Anna explains that she's a First Responder trained to give emergency medical care. Relieved, the father asks her to look at the boy's wound.

As Anna reaches for her kit, the boy sits down on the sand. "Tell me what happened," she says. When he responds, she notes that he is shy but alert. His color seems okay too. Anna decides to look at the wound. Just as she bends down, the boy lifts his foot and the towel falls away. Suddenly the gash on top of the foot sprays blood onto her hands and arms. Embarrassed and panicky, she elevates the limb, grabs a few dressings, and applies direct pressure to the wound. Blood quickly saturates the pads and covers her fingers.

Just then another lifeguard approaches. "Yow! Anna," he cries, "where are your gloves? I'm gonna call 9-1-1."

Meantime Anna has the father hold the limb while she applies direct pressure to the wound. Once the bleeding is in control, she applies a bulky dressing and bandages it in place. By the time the EMTs arrive, the father has already decided to drive the boy to the hospital himself. He signs a refusal form, and he and the boy leave the beach together.

A week or so later, Anna receives a call from the local infection control officer. He tells her that she'll need to be tested. Anna feels her heart stop in her chest. She continues to listen. "The ten-year-old boy you helped last week," he tells her, "has tested positive for HIV. "

LEARNING OBJECTIVES

In the early days of EMS it was almost a rite of passage for new workers to get splattered with blood. Gloves, masks, and other equipment often were missing from a First Responder's jump kit. But those days ended with the spread of HIV and AIDS.

Today we face a variety of diseases, including life-threatening strains of hepatitis and resistant strains of tuberculosis (TB). As a First Responder, you risk exposure to those diseases every time you care for a sick or injured patient. This chapter will help you understand your risks. It also will describe proven ways of protecting yourself.

By the end of the chapter, you should be able to:†

- 1-2.8 Discuss the importance of body substance isolation (BSI). (pp. 45-46)
- 1-2.9 Describe the steps the First Responder should take for personal protection from airborne and bloodborne pathogens. (pp. 46-49)

INFECTIOUS DISEASES

An infectious disease is one that can be passed on from person to person. This is done by way of tiny organisms we call germs or **pathogens**. Pathogens may be found in body fluids, including saliva, mucus, blood, and urine. A sick person's body fluids spread disease by way of

- Droplet infection, such as through sneezing or coughing.
- Blood-to-blood contact, such as blood transfusions.
- Body fluid contact with another person's mucous membranes or open wounds.

Some pathogens like hepatitis B are passed on only by way of blood. Others like HIV can be found in all the fluids of a sick person's body, even breast milk. However, HIV and AIDS are not as common a risk to health care workers as hepatitis. About 8800 health care workers contract hepatitis B each year. Two hundred of them ultimately will die from hepatitis-related complications.

†Numbered objectives are from the 1995 U.S. DOT "First Responder: National Standard Curriculum."

The problem with caring for patients who may have an infectious disease is that they may not appear to be sick at all. Another problem is that they may have a variety of medical problems that mask the signs and symptoms of infection. So, the only sure way to protect yourself is to assume that all patients have infectious diseases and that all body fluids are infectious.

PROTECTING YOURSELF

The U.S. Occupational Health and Safety Administration (OSHA) sets the standards for infection control methods. Their methods for preventing the spread of bloodborne pathogens are known as **universal precautions**. These include rescuer strategies such as cleaning, disinfecting, and sterilizing equipment, as well as system-wide strategies such as mandating training for workers most at risk.

> **STREET NOTES**
>
> Always assume that all body fluids are infectious.

The U.S. Centers for Disease Control (CDC) also publish guidelines. They ask us to assume that all body fluids are infectious and recommend the use of barrier devices such as latex gloves for all contact with patients. Their guidelines are called **body substance isolation (BSI)**.

In general, to protect yourself against infectious disease you should:

- *Wash your hands aggressively.* This may be the number one method of preventing the spread of disease. Wash often, and always wash after a call. Use plenty of soap and water. Brush under your fingernails, and scrub all exposed skin (Figure 5-1).
- *Keep your equipment clean.* Wash and disinfect all equipment that has been exposed to body fluids. Use soap and water, followed by a wipe down with a 10% bleach solution. Remember that blood often will be hidden in Velcro fasteners and on the inside of carrying cases. If you can't disinfect equipment properly, throw it away.
- *Discard contaminated materials.* Secure them in plastic bags that have been clearly labeled (Figure 5-2).
- *Use masks and other barrier devices* (Figure 5-3).

  Masks. Disposable surgical masks will protect you from blood splatter. When placed on your patient, they also help to prevent the spread of airborne pathogens. When you suspect tuberculosis, wear a high efficiency particulate air (HEPA) respirator (Figure 5-4). It will keep you from inhaling the infected spray from a patient's sneeze or cough.

Eye protection (Figure 5-5). Wear goggles or safety glasses if there is a risk of being splattered with blood or other body fluids. If you wear prescription glasses, attach removable side shields.

Gloves. Disposable latex or vinyl gloves should be worn when there is any risk of contact with body fluids. To make sure they don't forget, most EMS workers put on gloves the moment they arrive on the scene. Consider wearing two pairs at once.

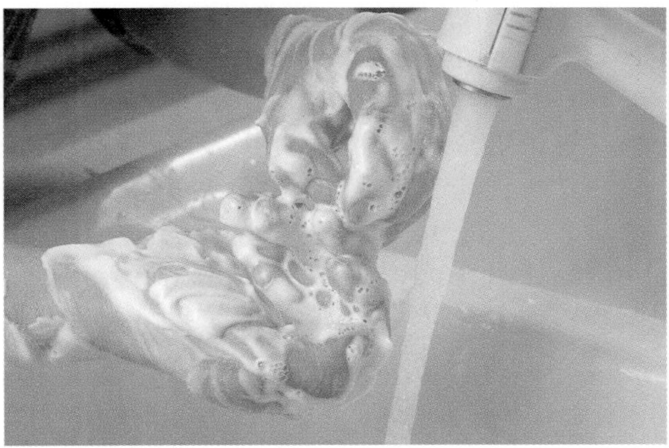

Figure 5-1
Handwashing may be the most important way of preventing infection.

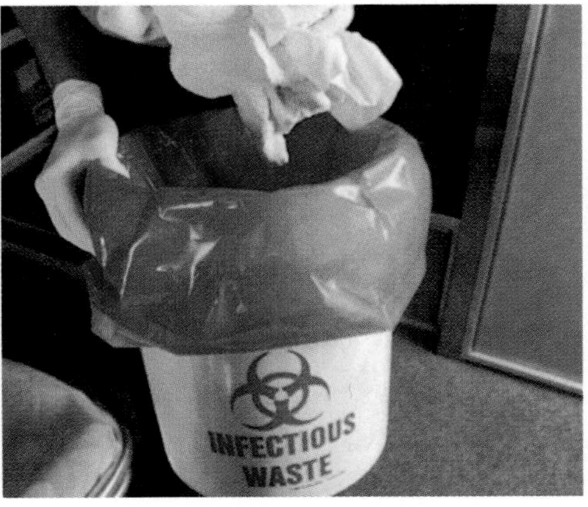

Figure 5-2
Dispose of all contaminated materials properly.

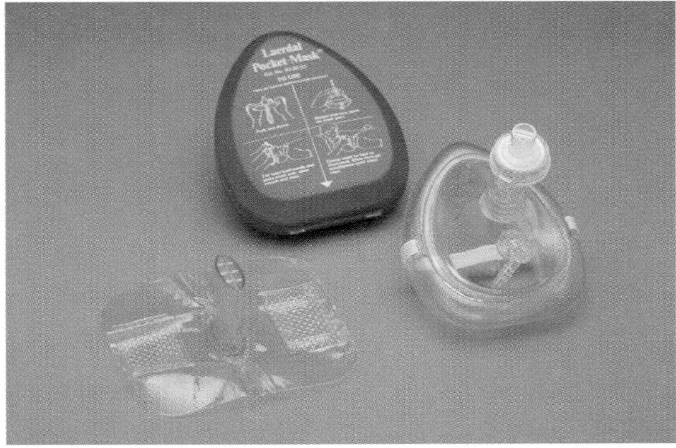

Figure 5-3
Masks and other barrier devices prevent direct contact with body fluids.

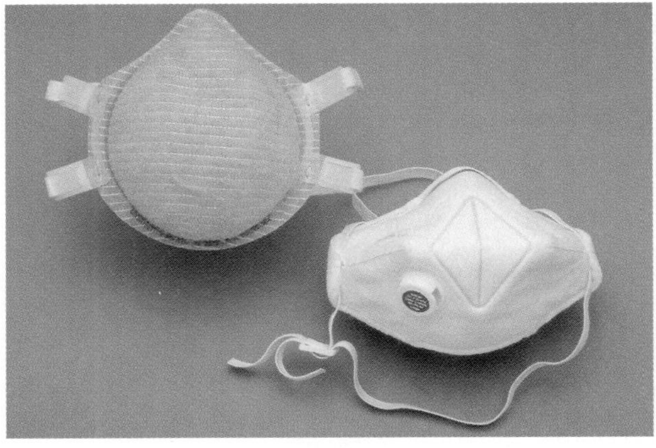

Figure 5-4
Use a HEPA respirator with suspected TB patients.

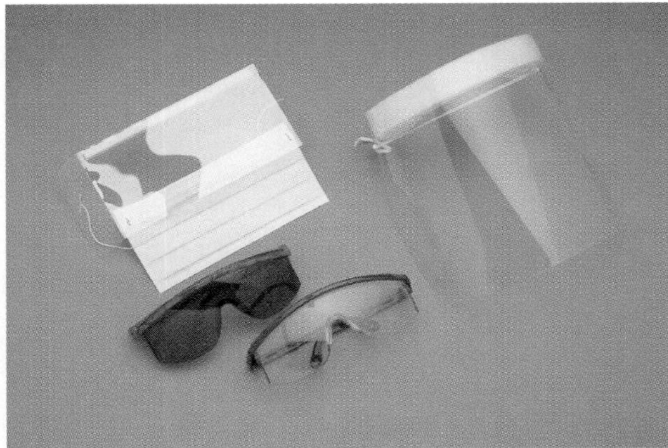

Figure 5-5
Types of protective eye wear.

If you have blood on the outside pair, you'll be able to remove them while the inner pair continues to protect you from exposure. Wear a new pair of gloves for each patient. When sharp objects are on the scene or when you are involved in an extrication, also wear heavy leather work gloves.

Gowns. Disposable gowns should be worn when there is a risk of major splash contamination, such as in childbirth or major trauma. Keep an extra uniform with you too.

- *Maintain current immunizations.* Be sure you are immunized against tetanus and hepatitis B, and get tested annually for TB. Many EMS systems also require annual flu shots and vaccinations against measles.

The key to protecting yourself is to assess infectious risks during the scene size-up. Most health care workers expose themselves to infection because they are either careless or unprepared.

TABLE 5-1 PRECAUTIONS AGAINST INFECTIOUS DISEASES

COMMON INFECTIOUS DISEASES	ROUTES OF TRANSMISSION	EMS PRECAUTIONS
HIV/AIDS	Blood and other body fluids, direct blood-to-blood contact	Masks, gloves, protective eyewear, gown, bandages on all open sores and wounds. Avoid mouth-to-mouth ventilation.
Hepatitis A, B, C, D	Blood, stool, and other body fluids, direct contact or on contaminated objects	Masks, gloves, protective eyewear, gown, bandages on all open sores and wounds. Avoid mouth-to-mouth ventilation. Also get vaccination; or get HBIG within two weeks of exposure and again one month later.
Tuberculosis	Oral or nasal secretions, airborne or on contaminated objects	HEPA filter or HEPA respirator. Masks with HEPA filter or HEPA respirator, gloves, protective eyewear. Avoid mouth-to-mouth ventilation.
Meningitis	Oral or nasal secretions	Masks, gloves, protective eyewear. Avoid mouth-to-mouth ventilation.
Measles	Oral or nasal secretions, airborne droplets or direct contact	Masks, gloves, protective eyewear. Avoid mouth-to-mouth ventilation. Get vaccination.
Influenza (flu)	Oral or nasal secretions, airborne droplets	Masks, gloves, protective eyewear. Avoid mouth-to-mouth ventilation. Get annual vaccination.

It's not enough that you understand how to take precautions. Be sure you also know when to take them!

REPORTING EXPOSURE

A rescuer's face is splashed with blood, much like Anna was splashed in the scenario at the beginning of the chapter. Another performs mouth-to-mouth resuscitation on a patient with meningitis. Still another finds that her hands are drenched in a patient's urine. Which instance should be reported as exposure to an infectious disease?

That depends on your state laws and local protocols. However, it's important for you to report to your supervisor any possible exposure to a disease. Create a paper trail that documents the type of exposure and describes the call. Your infection control officer will work with staff at the receiving hospital to determine the next course of action.

CONCLUSION

During your career as a First Responder, you will care for patients who suffer from infectious diseases. Sometimes you'll know it. Sometimes you won't. Remember that most infectious exposures occur when rescuers rush into calls headlong without weighing the risks. So always assume that all body fluids are infectious, and always strictly follow all appropriate precautions.

KEY TERMS

You may wish to use this list to review your understanding of key terms introduced in the chapter.

body substance isolation (BSI) standards and methods used to prevent infections transmitted by any body fluid.

pathogens microorganisms that produce disease.

universal precautions standards and methods used to prevent infection by bloodborne pathogens.

APPLICATION QUESTIONS

You may wish to use these questions to review your understanding of the chapter. For answers with page references, see Appendix 2.

1. You have arrived at the scene of a motor vehicle crash. You notice that one of your coworkers is not wearing protective gloves while managing a bleeding patient. How could you handle this situation?

2. You have responded to a childbirth in progress. Describe the personal protective equipment you will put on before caring for the patient.

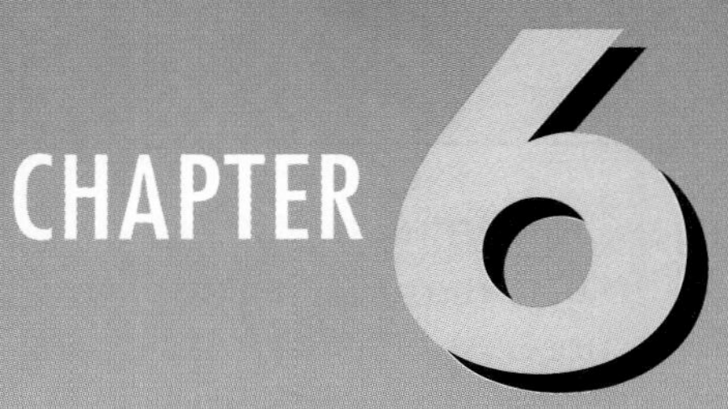

CHAPTER 6 LIFTING AND MOVING

FIRST RESPONSE

It's 5:00 a.m. and Chris Atkins, a volunteer firefighter, is driving to work when he witnesses a car crash. Seconds later, he passes the vehicle and pulls over to the shoulder of the road. He approaches the crumpled remains of a sedan, front end buried in the shattered trunk of a giant oak. Smoke is rising from the engine. The odor of fuel is strong, and there are muffled cries coming from inside the car.

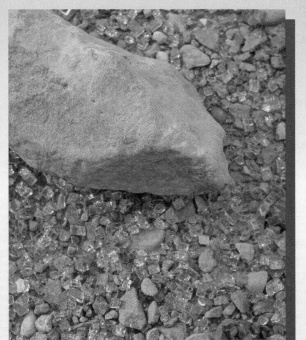

Chris radios EMS dispatch and is told fire rescue will arrive in minutes. He grabs his turnouts and jump kit. At the car he finds the doors and windows jammed shut. He can see the blood-streaked faces of three people inside, even though the smoke is getting thicker. "Get down! Cover your faces," Chris shouts. "I'm going to break the glass." Chris bashes in a side window with a rock. Immediately a 15-year-old female thrusts herself through the opening and tumbles out of the car. Another follows right behind her.

"I can't get out. My leg is broken," shouts the remaining teenager. Chris follows the young man's eyes to the front of the car. A plume of yellow flame is licking the underside of the buckled hood.

Chris breaks the window on the driver's side. He loops his arms under the patient's armpits and clasps them around his chest. "Push with your good leg, buddy. I'm going to pull you out the window." The patient nods and frantically pistons against the dashboard with his good leg. Chris strains backward, grunting, heaving, pulling as hard as he can. Slowly the patient emerges, screaming from the knifing pain in his leg. Chris drags him from the car as flames spread to the passenger compartment. Within moments the entire vehicle is engulfed in fire and smoke.

In an hour or so, Chris is among the last on the scene. Finally getting back into his car, he feels a sharp tinge in his lower back. "Oh, no," he murmurs to himself, "guess I'll be seeing the doctor too."

LEARNING OBJECTIVES

In the scenario on the previous page, Chris injured his back when he moved a patient during a life-threatening situation. In most cases, however, you'll be able to prevent career-ending back injury by using the correct techniques for lifting and moving. Many First Responders are injured every year because they attempt to lift or move patients improperly. Back injuries are the most common on-the-job injury. They also cause more permanent problems for EMS workers than any other injury.

By the end of the chapter, you should be able to:†

- 1-5.1 Define body mechanics. (pp. 52-53)
- 1-5.2 Discuss the guidelines and safety precautions that need to be followed when lifting a patient. (p. 53)
- 1-5.3 Describe the indications for an emergency move. (p. 54)
- 1-5.4 Describe the indications for assisting in nonemergency moves. (pp. 55-58)
- 1-5.5 Discuss the various devices associated with moving a patient in the out-of-hospital arena. (pp. 59-61)

* Correctly position patients according to their complaints and mental status. (pp. 58-59)

BODY MECHANICS

The term **body mechanics** refers to the study of how the body moves. It can help you to identify the best ways to lift, carry, push, pull, and reach for heavy objects without injury (Figure 6-1).

A key to good body mechanics is correct alignment of the spine. Maintain the normal curve of your back whenever you lift an object. Don't slump forward or lean back. Use your back and stomach muscles to support your spine. Then let the strong muscles of your legs, thighs, and buttocks do the work of lifting. Be sure your feet are firmly planted a comfortable distance apart. Don't twist. Remember—the farther away the weight is from your body, the harder your muscles have to strain. So keep the object close to you, and lift in several short moves, not one long one, whenever possible.

Another important rule of good body mechanics is to know your limits. If your patient is too heavy, get help! Then work as a

†Numbered objectives are from the 1995 U.S. DOT "First Responder: National Standard Curriculum." Asterisks indicate supplemental material.

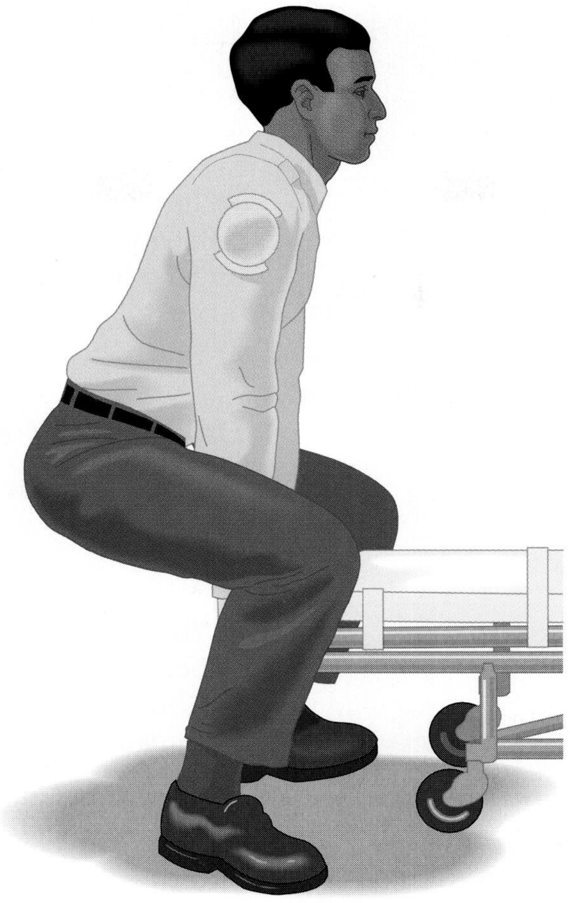

Rules of Lifting
- Know the weight.
- Know your physical limitations
- Keep your back locked in normal inward curve.
- Use leg, abdominal, and back muscles.
- Keep the weight close to your body.
- Communicate with your partner.

Figure 6-1
Basic rules of good body mechanics.

team. You can drop a patient or injure yourself badly if everyone isn't in on the same game plan. So talk with your partners about a lifting strategy. Decide who lifts which part of the patient, where you'll place him after the move, and how many moves it'll take to get there. Agree on a count-off procedure ("I'll say, one-two-three and then we'll lift"). Usually, the rescuer at the patient's head leads the effort and counts off.

Practice the techniques of good body mechanics until they become automatic. Once they're yours, you'll be able to lift and move safely, even in life-threatening emergencies.

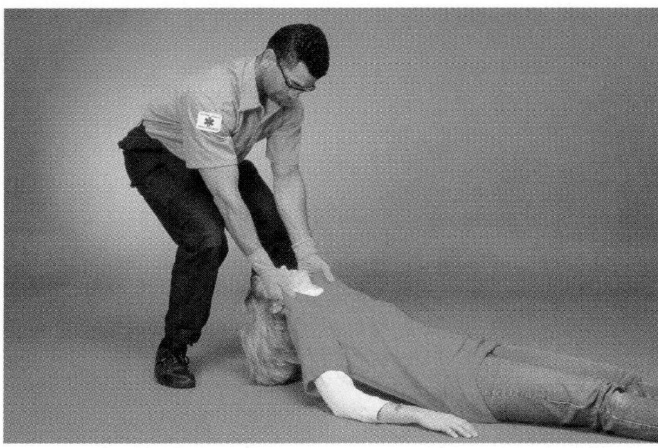

Figure 6-2
Shirt drag.

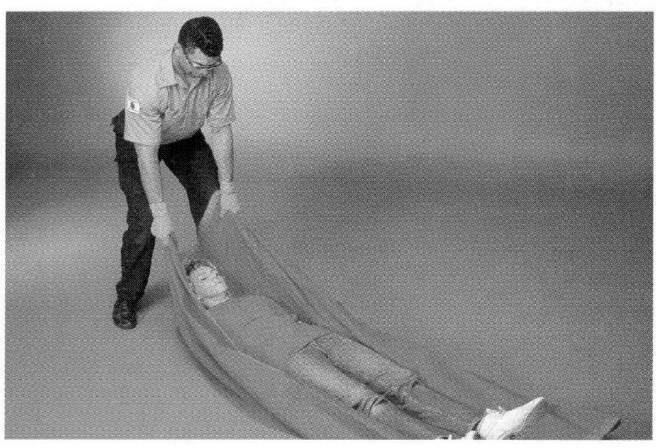

Figure 6-3
Blanket drag.

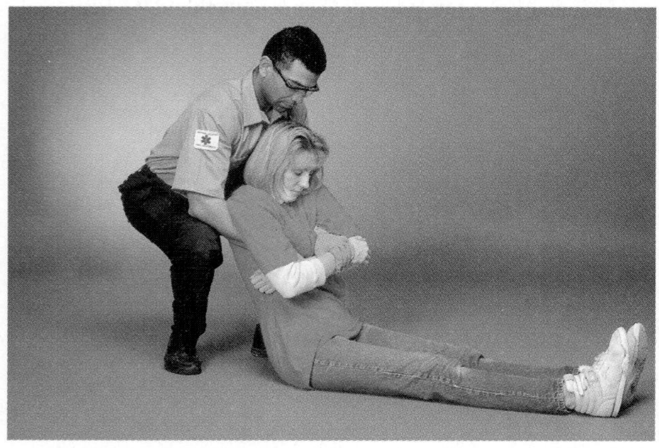

Figure 6-4
Shoulder drag.

MOVING A PATIENT

As a First Responder, you'll move patients who are in immediate danger, position patients to prevent further injury, and help other EMS workers to move patients. The following text explains the conditions under which each type of move may be made.

EMERGENCY MOVES

In general, a patient should be moved immediately only when the following conditions exist:

- There's immediate danger to the patient because of fire or danger of fire, explosion or danger of explosion, or other life-threatening hazards.
- You're not able to gain access to other patients who need life-saving care.
- You're not able to provide life-saving care to your patient because of his or her location or position.

Such a move is called an **emergency move**. Its greatest danger is the possibility of causing further injury to your patient's spine. However, realize that protecting a patient's spine won't matter if he dies from a blocked airway or in a car fire. In an emergency, make every effort to protect the spine by pulling your patient in the direction of the long axis of his body.

Three emergency moves to use when patients are at ground level are the *shirt drag*, *blanket drag*, and *shoulder drag*. In the shirt drag, pull the patient's clothing in the neck and shoulder area (Figure 6-2). In the blanket drag, place the patient on a blanket and drag the blanket (Figure 6-3). For the shoulder drag, get behind the patient, put your hands under the armpits, and grasp the patient's forearms (Figure 6-4).

Direct Ground Lift

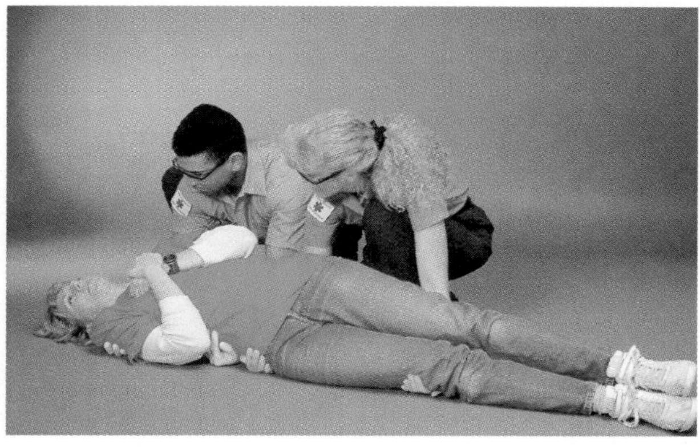

Figure 6-5a
Rescuers get in position.

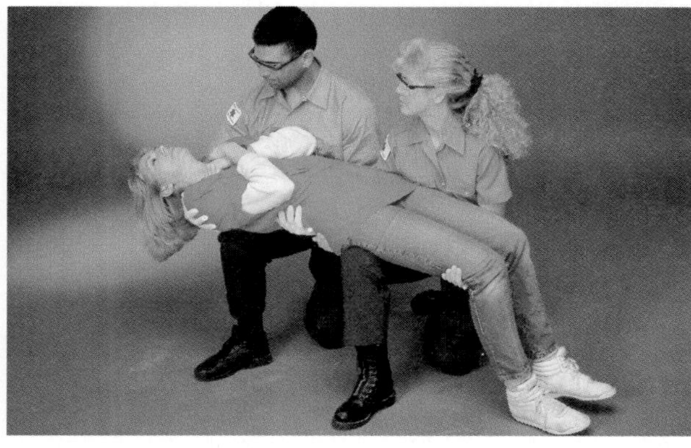

Figure 6-5b
On signal from the rescuer at the head, both lift the patient to their knees.

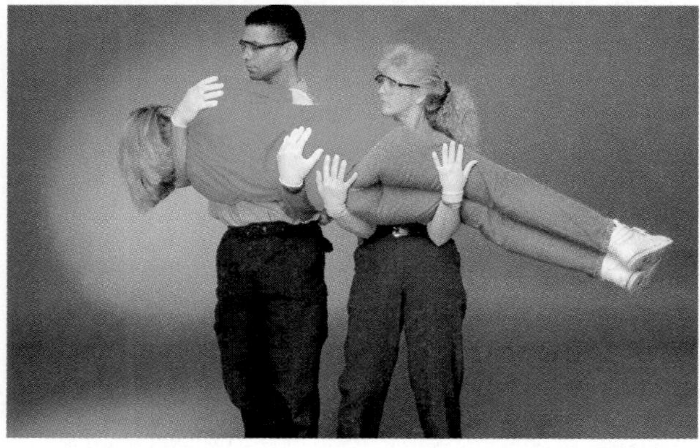

Figure 6-5c
On signal they roll the patient towards their chests, stand, and are ready to move the patient to the stretcher.

NONURGENT MOVES

In general you should assist other rescuers with **nonurgent moves**. They include the *direct ground lift*, the *extremity lift*, the *direct carry*, and the *draw sheet move*. Nonurgent moves are most often used to move a patient from a sitting or lying position to a stretcher. So before moving a patient, prepare the stretcher. Be sure the stretcher straps are unbuckled. If there are blankets on the stretcher, they should be pulled back. Lower the rails if it has them, and adjust the height.

> **Remember** *Keep your patient—and your back—safe! Make nonurgent moves in several short steps, and clearly communicate the plan for the move with the other rescuers.*

DIRECT GROUND LIFT

The direct ground lift is a good move to perform for lifting a patient with no suspected spine injury. It requires at least two rescuers (Figure 6-5).

1. Two rescuers line up on one side of the patient. Each kneels on a knee, preferably the same one.
2. Place the patient's arms on his or her chest.
3. The rescuer at the head places one arm under the patient's neck and shoulder, cradling the head. The other arm is placed under the patient's lower back. The second rescuer places one arm under the patient's knees and one arm above the buttocks.
4. On signal from the rescuer at the head, both lift the patient to their knees.
5. On signal they roll the patient towards their chests.

6. On signal the rescuers stand and move the patient to the stretcher.

7. To lower the patient to ground level, the steps are reversed.

If a third rescuer is available, he should place both hands under the patient's waist. To make room for the added help, the first rescuer then should have one arm at the middle of the patient's back.

EXTREMITY LIFT

The extremity lift is a two-rescuer lift that can be performed on patients with no suspected spine injury and no suspected leg or arm injury (Figure 6-6).

1. One rescuer kneels at the patient's head. The other kneels at the patient's knees.
2. The rescuer at the head works one hand under each of the patient's shoulders and grasps the patient's wrists.
3. The other rescuer slips one hand under each of the patient's knees.
4. On signal, both rescuers move up to a crouching position.
5. On signal, both rescuers stand up and move the patient to the stretcher.

Extremity Lift

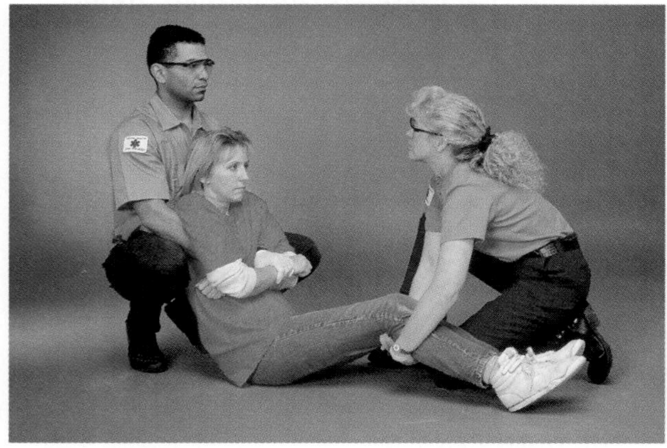

Figure 6-6a
Rescuers get in position.

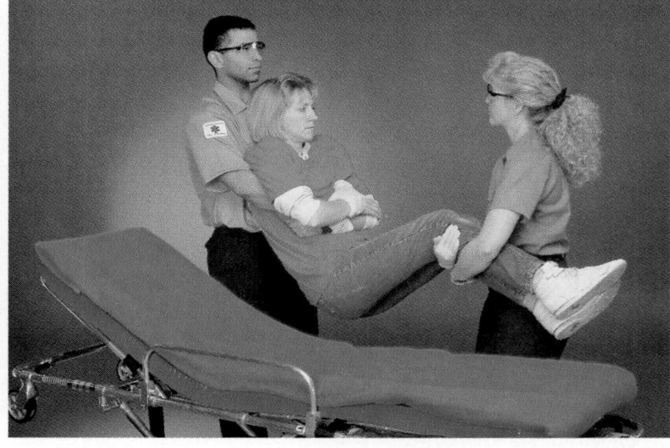

Figure 6-6b
On signal, both rescuers move up to a crouching position, stand, and are ready to move the patient to the stretcher.

Direct Carry

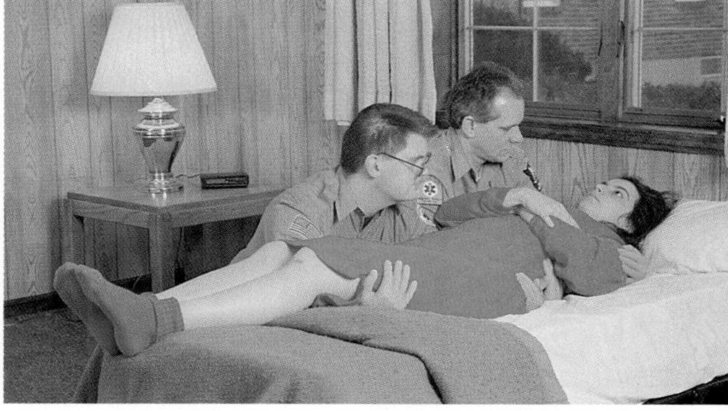

Figure 6-7a
After placing the stretcher at the foot of the bed, rescuers get in position.

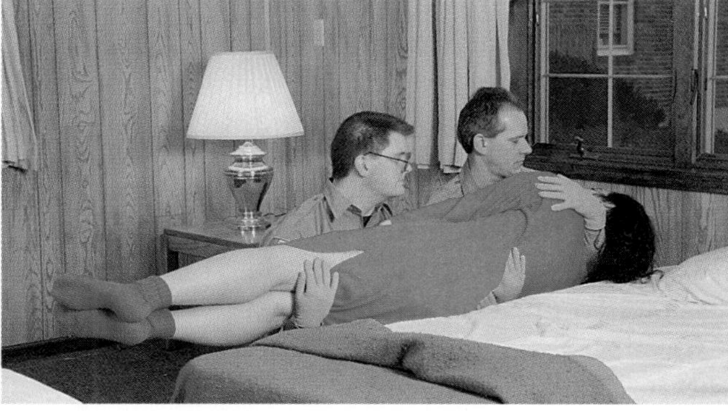

Figure 6-7b
On signal, both rescuers slide the patient to the edge of the bed, lift, and then curl the patient to their chests.

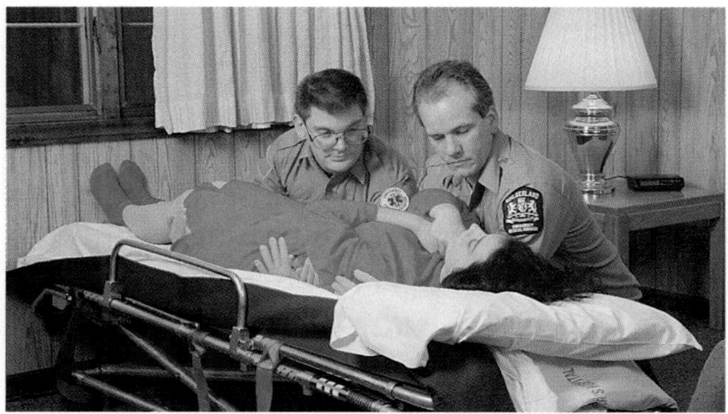

Figure 6-7c
On signal they have rotated and are ready to move the patient to the stretcher.

Direct Carry

The direct carry is a good two-rescuer technique for moving a patient from a bed to a stretcher (Figure 6-7). The patient should have no suspected spine injury.

1. The stretcher is placed at the foot of the bed.
2. Both rescuers stand at the side of the bed, facing the patient.
3. The first rescuer slides one arm under the patient's neck and cups the patient's far shoulder.
4. The second rescuer slides one arm under the patient's hip. He lifts slightly, so that the first rescuer can slide an arm under the patient's back.
5. The second rescuer then slides his free arm under the patient's calves.
6. On signal, both rescuers slide the patient to the edge of the bed, lift, and then curl the patient to their chests.
7. The patient is then moved to the stretcher and placed on it.

Draw Sheet Move

This is an effective two- or three-rescuer method of moving a patient who is already on a sheet in a bed (Figure 6-8). The patient should have no suspected spine injury.

1. One rescuer loosens the bottom sheet of the bed. The other rescuer positions the stretcher next to the bed.
2. The first and second rescuers position themselves across the stretcher from the patient. If there's a third rescuer, he or she should get on the other side of the bed, facing the patient.
3. The first and second rescuers reach across the stretcher to grab the sheet at

Draw Sheet Method

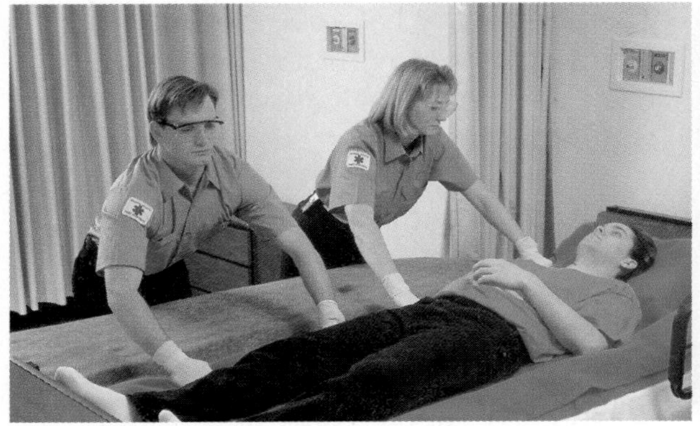

Figure 6-8a
After placing the stretcher next to the bed, rescuers get in position and grab the sheet.

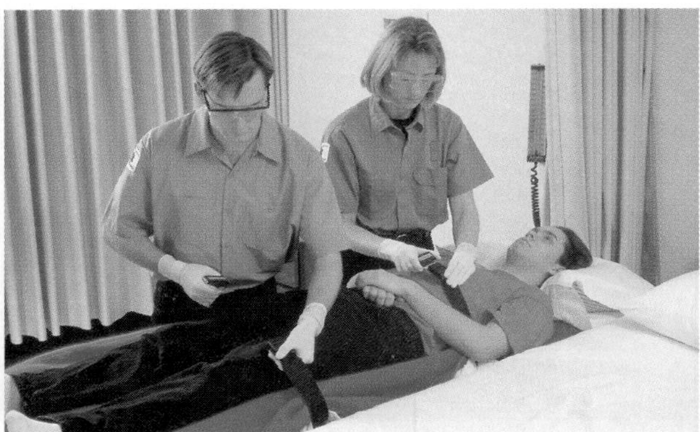

Figure 6-8b
On signal, they lift the patient over the gap and slide the patient onto the stretcher.

the patient's head, chest, hips, and knees. If there's a third rescuer, he or she should grasp the sheet at the patient's shoulders and hips.

4. On signal from the rescuer at the head, the rescuers should lift and slide the patient onto the stretcher.

Note that between the bed and the stretcher there's usually a small gap and some rough terrain (bed rails and stretcher frame). Be sure to lift the patient over this gap as you slide him toward the stretcher.

PATIENT POSITIONING

Unless there is an immediate danger at the scene, patients should not be moved until the EMTs arrive to evaluate and stabilize them. However, in some cases a patient's emergency care will include proper positioning. To decide on a best position, you'll have to answer questions such as: What is the patient's chief complaint? What position will help the patient? What position will the patient tolerate?

Throughout the textbook, we'll address positioning when we talk about specific problems and complaints. Briefly, the positions a First Responder may consider include:

- *Recovery position.* The patient is lying on his side. This allows for drainage from the mouth and keeps the tongue from falling back and blocking the airway. Use it to help unresponsive, breathing patients who are not injured. It also may be helpful for breathing patients after artificial ventilation or CPR.

- *Supine position.* The term *supine* means lying on the back with the face upward. All unresponsive patients who need artificial ventilation or CPR must be placed in this position first.
- *Position of comfort.* Patients who have no spinal injury, but who have pain, difficulty breathing, or nausea and vomiting may assume any position that makes them comfortable. Many short-of-breath patients, for example, will want to stay in an upright sitting position.
- *Shock position.* The patient is lying on his back with legs elevated eight to 12 inches. This position will help manage shock in patients who are immobilized as well as in patients who have no suspected spinal injury. (You'll learn more about shock in Chapter 12.)

EQUIPMENT FOR MOVING PATIENTS

In general you should not move patients. In unsafe conditions you may be forced to make an emergency move. However, the rest of the time you'll only move patients to help EMTs put them in stretchers and into an ambulance. Then you'll probably use a variety of equipment.

Stretchers or cots are lightweight (Figures 6-9 and 6-10). The wheeled stretcher is the standard carried on all ambulances (Figure 6-11). The stair chair is ideal for patients who must be kept in a sitting position. It also is used to move patients through tight doorways and down curved stairways (Figure 6-12).

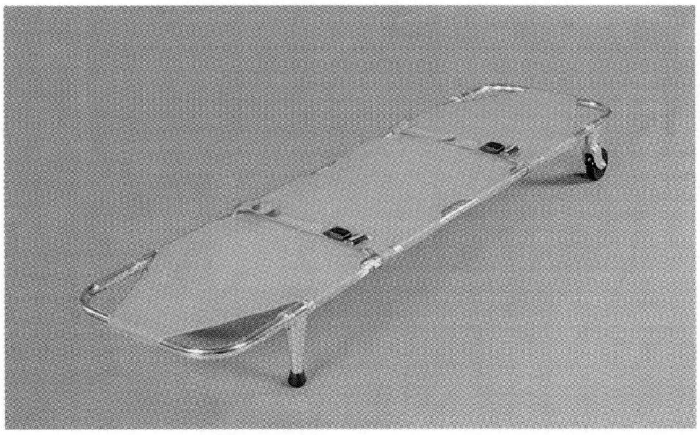

Figure 6-9
Portable metal stretcher.

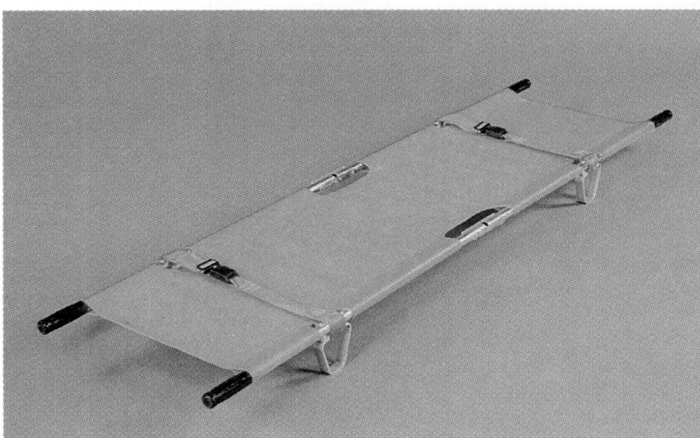

Figure 6-10
Portable pole or canvas stretcher.

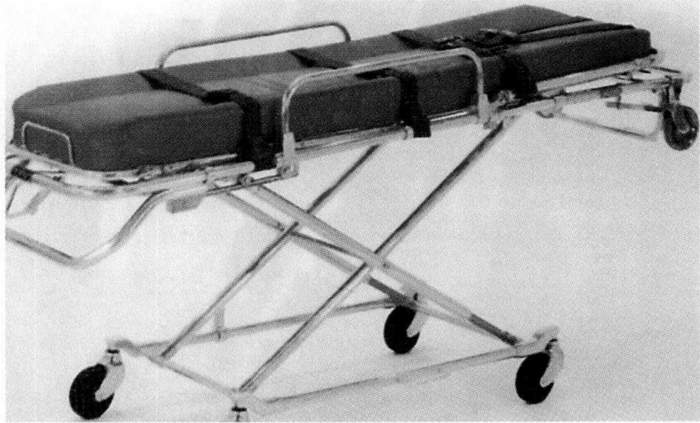

Figure 6-11
Wheeled stretcher.

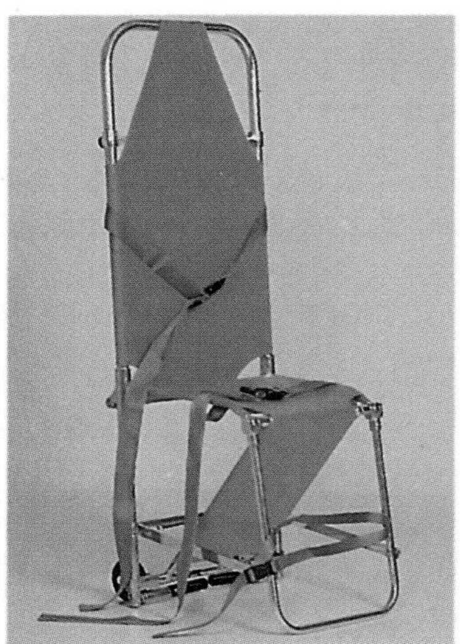

Figure 6-12
Stair chair.

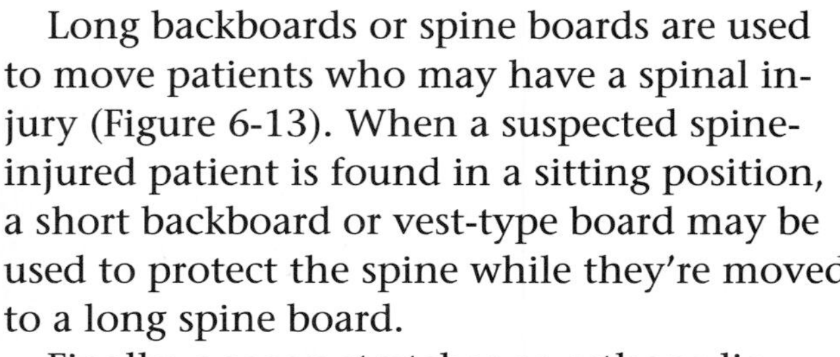

Long backboards or spine boards are used to move patients who may have a spinal injury (Figure 6-13). When a suspected spine-injured patient is found in a sitting position, a short backboard or vest-type board may be used to protect the spine while they're moved to a long spine board.

Finally, a scoop stretcher or orthopedic stretcher is used to move patients with curved spines or hip injuries (Figure 6-14). This device is concave and easier on backs than a long backboard. It also can be broken into halves and reconnected after being carefully fitted beneath a patient.

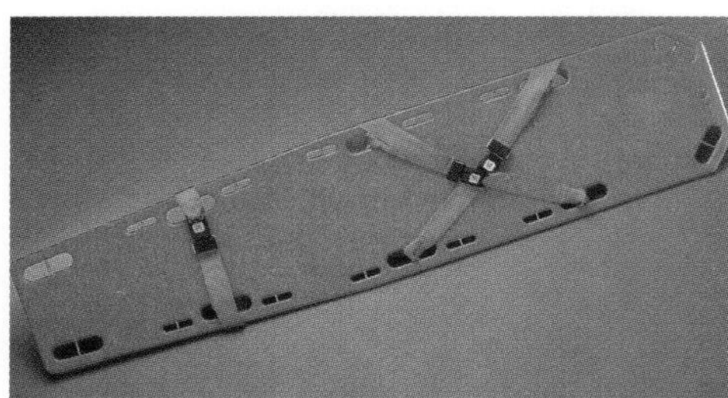

Figure 6-13a
Long backboard.

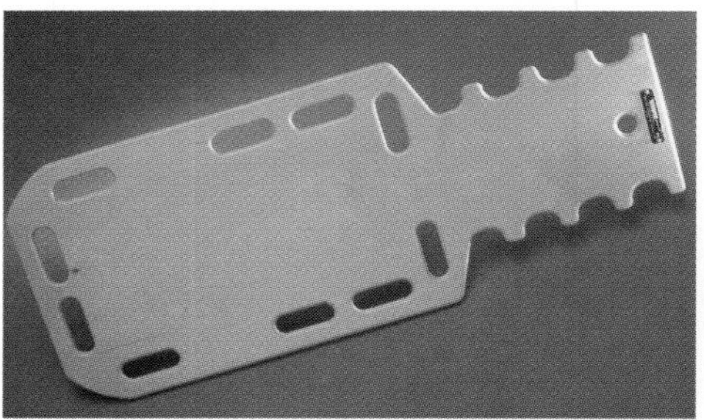

Figure 6-13b
Short backboard.

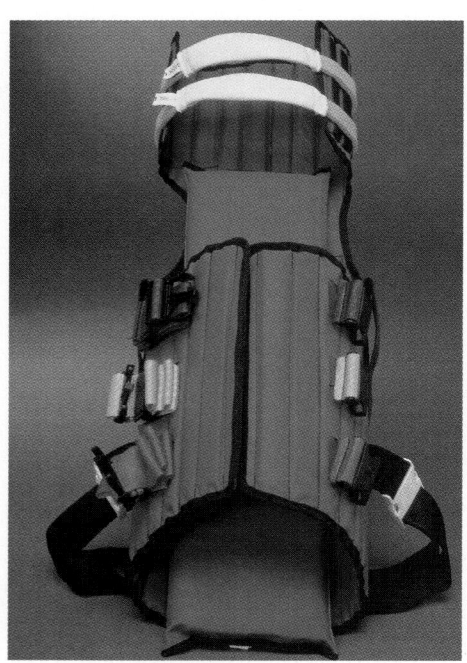

Figure 6-13c
Vest-type backboard for adults.

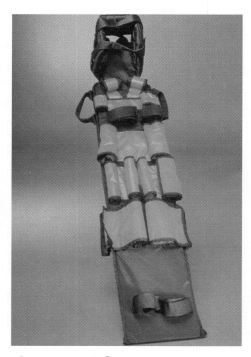

Figure 6-13d
Vest-type backboard for infants.

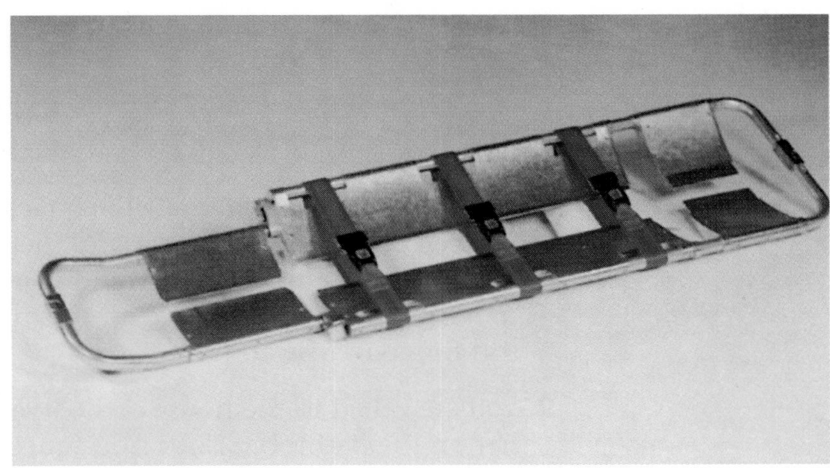

Figure 6-14
Scoop stretcher.

CONCLUSION

As a First Responder, you'll only move patients who are in immediate danger. You'll help other EMS workers to move patients after they've been examined and stabilized. You'll also position patients to prevent further injury when appropriate. But remember to do all this lifting and moving with your own safety in mind!

Follow the rules of good body mechanics to protect yourself from back injuries. When you help other rescuers, work as a team and communicate well during lifting and moving procedures. Remember—you won't be able to care properly for your patients if you're injured in the process.

KEY TERMS

You may wish to use this list to review your understanding of key terms introduced in the chapter.

body mechanics application of the study of muscles and body movement to using the body and to preventing and correcting problems related to posture and lifting.

emergency moves techniques for moving a patient when there is immediate danger due to hazards, when the rescuer is unable to gain access to other patients who need life-saving care, and when the rescuer is unable to provide life-saving care to the patient because of his or her location or position.

nonurgent moves techniques for moving patients when there is no immediate danger.

APPLICATION QUESTIONS

You may wish to use these questions to review your understanding of the chapter. For answers with page references, see Appendix 2.

1. You find a 44-year-old male lying face down on the ground, wedged between a dumpster and the wall of a building. You see no signs of breathing. Would you perform an emergency move or a nonurgent move on this patient? Explain the reason for your answer.
2. You are called to the house of a 63-year-old female. You find her on the bathroom floor. You squeeze in next to her and find that her airway, breathing, and circulation appear to be normal. She has a large bruise on her forehead and is complaining of neck pain. You consider using a shirt drag to pull her out of the bathroom so you can examine her more thoroughly. Should you do it? Why or why not?
3. What are the four or five questions you and other rescuers need to answer in order to work together to move a patient?

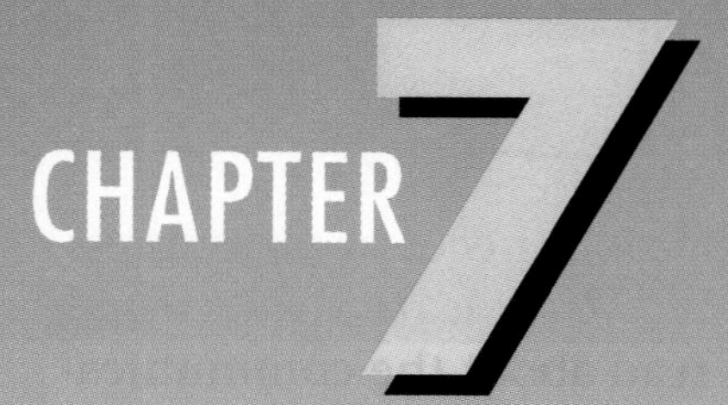

CHAPTER 7 PATIENT MANAGEMENT STRATEGIES

FIRST RESPONSE

Christine and Jake have handled many car crashes in their careers. When they arrive at the scene of this one, they realize they have a challenge on their hands. There appear to be no scene hazards, but there's a blizzard of screaming voices, panicked onlookers, and good Samaritans tripping over one another trying to lend a hand.

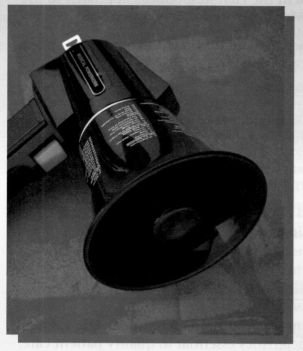

After spending precious seconds pushing only a few feet into the crowd, Christine and Jake stop. "This isn't working," Jake shouts. "There are too many people, too much noise. Where are the patients?" Christine doesn't know either. "We've got to get this scene under control!" They step back to the rescue vehicle, and Jake switches on the PA system. He directs the crowd to move back from the crash site.

Once they get to the patients, Jake continues to handle the crowd while Christine moves in to triage the patients. Jake soon joins her. They find that one patient is in serious condition. The other two have no life-threatening injuries, but they have lots of bumps, cuts, and scratches. Christine reports to EMS dispatch as soon as she can to request additional resources. With extra help on the way, they can reassess the patients, monitor for changes, and check their interventions.

It isn't long before the EMTs arrive. After giving them injury reports, Christine and Jake help them prepare the patients for transport. Later, when the scene has been cleared, they sit on the back bumper of their vehicle, sweaty and tired. "I'm beat," Jake says. "That call really worked us hard. Until we got ourselves organized, that tiger really had us by the tail."

Christine nodded in agreement. "Getting organized and prioritizing the important jobs first, that's the way to avoid falling on your face." Both First Responders agree that this call would be one for the books.

care decisions. An example of a key knowledge would be understanding that you must see adequate chest rise to confirm that you are rescue breathing for a patient correctly.

The grieving process.

LEARNING OBJECTIVES

This chapter will introduce you to the skills necessary to successfully run calls and take care of patients. You'll learn the attributes

FIRST RESPONDER COMMUNICATION SKILLS

Managing the terminally ill patient also can be difficult. Dealing with one's own mortality often involves a grieving process.

Finally, be aware that calls in which death occurs may be dangerous. People close to the dead patient may become irrational, even violent. Carefully assess each scene for safety. If necessary, leave. Do not re-enter the scene until it is secure.

THE PATIENT

As a First Responder, you'll care for a wide range of patients. You also can expect a wide range of responses including pain, fear, despair, and anger. So unless you've developed effective ways to communicate, finding out what medical care each patient needs can be difficult. When devising a communication strategy for your patient, ask yourself three questions:

- What does my patient think and feel?
- What does my patient need?
- What do I need to get done as a First Responder?

Answering those questions will help you to develop a communication strategy that will meet both your patient's needs and your needs. This questioning approach also will help you to communicate specific problem-solving strategies to your patient. Remember that you'll often help people who feel out of control and frightened.

Think of an office worker who is in a car crash while on the way to work. In addition to being scared and hurt, she's probably worried about the damage to her car, about being late for work, about getting word to her family, and about a dozen other problems. In order to do your job, you may need to address some of those concerns, like this:

> Beth, the first thing we need to do is make sure you're okay. You said your back feels funny. So, first we're going to protect your head and neck with this equipment. Then the EMTs will transport to the hospital, where a doctor will make sure you're okay. The hospital will make your phone calls so that work and your family won't worry. Finally, a police officer will go to the hospital to interview you about the crash. He or she will tell you where your car will be towed. For now, let's take care of you so that you can take care of all the other issues. Okay?

STREET NOTES

Arguing with or confronting a patient usually fails to improve the situation. It's like pouring kerosene on a fire. Honest, gentle, nonjudgmental communication works best as a rule.

Don't be afraid to try different communication strategies. Some patients will require a gentle approach. Others may respond to reasoning. Still others may require a firm stance. The following paragraphs describe strategies for some specific types of patients.

Infants and Children

Communication with children should be based on their age and level of development. For example, infants respond to the tone of your voice and the warmth of your touch. School-age children appreciate it if you don't loom over them. Kneel, if necessary, to talk to them at their eye level. Also try to anticipate a child's fears. If a procedure will hurt, don't lie about it. Reassure the child by telling why it's necessary and how you'll proceed. Rely on praise rather than threats to get a child to follow directions. As a rule, encourage a parent or guardian to stay while you assess the patient. You'll find that a child is more likely to allow you to complete an exam when in the parent's arms.

The Elderly Patient

Always show respect for elderly patients by addressing them as "Mr.," "Mrs." or "Ms." Don't assume that all elderly patients are confused, hard of hearing, or blind. Assess their mental status just as you would any other patient. Many older patients will be overwhelmed by an emergency. You may need to slow down a bit when explaining or carrying out emergency care. Don't rush them for answers to your questions. Wait. Give them a chance to gather their thoughts and respond. You'll also find that elderly patients will greatly appreciate you tending to such things as locking the front door, getting word to a relative, and so on.

The Assaulted Patient

Patients who have been physically assaulted need a gentle, supportive approach. Many will not want to be touched. Sexual assault patients in particular may not want to discuss the assault at all. Limit your questions to determining the extent of the patient's injuries. If you're managing a female patient who has been sexually assaulted, consider having a female rescuer care for her. However, according to experts more important than gender is the First Responder's ability to be caring and concerned.

The Altered Mental Status Patient

Altered mental status patients range from slightly confused to unresponsive. As a rule, they require clear, simple communication. However, you may need to repeat your questions more than once. Do so patiently. Work slowly. Realize that their perceptions are altered, and you may get only irrational responses. If you see a potential for violence, call the police for help immediately.

The Combative Patient

Combative patients often perceive others—especially someone in a uniform—as a direct threat. So talk to them quietly. Move slowly. Adopt a body position that is nonthreatening, and avoid getting too close. If your patient appears to be rational, try to determine the cause of the behavior. Talking about it may help lessen the patient's fears or anger. Most important, remember always to place your safety and the safety of other rescuers first. Stay away from a combative patient if there is any indication that you may be attacked. Call the police for help. Do not approach the patient until the scene and, if necessary, the patient are secure.

Patients with Physical or Mental Disabilities

Physically handicapped patients may need you to make an extra effort to communicate effectively. For example, when you speak to hearing impaired or deaf patients, be sure they can see your lips (Figure 7-2). If they speak American Sign Language and you don't, try to find a relative or bystander who can interpret for you. Also consider writing notes on a pad.

Many people tend to shout when they realize they're talking to someone who's blind. Don't. Speak in your normal tone of voice. During assessment and treatment, take extra care to describe to blind patients exactly what you're going to do before you do it. If you have to walk away, be sure you tell them where you're going, why, and when you'll return. While waiting for the ambulance, you may find that keeping your hand lightly on the patient's shoulder will help to calm and reassure him or her.

Some of your patients will be unable to walk or move independently. They may have cerebral palsy or muscular dystrophy. They may be paralyzed because of a spine injury. Whatever the reasons, communicate with these patients just as you would with any other. If the patient has speech problems, stay calm and try to enlist the help of the patient's family or friends. Asking questions that require a "yes" or "no" answer also may be helpful.

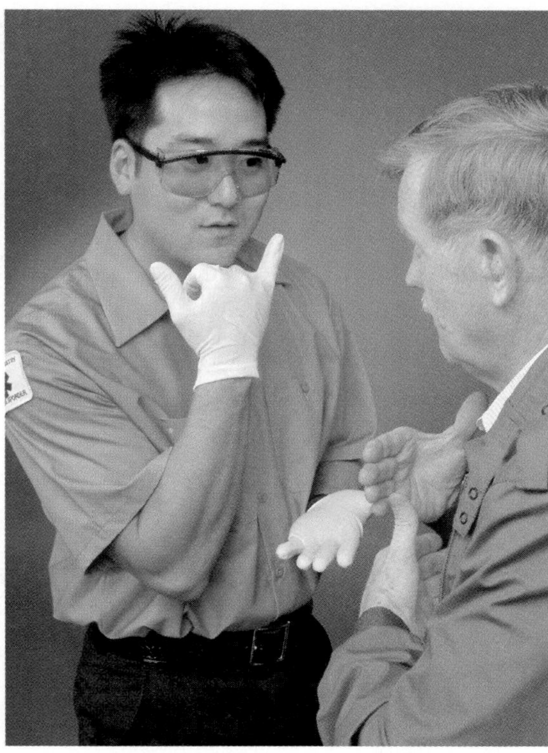

Figure 7-2
Communicate effectively with all patients.

Another example is the patient with Down's syndrome. Because of a low I.Q., this patient may not fully understand the emergency and become quite frightened. Do everything you can to avoid being perceived as a threat. Be kind and reassuring. Engage the patient's parents or caregiver in helping to keep the patient calm. Slow down the pace of your questions. Wait for the patient to respond, and listen carefully to the answers. They will help to tell you how much the patient understands and what you need to reexplain.

THE EMS CALL

Based on the scenario at the beginning of the chapter, the following will help you walk through what typically goes on before and after an EMS call. Immediately following this very general description, you'll find a specific five-step approach to patient management.

PREPARATION

Christine and Jake have just arrived for their shift in a fire rescue unit. They are volunteers and pull three 24-hour shifts per month. As soon as they arrive at the station, they begin to pre-

STREET NOTES

You've got to respond to a call in minutes. So keep your unit stocked and in top condition at all times.

pare for their first call. They make sure the unit is stocked with medical equipment such as airways, ventilation devices, a suction unit, and basic wound care supplies. They confirm that the unit is stocked with all nonmedical supplies as well, including street maps and safety equipment. They also make sure their radio, emergency lights, PA system, and window defrosters are working.

Both Christine and Jake are in uniform, ready to respond to an emergency immediately. They maintain readiness throughout their shift.

DISPATCH

Several passersby witness a car accident and dial 9-1-1 on their cellular phones. Their calls are routed to the regional dispatch center, which handles all such calls 24 hours a day. A trained dispatcher answers, gathering as quickly as possible critical information such as:

- The nature of the call.
- The name, location, and call-back number of the caller.
- The location of the patients.
- The number of patients and the severity of their injuries.
- Any other special problems EMS workers may need to know, such as downed power lines or other hazards.

EN ROUTE TO THE SCENE

Christine and Jake are told the nature and location of the call, as well as other pertinent information. Because they stay in radio contact with the dispatcher, they learn that there's at least one major trauma patient among a total of three patients. In response Christine and Jake ask for a medical helicopter and another First Responder unit. They want enough help on scene to provide patient care and to prepare a landing zone for the helicopter.

Jake and Christine also discuss the roles each will take. They decide that Jake will assist with overall scene management, and Christine will assess and treat patients.

ARRIVAL AT THE SCENE

After notifying dispatch that they've arrived on scene, Jake and Christine begin scene size-up. They check the scene for safety and put on protective gloves. They see that the utility pole involved in the crash doesn't appear to be damaged. There are no downed power lines or other hazards.

As Christine begins to assess the three patients, Jake moves the remaining bystanders away from the car. He also sets out flares, calls for additional EMS units, and identifies a spot for the helicopter to land. He notes the mechanism of injury and then finds Christine. She has been performing **triage** (ranking the patients by the severity of their injuries). There is one **critical patient** (a seriously ill or injured patient). The other two have only minor injuries.

TRANSFERRING PATIENTS TO OTHER EMS CREWS

Soon the responding units arrive. Christine gives patient reports to the EMTs and assists with getting the patients ready for transport. Other rescuers set up the landing zone for the helicopter. Then the critical patient is transferred to the arriving helicopter crew and flown off to a trauma center. The two other patients are loaded into the ambulances and transported to the local hospital.

POST-RUN DUTIES

After the call, Christine and Jake clean off or discard used equipment. Then they notify dispatch that they're available for another call and return to the station to restock the disposable supplies. Their last job is to file the patient care report.

A FIVE-STEP APPROACH TO PATIENT MANAGEMENT

Once you arrive at the scene of the emergency, use the following five-step approach to patient management. The five steps include: scene size-up, initial assessment and treatment, the physical exam and treatment, ongoing assessment and treatment, and patient hand-off. Follow the steps in order. They'll help you to manage the call in the safest and most effective way.

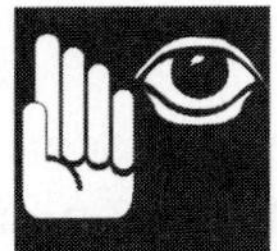

SCENE SIZE-UP

An accurate scene size-up keeps you and other rescuers safe. It also provides you with important information about the patients. Perform it as soon as you arrive at the scene. It includes the following tasks:

- Identify any scene hazards, and take BSI precautions.
- Note the cause of the emergency. Look at the scene as a whole and note clues.
- Obtain an accurate patient count and, if there is more than one patient, observe which one needs the most urgent care.
- Call for specialized or additional resources if needed.

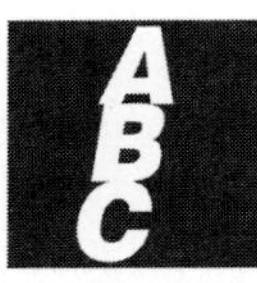

INITIAL ASSESSMENT AND TREATMENT

Once you ensure the scene is safe, begin an initial assessment. It includes a general impression of the patient's mental status and an assessment of the patient's airway, breathing, and circulation (ABCs). If you discover any life threats, such as blocked airway, bleeding, or shock, treat them immediately. Don't move on to the next step until this is done.

THE PHYSICAL EXAM AND TREATMENT

This step includes getting the patient's medical history, performing a head-to-toe examination, assessing vital signs, and treating the patient's wounds or illness.

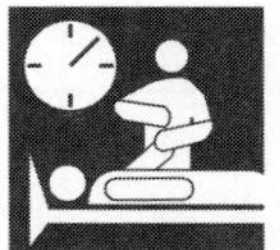

ONGOING ASSESSMENT AND TREATMENT

If the EMTs have not yet arrived, monitor your patient's condition closely until they do. Re-check the patient's airway, breathing, and circulation (ABCs) continually so that life-threatening changes can be treated immediately. Check all your interventions (artificial airways, oxygen mask, bandages, and so on) to be sure they are performing as they should.

PATIENT HAND-OFF

This final step includes both spoken and written reports to the transporting EMTs. In your reports communicate patient assessment findings and treatment so the EMTs can take over the patient's care appropriately.

CONCLUSION

In this chapter we've told you that successful patient management relies on First Responder characteristics and skills, good communication, and a basic five-step plan. We'll let a First Responder tell you how this approach to patient management helps him: "I walk into calls with this five-step plan burned into my brain. It helps me to organize patient care from beginning to end. Also, if I get turned around, I just have to tick off each of the steps in my mind to get back on track."

KEY TERMS

You may wish to use this list to review your understanding of key terms introduced in the chapter.

critical patient a seriously injured or ill patient; a patient in crisis.

triage the process of ranking patients according to the severity of their injuries, so that the most seriously injured patients are treated first.

APPLICATION QUESTIONS

You may wish to use these questions to review your understanding of the chapter. For answers with page references, see Appendix 2.

1. You have responded to a call for a "baby not breathing." You find a six-month-old that has been dead for some time. Your protocols tell you not to attempt to resuscitate this infant. Describe how you will communicate this information to the parents.

2. You have responded to a call for a "man down." You find an intoxicated 47-year-old male lying in the street. You move to assess him, and he sits bolt upright and shouts, "Get away from me. Leave me alone!" What should you do?

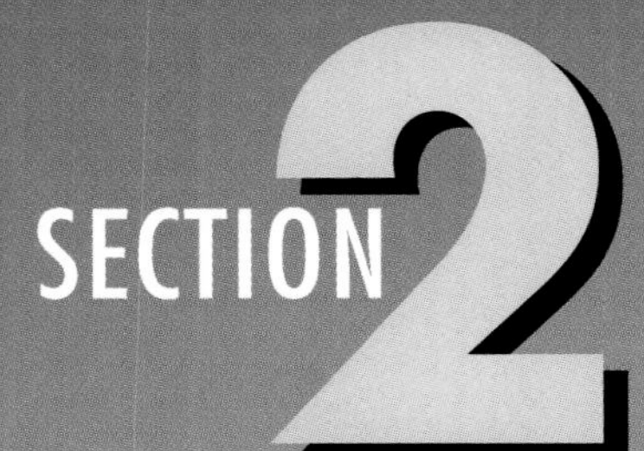

FIRST RESPONDER SKILLS

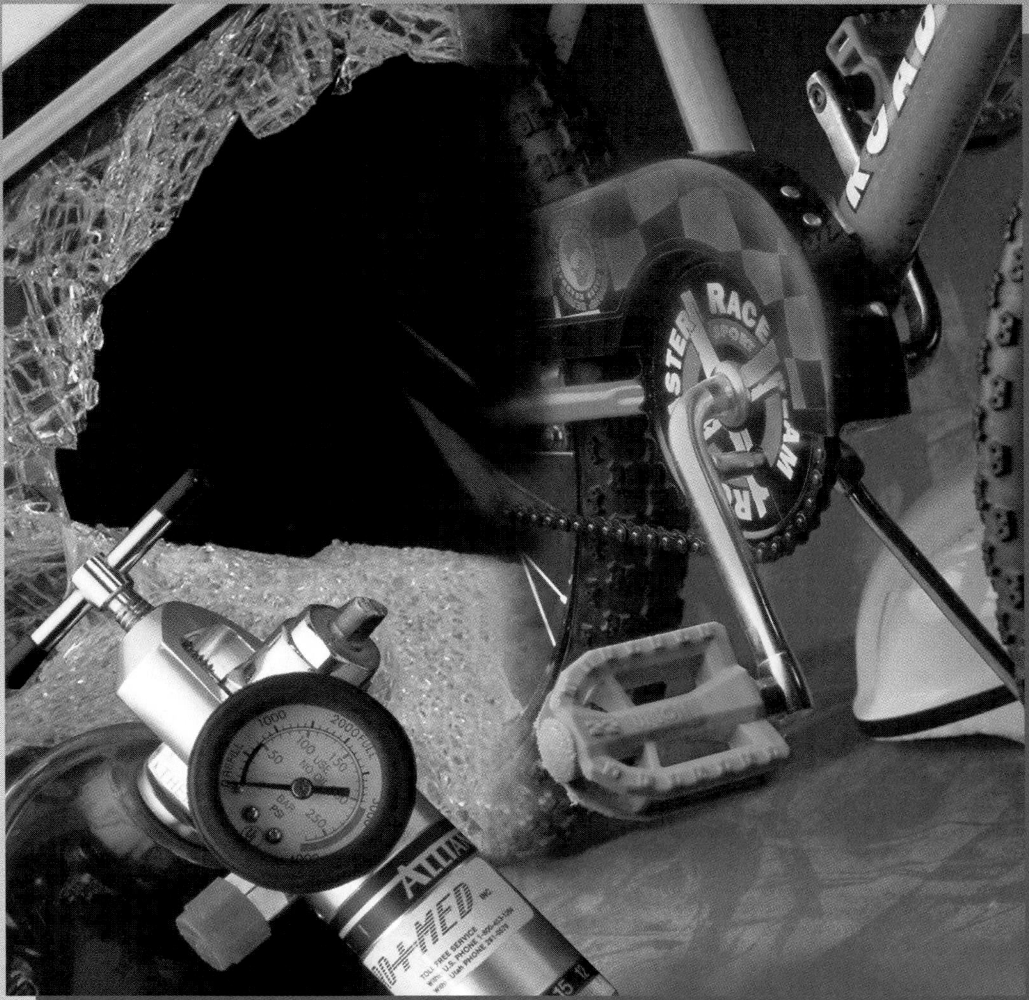

What happens in the field? What do I do if the patient isn't breathing or is losing too much blood? What if the patient can't tell me what's wrong? What if there's more than one patient? Section 2 will help you find the answers to these questions. It'll walk you through each of the five steps of patient management.

You'll see how to size up a scene for hazards. You'll learn how to recognize and treat a patient's life-threatening problems. You'll also find the elements of a good patient history, how to perform a thorough head-to-toe exam, and what to report to the EMTs who must take over patient care.

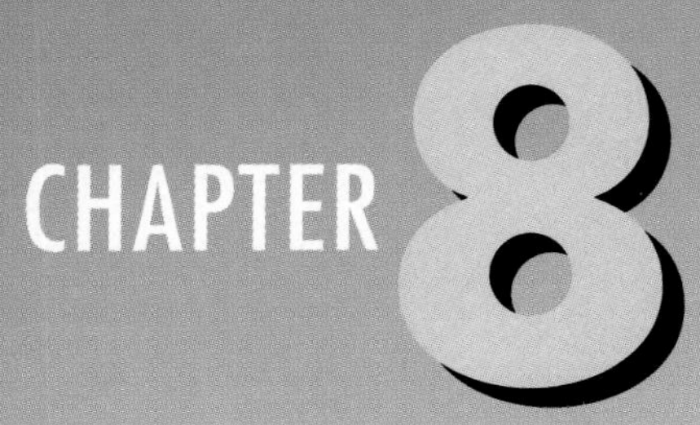

CHAPTER 8 SCENE SIZE-UP

FIRST RESPONSE

The Friday night party at Billy's Tavern is getting louder by the minute. Tanya, an off-duty police officer, already has seen the bouncer confiscate a baseball bat and usher two rowdies to the door. Suddenly she hears breaking glass and a drunken howl. A fight? As she makes her way to investigate, she hears the *pop pop pop* of semiautomatic handguns.

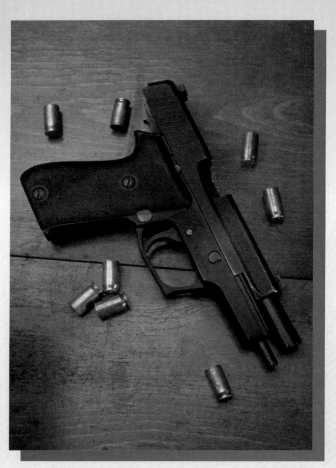

People flee in all directions, diving behind tables, the chairs, anywhere to get out of the line of fire. Tanya remembers she's unarmed, and she has no idea where the shooters are. So she stays put until the police arrive.

Within moments of their arrival, the police confirm that one gunman has fled the scene and the other is dead. Six bystanders have been shot. They start moving the crowd away from the victims immediately. After recognizing Tanya, one of the police officers asks her to help care for the shooting victims.

"Sure," she says. "Do you have your jump kits?" The police officer nods.

One officer hands her a pair of protective gloves. "Let's go," he says. Tanya and another police officer follow. Just then a second police unit arrives. Those officers maintain the security of the scene while Tanya and her new partners begin triage.

In minutes they update EMS dispatch: "We've got two high priority patients and two low priority patients. We've also got two we're triaging out. They're dead on scene. We need two additional ground ambulances, an extra fire engine, and the Life Star helicopter at St. Agnes sent this way."

Once scene size-up is complete, Tanya and the other two First Responders focus on assessment and care of their patients.

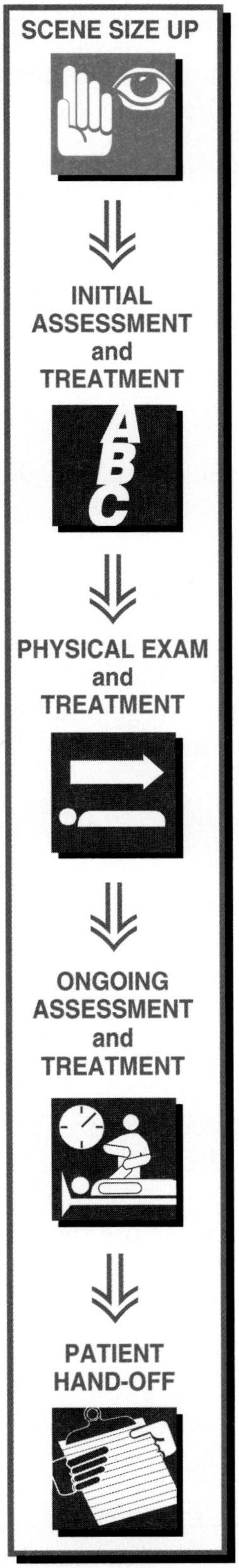

SCENE SIZE UP

INITIAL ASSESSMENT and TREATMENT

PHYSICAL EXAM and TREATMENT

ONGOING ASSESSMENT and TREATMENT

PATIENT HAND-OFF

LEARNING OBJECTIVES

Your scene size-up is the first critical step to take when caring for patients in the field. It will allow you to identify scene hazards and the types of resources needed to manage the emergency. Performed correctly, it also will provide you with valuable clues to the causes of your patient's injury or illness.

By the end of the chapter, you should be able to:†

- 1-2.7 Explain the need to determine scene safety. (pp. 80-81)
- 1-2.10 List the personal protective equipment necessary for each of the following situations (pp. 81-83):
  - Hazardous materials
  - Rescue operations
  - Violent scenes
  - Crime scenes
  - Electricity
  - Water and ice
  - Exposure to bloodborne pathogens.
  - Exposure to airborne pathogens.
- 3-1.1 Discuss the components of scene size-up. (p. 80)
- 3-1.2 Describe common hazards found at the scene of a trauma and a medical patient. (pp. 81-83, 86)
- 3-1.3 Determine if the scene is safe to enter. (pp. 80-87)
- 3-1.4 Discuss common mechanisms of injury/nature of illness. (pp. 87-88)
- 3-1.5 Discuss the reason for identifying the total number of patients at the scene. (pp. 90-93)
- 3-1.6 Explain the reason for identifying the need for additional help or assistance. (pp. 82, 83, 86, 93-94)
- 7-1.3 Discuss the role of the First Responder in extrication. (pp. 93-94)
- 7-1.4 List various methods of gaining access to the patient. (p. 93)

†Numbered objectives are from the 1995 U.S. DOT "First Responder: National Standard Curriculum."

- 7-1.5 Distinguish between simple and complex access. (p. 93)
- 7-1.6 Describe what the First Responder should do if there is reason to believe that there is a hazard at the scene. (pp. 83-87)
- 7-1.7 State the role the First Responder should perform until appropriately trained personnel arrive at the scene of a hazardous materials situation. (pp. 83-85)
- 7-1.8 Describe the criteria for a multiple-casualty situation. (pp. 90-91)
- 7-1.9 Discuss the role of the First Responder in the multiple-casualty situation. (pp. 90-93)
- 7-1.10 Summarize the components of basic triage. (pp. 90-91)

COMPONENTS OF SCENE SIZE-UP

Scene size-up is made up of four basic parts: scene safety, **mechanism of injury** (forces that cause that injury) or **nature of the illness**, basic triage, and access and extrication. In general, scene size-up can be performed by answering these questions:

- *Scene safety*. Is the scene safe? If not, what needs to be done to make it safe?
- *Mechanism of injury or nature of illness*. What is the problem? What are the clues to the who, what, when, where, why, and how of the problem?
- *Patient triage*. How many patients are there? If more than one, which patients need the most urgent care?
- *Access and extrication*. Is there appropriate access to the patient? Are specially trained personnel needed?

Jumping in without performing scene size-up is the most common error made in the field. *Never skip this step*. There's nothing more important to the success of the call than scene size-up. It will keep you organized. It will keep you from losing precious time. Most important, it will help keep you, other rescuers, patients, and bystanders safe.

SCENE SAFETY

Any emergency scene may be hazardous to you. It could be the site of an overturned car that is too unstable for you to approach. It could be a toxic waste spill or a violent criminal who is hiding.

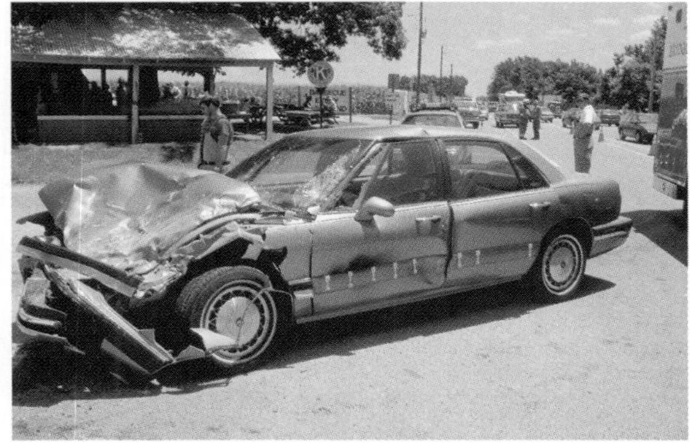

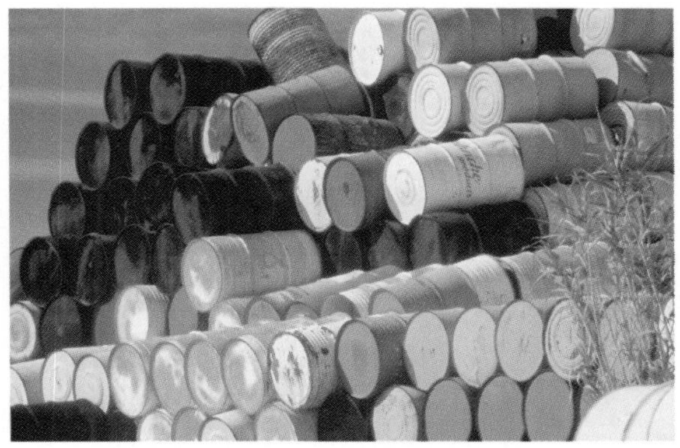

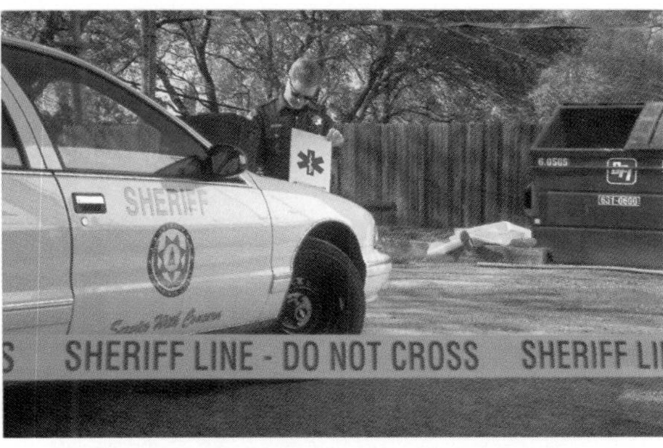

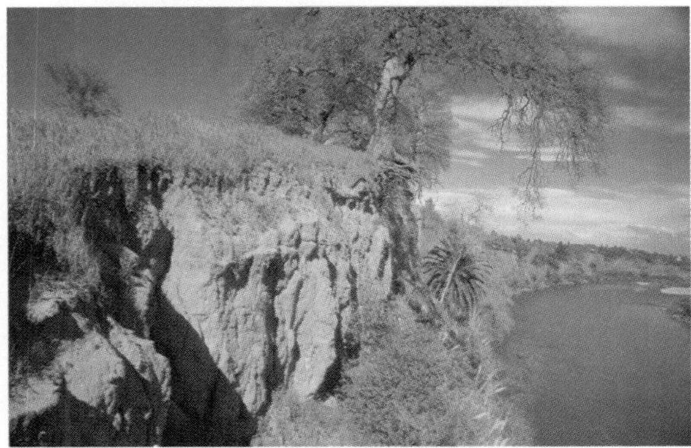

Figure 8-1
There may be hazards at any emergency.

It also could be hazardous just because the ground is sloped or wet and icy (Figure 8-1).

Safety is your highest priority. Plan for it. Start to develop questions as soon as dispatch gives you the basic call information. Here are some examples:

> "Rescue 21, respond to an assault victim at 724 Overton Drive." *Is the assailant still on the scene? Will he or she return to the scene?*
>
> "Rescue 21, respond to reports of a head-on collision at Highway 4 at Willow Pass." *Is the collision in the road? Is there a fuel spill? Downed power lines? Broken glass and sharp metal?*
>
> "Rescue 21, respond to a poisoning at 454 Cherry Avenue." *Did the patient ingest something? If it's an inhaled poison or a contact poison, will it be a danger to rescuers?*

Keep your questions in mind as you arrive on scene. The answers will tell you what safety precautions you should take. As you pull up, keep your eyes moving and take in the entire scene. Look for signs of any type of hazard. Don't forget that the environment you step into may be dangerous too. Note that if the scene is not safe for you, it isn't safe for other rescuers, the patients, or bystanders. The bottom line about scene safety is this: *If it's not safe, then make it safe. Otherwise, do not enter!*

BSI AND OTHER PRECAUTIONS

Always take BSI precautions. As you read in Chapter 5, infectious diseases are one of the top threats to EMS worker safety. Don't risk getting so involved with your patient that you forget to protect yourself. Put on your gloves, eye wear, and all other appropriate personal protective equipment *before* treating your patient (Figure 8-2).

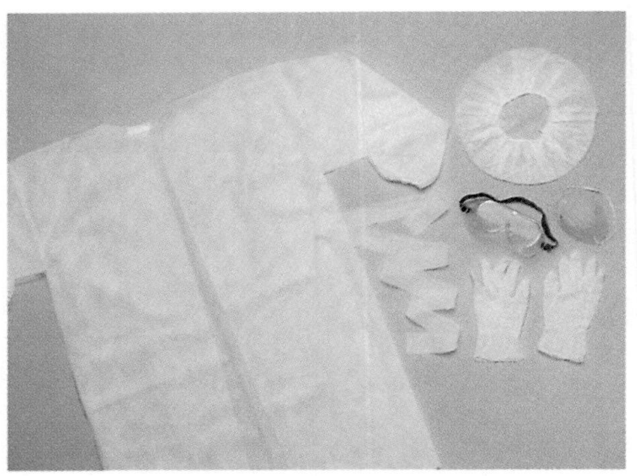

Figure 8-2
An infection control kit.

> **STREET NOTES**
> Glove up, gown up, mask up! Take all necessary BSI precautions before you get to the patient.

In general you should call for specialized personnel to handle other hazards, such as fires and complex rescues. They will have the appropriate clothing and equipment necessary to do their jobs safely. Some examples of specialized protective equipment are (Figure 8-3):

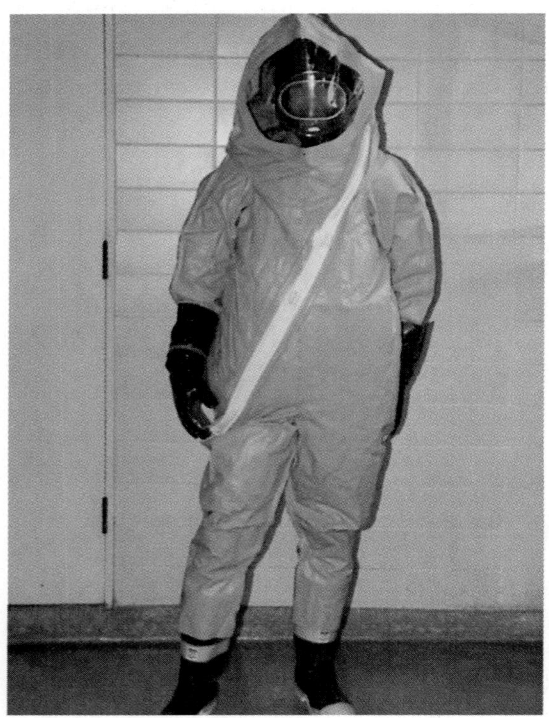

Figure 8-3a
Protective suit for a hazardous materials emergency.

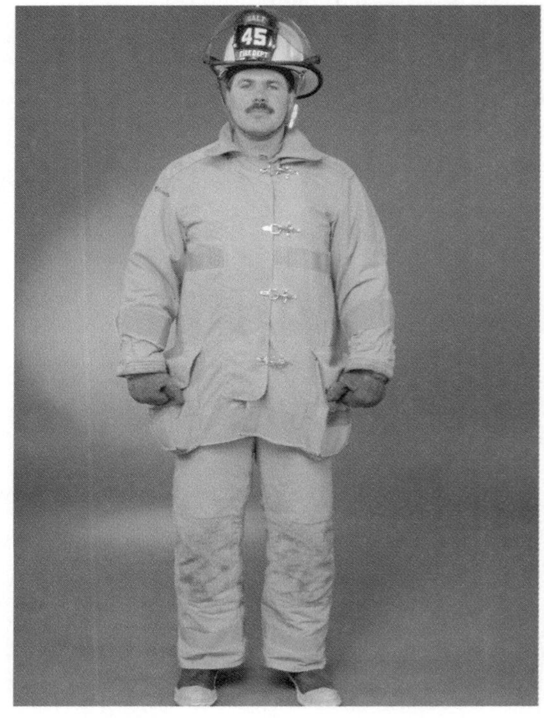

Figure 8-3b
Typical turnout gear.

- Chemical-resistant jumpsuit, for hazardous materials accidents.
- Turnout gear for rescue operations.
- Body armor or bullet-proof vest for crime or violent scenes.
- Personal floatation device for water rescues.
- Cold-water immersion suit for ice rescues.

Note that ordinary equipment will not protect you from electrical hazards. Downed power lines, electrocuted patients, and other electricity related emergencies pose extreme danger to rescuers. Stay clear of the scene until power company specialists assure you that the power is off and the scene is safe.

HAZARDOUS MATERIALS

Hazardous materials, or **hazmats**, are substances that can injure people or damage property if not handled correctly. They include solids, liquids, and gases. They're toxic, flammable, or reactive. To help control the risks of transporting and storing hazmats, the federal government has developed strict safety regulations. (See OSHA publication 29 CFR 1910-120, "1989 Hazardous Waste Operations and Emergency Response Standards.")

All vehicles that carry hazmats must display warning labels or placards (Figures 8-4 and 8-5). That's why one of the best pieces of equipment a First Responder can have is a pair of binoculars. Use them to read the labels and placards from a distance. Then refer to a book you should carry with you at all times. It's the U.S. Department of Transportation publication RSPA-P-5800.6, "1993 Emergency Response Guidebook: A Guidebook for First Responders During the Initial Phase of a Hazardous Materials Incident." It will tell you what the hazmat is, what to do about it, and what emergency medical care to provide.

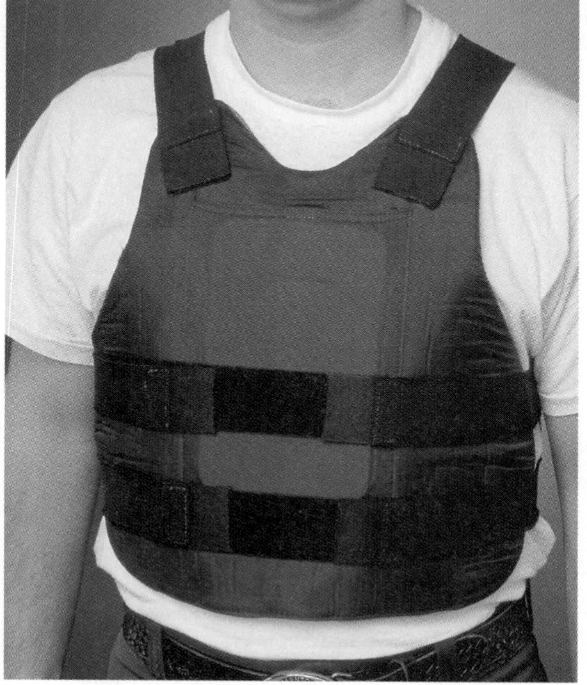

Figure 8-3c
Body armor.

Remember *Never enter a hazardous materials scene unless you are properly trained and fully protected by specialized equipment.*

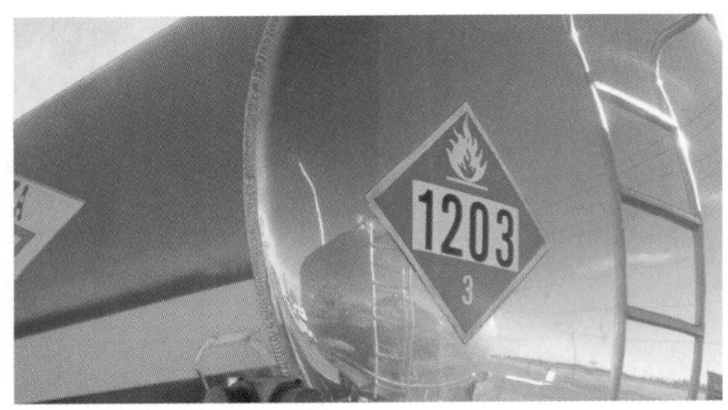

Figure 8-4
Warning placard.

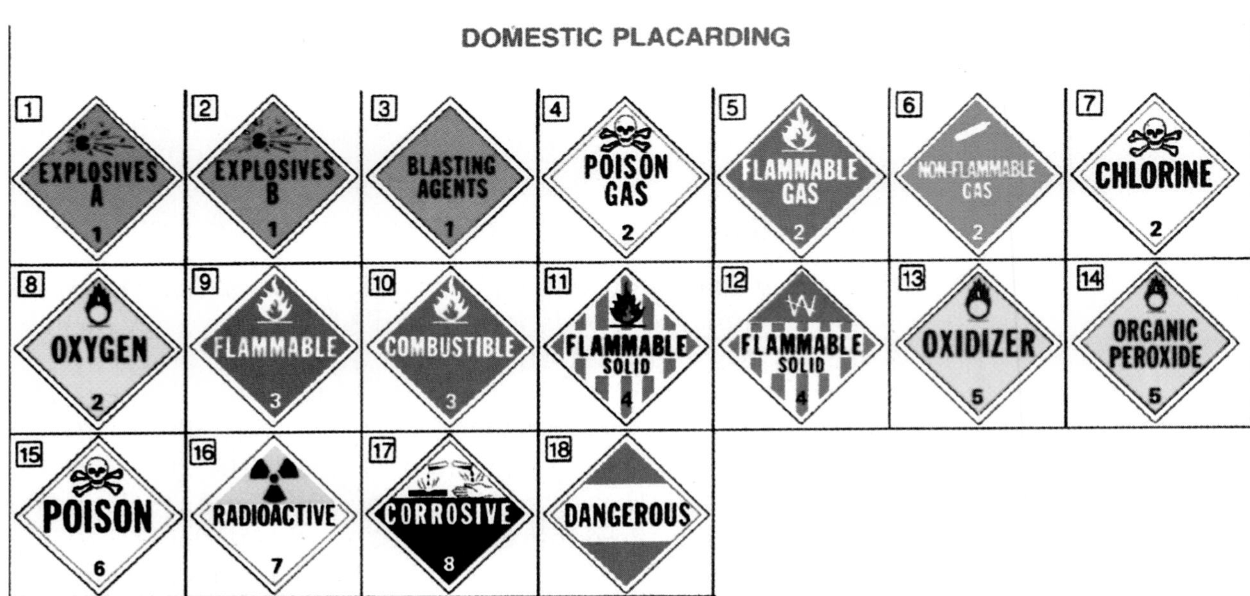

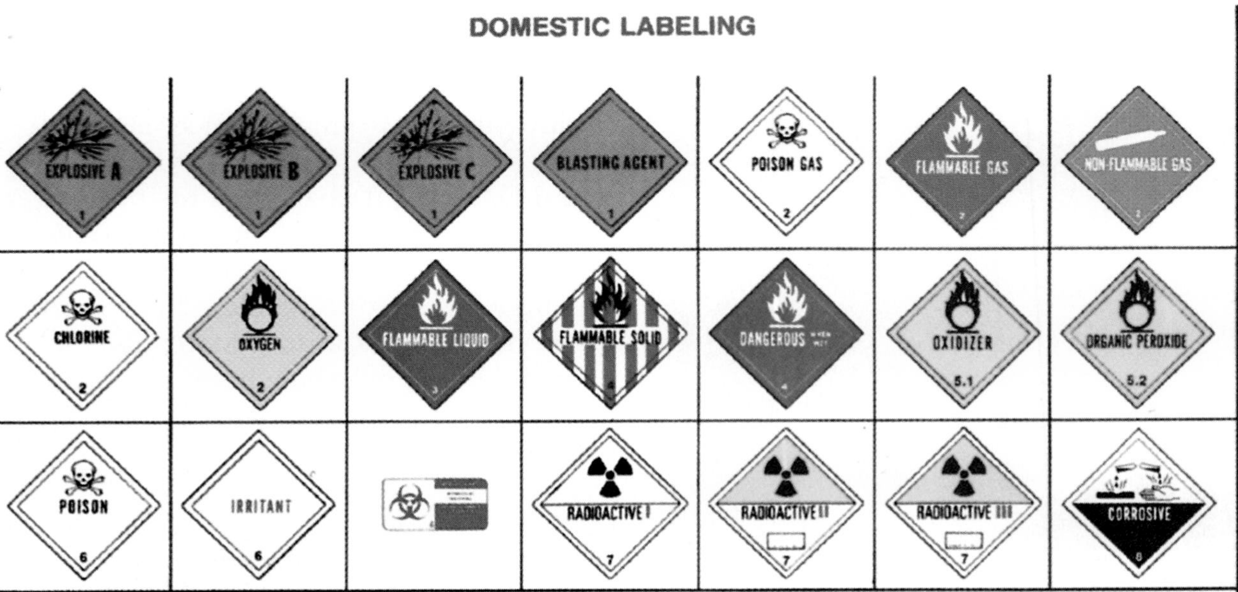

Figure 8-5
Examples of warning labels.

When you first approach a hazmat emergency, look at it through your binoculars (Figure 8-6). If you can cover its image with your thumb, you're probably at a safe distance. Be sure to station yourself uphill and upwind from the scene. Report to dispatch, and turn the call over to the local hazmat team. They are specially trained and equipped to handle the emergency safely. Don't try to handle a hazmat emergency yourself. Your role is to isolate the area, deny others entry, and avoid contact with the substance.

Provide medical care to hazmat victims only after the scene is safe, hazmat containment is complete, and your patients have been properly decontaminated. Don't allow transport of a contaminated patient. It will only serve to spread the problem to ambulance and hospital personnel.

Here are some key questions to answer when arriving at the scene of a hazmat incident:

- Am I parked uphill and upwind?
- Can I cover the incident with my thumb?
- What is the hazardous material?
- Have I denied access to bystanders?
- Have I activated a hazmat team?
- Have my patients been decontaminated before I handle them?

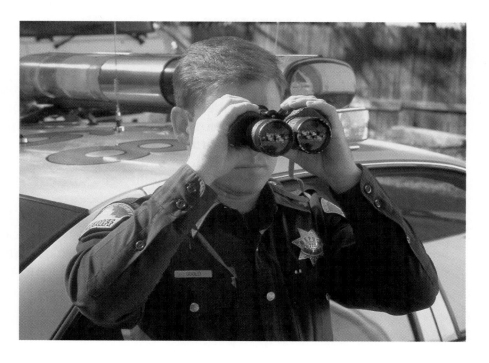

Figure 8-6
Use binoculars to observe a hazmat emergency from a safe distance.

MOTOR VEHICLE CRASHES

Vehicle crash scenes can be dangerous because they usually occur on or near roadways. Each year EMS workers are killed by oncoming traffic while helping crash victims. Flares, barricades, even rescue vehicles can be effective deterrents. Other threats at the scene of a vehicle crash include sharp metal and glass, downed power lines, fire, and explosion from ruptured fuel lines.

Call for specialized rescue teams to extricate pinned patients or patients in unstable vehicles. If you're asked to help, be sure you wear personal protective equipment appropriate to the emergency. That is, if the crash involves only a minor fender bender, you only may need to wear protective gloves when you have contact with the patients. If the crash involves a great deal of broken glass, twisted metal, and so on, consider firefighter's turnouts, sturdy boots, heavy rescue gloves, helmet, and face shield. You also should have reflective patches on your clothing.

Here are important questions to answer when arriving at a vehicle crash scene:

- Is there a threat of fire, explosion, electrocution, or hazardous materials exposure?
- Is the vehicle stable?
- Is the scene safe from oncoming traffic?
- Am I wearing the proper personal protective equipment?

VIOLENCE

Enter the scene of a violent crime only after the police have told you that it's secure. Then, don't disturb crime scene evidence unless you must do so to provide patient care.

Always be alert to threatening behaviors in your patient. Watch for hostile body posture, facial expressions, or language. Stay out of arm's reach, and present less of a target by standing to your side. Plan an exit route before approaching the patient. If you sense any possibility of a threat, don't block the patient's exit from the scene. Leave the management of violent patients to law enforcement officers. If your patient becomes violent during the course of treatment, back away and call the police. "Abandonment" doesn't apply when your own life is in danger.

Questions to answer when managing a potentially violent patient include:

- Does the patient appear threatening? Is the patient's language threatening? Expressions? Tone of voice?
- How close am I to the patient? Am I out of arm's reach?
- Have I reduced my size as a target by presenting a side profile?
- Do I have an escape route?

MECHANISM OF INJURY/NATURE OF ILLNESS

Once you are sure the scene is safe, your next job is to look for the cause of the patient's emergency. Ask the patient or the patient's family why EMS was called. Then evaluate the mechanism of injury (the forces that caused the injury) or determine the nature of illness.

MECHANISM OF INJURY

The mechanism of injury (MOI) is the cause of a patient's injuries (Table 8-1). Recognizing the MOI will help you decide if the scene is safe and if it will stay safe. It also will give you a good idea of how serious the patient's injuries may be.

TABLE 8-1 COMMON MECHANISMS OF INJURY
Automobile crashes
Beatings and other physical abuse
Blast or explosion forces
Burns
Ejection from vehicles
Falls
Heat and cold exposure
Motorcycle crashes
Pedestrian-vehicle collisions
Recreational vehicle crashes
Sexual attacks and abuse
Shootings
Sports falls and collisions
Stabbings

For example, say you arrive at the scene of a motor vehicle crash and find the driver standing by his car. He looks a little unsteady but says that he feels just fine. However, when you look at his car, you see that the front end is crushed, the windshield is shattered, and the steering wheel is bent. Is the patient really "just fine"? Probably not. The forces that caused the damage to the car may have caused damage to your patient as well. Those forces are the *mechanisms of injury*.

When you identify the MOI, be sure to consider it carefully for specific clues to the patient's injuries. A fall onto a cement driveway, for example, won't produce the same injuries as a fall onto a pile of bush clippings. A patient's injuries from a vehicle rollover will vary greatly depending on whether or not the patient was wearing a seat belt.

STREET NOTES

When the mechanism of injury is significant, assume a patient is seriously injured until proven otherwise.

Vehicle collisions will be among your most frequent types of call. They usually involve significant MOIs. Always suspect at least three impacts in a vehicle collision: one to the car, one to the patient's body, and one to the organs inside the patient's body (Figure 8-7). Also, if you find a passenger is dead or seriously injured, assume that the others involved in the crash have been seriously injured too.

NATURE OF ILLNESS

When you find no sign of injury in the patient or at the scene, consider illness as the cause of the emergency. For example, say you respond to a report of a "woman down." The teenage son leads you to his breathing but unresponsive 42-year-old mother in her bed. There's no sign of violence or an accident anywhere. If the patient can't tell you what his or her problem is, question someone who might know. In this case ask the son, "Why did you call 9-1-1?" The son tells you that he can't wake up his mother, that he found an empty sleeping pill bottle, and that his mother had talked earlier about wanting to die. Now you have an idea about how to proceed.

Always look for clues that will help you to determine the nature of the patient's illness. Be sure to look for signs of the problem such as pill bottles, Medic Alert medallion, or oxygen tubing that could indicate a chronic condition.

CALLING 9-1-1

If it hasn't already been done, activate the EMS system as soon as you know the nature of the emergency. When you call 9-1-1 or

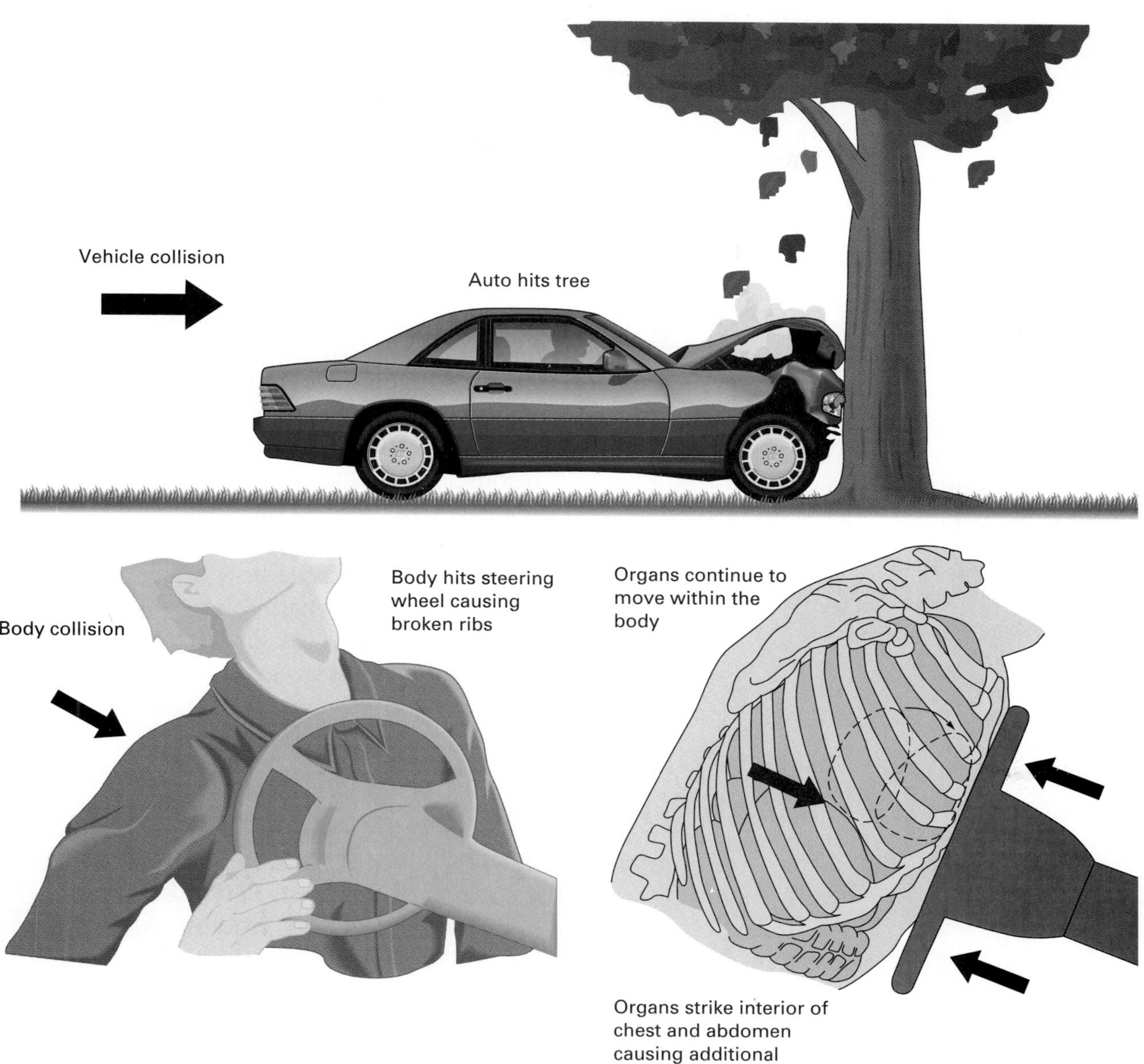

Figure 8-7
Suspect three impacts in any vehicle collision.

another emergency number, be sure to give the dispatcher the following information:

- Your name and call-back number.
- Location of the incident.
- What the emergency is and how serious it might be.
- Number of patients involved.

In many EMS systems the dispatcher is trained to provide medical assistance over the telephone. If during the scene size-up you can't determine if 9-1-1 is needed, continue with your assessments until you can.

MASS-CASUALTY INCIDENTS AND BASIC TRIAGE

Once you've assured scene safety and noted the mechanism of injury or nature of illness, you must ask two very important questions: *How many?* and *How bad?* If you have more than one patient, it's critical that you answer those two questions. By doing so, you can call for the right kind and the right number of additional resources. You'll also be able to prioritize your patients so that the most critical patients get care first.

After you determine how many patients you have and how badly they may be hurt, report to dispatch. Ask dispatch for additional resources as necessary. Then confirm that they're on the way to the scene.

STREET NOTES

Are all car crash victims still on the scene? An extra coat or a child's safety seat in the back of a crashed car may be a sign that a victim has wandered off.

TRIAGING PATIENTS

The term *triage* literally means "to sort." This critical part of scene size-up is done by sorting your patients very quickly according to the seriousness of their problems. Find out what triage system is used in your area. A typical one includes three levels:

- First (or highest) priority patients
  - Airway and breathing difficulties
  - Uncontrolled or severe bleeding
  - Decreased mental status
- Second priority patients
  - Burns without airway problems
  - Major or multiple painful, swollen, deformed extremities
  - Back injuries
- Third (or lowest) priority patients
  - Minor painful, swollen, deformed extremities

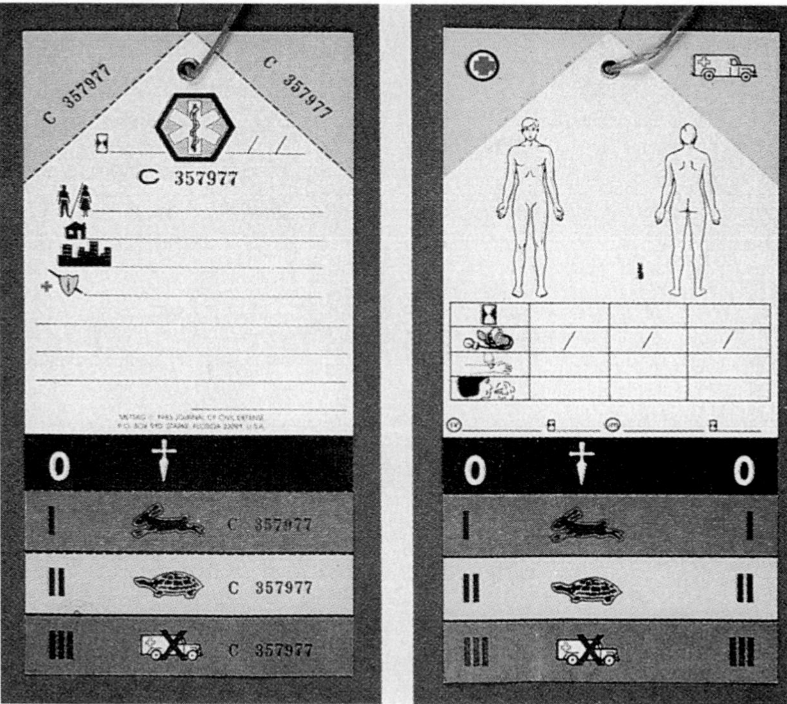

Figure 8-8
Typical triage tags.

- Minor soft-tissue injuries
- Death

In most cases you'll need very little time to determine the priority of your patient. Then, whenever possible, you should fill out a triage tag for each patient (Figure 8-8). Once triage is complete, you and other EMS workers will be able to see at a glance which patients to care for first and which should be sent first to the hospital. At this point, you also may need to update EMS dispatch and ask for additional resources.

MASS-CASUALTY INCIDENTS

A **mass-casualty incident** (MCI) or multiple-casualty situation (MCS) is an emergency that places a great demand on available equipment and personnel. Most First Responders will never run a mass-casualty call (Figure 8-9). However, you'll probably handle many calls that have more than one patient. Typically such calls are the result of car crashes.

If you're first to arrive at the scene of an MCI, confirm it with dispatch and request help. Establish a command post, check for hazards, and begin to triage your patients. Consider yourself the

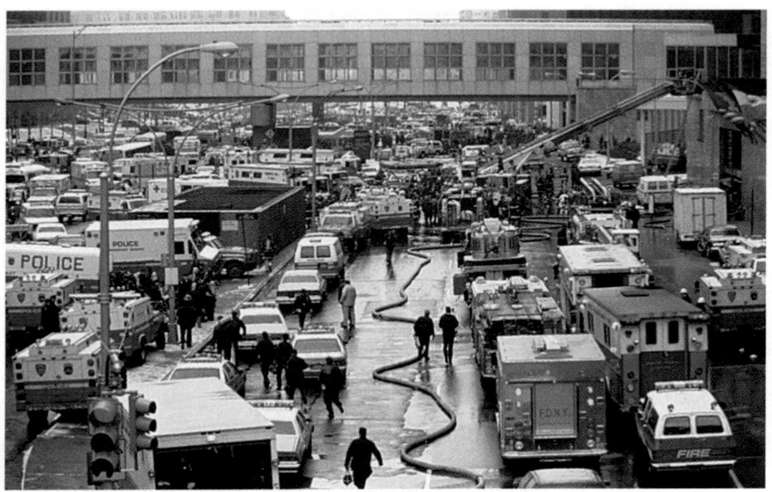

Figure 8-9
Mass-casualty incident at the World Trade Center in New York City.

triage officer until a rescuer with more training takes over. This officer also assigns and coordinates personnel, supplies, and vehicles. Usually most available resources go to the higher priority patients.

Figure 8-10 shows one example of the organization of a unified command. (A unified command includes all rescue services under one commander.) If you arrive at an MCI where incident

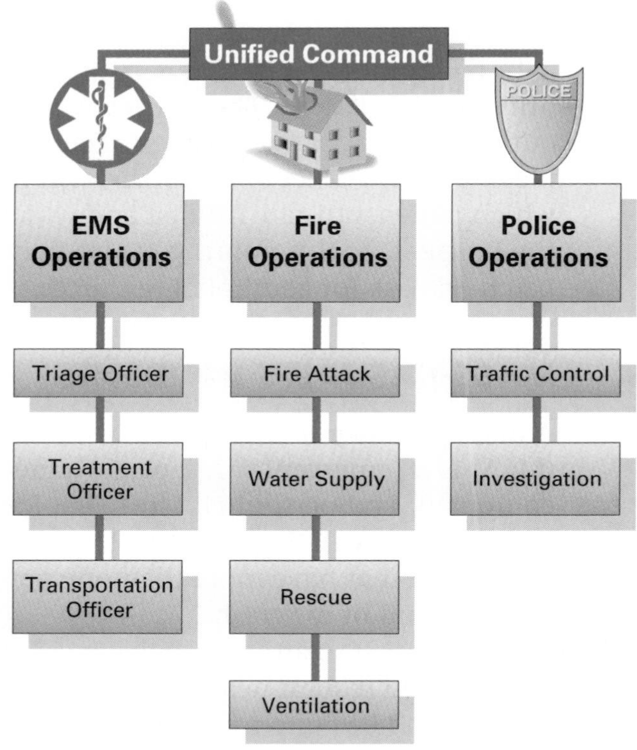

Figure 8-10
Example of a unified command structure.

command already is established, follow local protocols. Usually that means report to the command post, find the incident commander, and identify yourself and your level of training. He or she will give you directions and assign you to a task.

PATIENT ACCESS AND EXTRICATION

You must be able to get to your patient to provide effective emergency care. Sometimes that's easy. Sometimes it's not. There are two categories of access: simple and complex. **Simple access** does not require equipment. In many cases it'll include just opening a door or asking a patient to roll down a window (Figure 8-11). **Complex access** requires the use of hydraulic equipment and a variety of cutting and prying tools (Figure 8-12). It should be performed only by specially trained rescuers.

Extrication usually is performed after initial assessment and treatment. However, it may be necessary to extricate a patient first. In either case, begin to think about extrication as you conduct your scene size-up. The goal is to remove the patient from the car, building, or collapsed structure in a way that minimizes further injury.

Your top priority, of course, is your own safety and the safety of other rescuers. Always wear the appropriate personal protective equipment. Remember the importance of teamwork. It helps

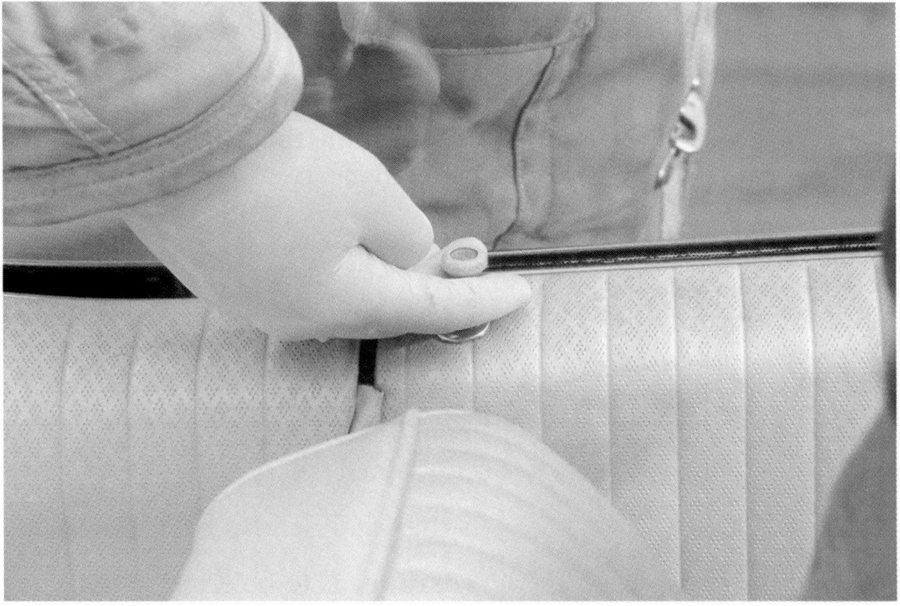

Figure 8-11
Simple access.

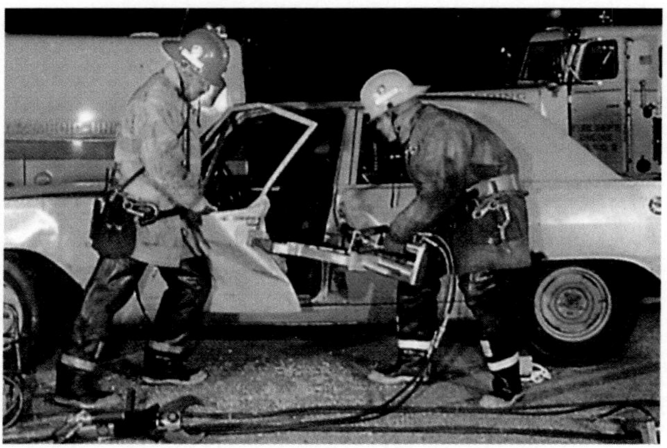

Figure 8-12
Complex access.

to assign a team leader to coordinate the moves, but it requires communication among all participants to assure success and safety.

During extrication, do all you can to protect the patient from broken glass, sharp objects, and other hazards including the environment. Explain unique aspects of the extrication to the patient and help to keep him or her calm.

CONCLUSION

Your scene size-up is the first critical step in caring for patients in the field. Performed correctly, it will provide you with valuable clues to the causes of the patient's emergency. It will allow you to identify scene hazards—from unsafe scenes to infectious risks—and to determine the necessary EMS resources needed to manage them effectively. In summary, scene size-up includes the following:

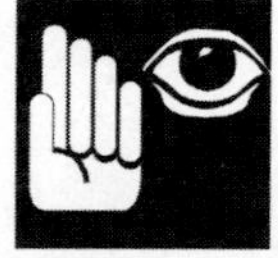

SCENE SIZE-UP

- Scene safety
  - Is the scene safe?
  - What needs to be done to make it safe?
- Mechanism of injury or nature of illness
  - What is the problem?

- What are the clues to the who, what, when, where, why, and how of the problem?

- Patient triage
  - How many patients are there?
  - Which ones need the most urgent care?
- Access and extrication
  - Is there appropriate access to the patient?
  - What additional resources are needed?

KEY TERMS

You may wish to use this list to review your understanding of key terms introduced in the chapter.

complex access access to a patient that requires specialized tools and training.

hazardous materials substances that can cause injury to a person or damage to property if not handled properly. *Also called* hazmats.

mass-casualty incident (MCI) an emergency in which the number of patients overwhelms the ability of the EMS system to manage it with a normal response. *Also called* multiple-casualty situation (MCS).

mechanism of injury (MOI) the forces that cause an injury to occur.

nature of illness the possible causes of a patient's illness.

scene size-up an assessment of the scene and its surroundings that includes scene safety, mechanism of injury/nature of illness, and access and extrication.

simple access access to a patient that does not require tools or training.

APPLICATION QUESTIONS

You may wish to use these questions to review your understanding of the chapter. For answers with page references, see Appendix 2.

1. You respond to reports of shots fired at an apartment building. The shooter has not been found. Occupants of the build-

ing see you parked down the street and run to your unit. They tell you a man has been shot in the parking lot and looks badly injured. What will you do?

2. You are at the scene of a vehicle crash. The cars and patients are in the middle of the roadway. What can you do to protect the scene from oncoming traffic?

3. Triage the following patients:

   a. A 42-year-old female with a badly broken lower leg (a large bone is protruding through the skin) and cuts and scrapes to most of her back.

   b. A 31-year-old male who is not breathing and has no pulse.

   c. A 69-year-old female with significant wounds to the chest and severe difficulty breathing.

   d. A 43-year-old male with minor cuts, scratches, and scrapes to his right arm and leg.

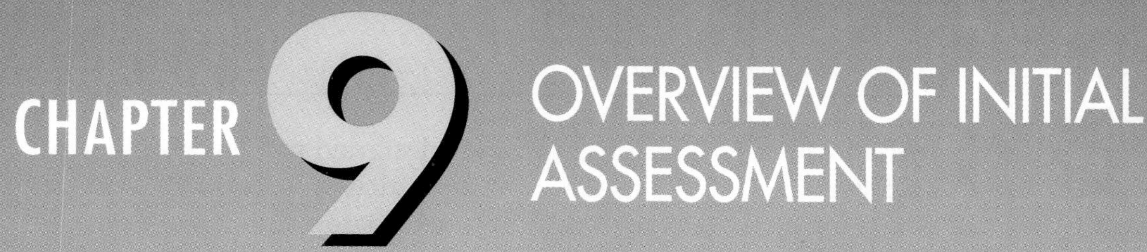

CHAPTER 9 OVERVIEW OF INITIAL ASSESSMENT

FIRST RESPONSE

Luis hears a loud crash as he exits the mini-market. An elderly man has tumbled off a curb and lies sprawled on the street. Luis sets down his bag of groceries and makes his way through a growing crowd of onlookers. "Someone call 9-1-1," yells a good Samaritan, "I think this guy's had a heart attack!" As the wide-eyed fellow readies himself to perform CPR, Luis sees the patient's chest rise. Is this guy still breathing?

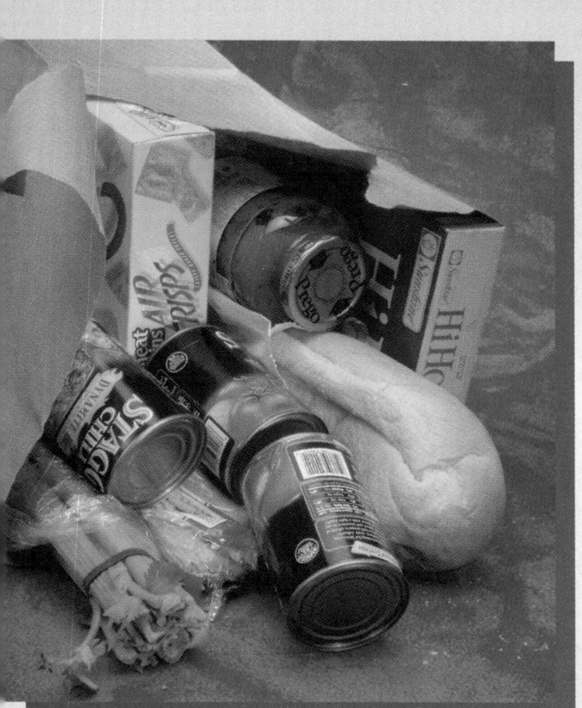

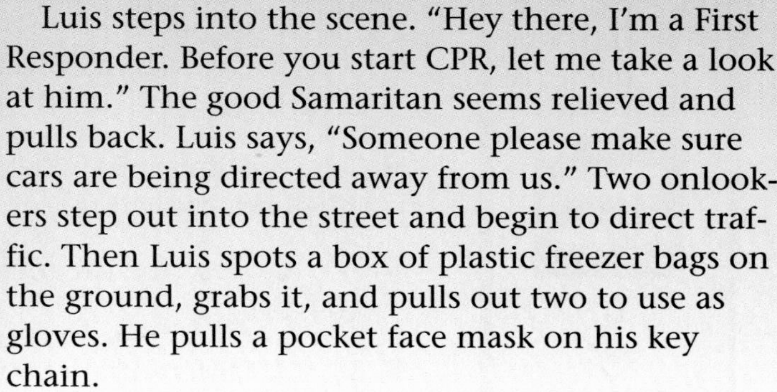

Luis steps into the scene. "Hey there, I'm a First Responder. Before you start CPR, let me take a look at him." The good Samaritan seems relieved and pulls back. Luis says, "Someone please make sure cars are being directed away from us." Two onlookers step out into the street and begin to direct traffic. Then Luis spots a box of plastic freezer bags on the ground, grabs it, and pulls out two to use as gloves. He pulls a pocket face mask on his key chain.

Luis begins the initial assessment of the patient. He notes a large bruise to the forehead. "I need someone to hold this man's head and neck." The good Samaritan steps forward. "I'll do it," he says. "My name is Ray." Luis shows him what to do.

"Sir," Luis calls to the patient, "are you awake?" No response. Luis gently rubs the man's sternum. Still no response. He moves to the patient's airway and hears snoring respirations. "A noisy airway is an obstructed airway," he murmurs. So Luis performs a maneuver to open it and immediately sees an improvement. He also notes that the patient has a strong, regular pulse and the skin is pale, warm, and dry. Just as he determines there is no major bleeding, the patient's eyes flutter open. "What happened?" the man whispers.

"Sir, please lie still," Luis responds. "Looks like you had a fall and bumped your head. We're taking care of you now and an ambulance is on the way." After making certain 9-1-1 was called, Luis gets the patient's permission to continue with patient assessment and treatment. In moments the Paramedics arrive to take over.

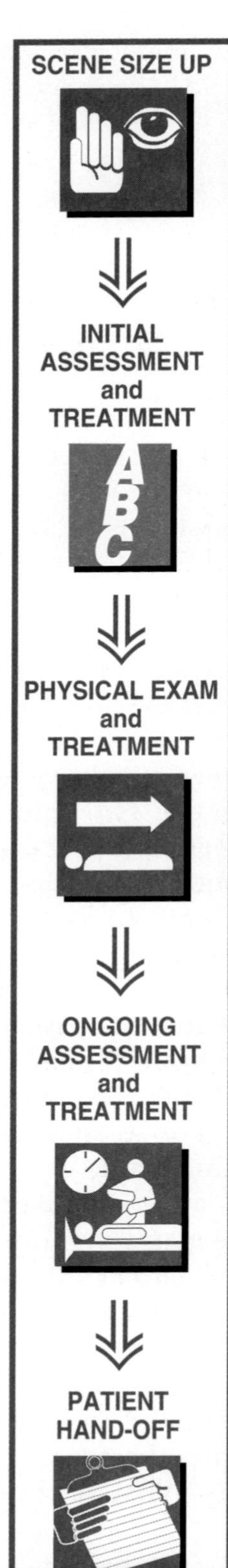

LEARNING OBJECTIVES

Initial assessment and treatment is designed to help you identify and treat life threats to your patient's airway, breathing, and circulation. It's also designed to help you determine if your patient is a high priority or low priority for transport.

This chapter will give you an overview of initial assessment. Each of the next three chapters will give you the details of assessing and treating life threats.

By the end of the chapter, you should be able to: †

- 3-1.7 Summarize the reasons for forming a general impression of the patient. (pp. 99-100)
- 3-1.8 Discuss methods of assessing mental status. (pp. 100-102)
- 3-1.9 Differentiate between assessing mental status in the adult, child, and infant patient. (p. 102)
- 3-1.10 Describe methods used for assessing if a patient is breathing. (pp. 102-104)
- 3-1.11 Differentiate between a patient with adequate and inadequate breathing. (p. 103)
- 3-1.12 Describe the methods used to assess circulation. (pp. 104-106)
- 3-1.13 Differentiate between obtaining a pulse in an adult, child, and infant patient. (pp. 104-105)
- 3-1.14 Discuss the need for assessing the patient for external bleeding. (p. 105)
- 3-1.15 Explain the reason for prioritizing a patient for care and transport. (p. 106)

* Explain how to make the transition from scene size-up to initial assessment. (pp. 98-99)

* Describe the information necessary to give a responding EMS unit an update on a patient's status. (pp. 106-107)

APPROACHING YOUR PATIENT

Put yourself in Luis's shoes, the First Responder in the scenario at the beginning of the chapter. You hear a loud crash and see a man fall. "Is the scene safe?" you ask yourself. In this case, you're

†Numbered objectives are from the 1995 U.S. DOT "First Responder: National Standard Curriculum." Asterisks indicate supplemental material.

able to make it safe. Then you look for the mechanism of injury or clues to the nature of the patient's illness. Finally, you make sure that there's only one patient, find no access or extrication problems, and verify that 9-1-1 was called. This has taken less than a minute.

You're ready to move to the next step in your emergency care plan—**initial assessment and treatment**. This step is meant to help you find and treat life-threatening problems first. Taking a total of about one minute, the initial assessment consists of:

- Forming a general impression of the patient's condition.
- Assessing the patient's mental status.
- Assessing the status of the patient's ABCs—airway, breathing, and circulation.
- Determining the patient's priority for transport.

FORMING A GENERAL IMPRESSION

Imagine you're still in Luis's shoes. You note your general impression of the patient, who is a middle-aged male. His body is sprawled face down in the street, with groceries scattered around him. He doesn't look like he tried to break his fall, so chances are he took a very hard blow when he hit the concrete. He can't describe his **chief complaint** (what the patient identifies as the problem). But you see a bruise to the forehead. Finally, you note that he's not moving. Your general impression of this patient is that he is unresponsive and that he may have significant injuries.

Forming a general impression is based on your immediate assessment of the following (Figure 9-1):

- The mechanism of injury or nature of illness.

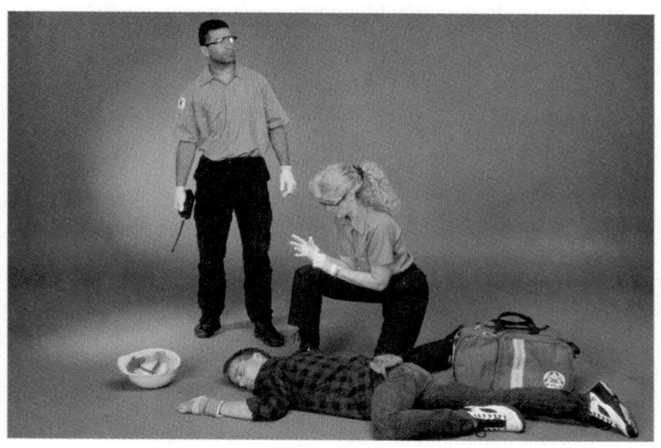

Figure 9-1
Starting forming a general impression of the patient as soon as you enter the scene.

- The patient's chief complaint.
- The patient's sex and approximate age.
- The patient's body posture.
- The patient's overall level of distress.

This is all done in a matter of seconds. Your immediate evaluation of the mechanism of injury or nature of illness also tells you if your patient is a **trauma patient** (injured) or a **medical patient** (ill). If it's unclear, assume the patient is a trauma victim.

Listen to the patient's chief complaint. At the same time, look at the patient's posture. Is he standing and does he appear to be strong and steady? Is he sprawled on the ground or slumped in a chair? These observations all contribute to your impression of the patient's overall level of distress.

Experienced rescuers will tell you that forming a general impression is very much like getting a "gut feeling." This feeling, or intuition, actually has been proven to be an accurate measure of how sick or injured a patient really is. Think of an extremely short-of-breath patient who has chronic breathing problems. You approach her and note that she's sitting with 30 feet of home oxygen tubing coiled at her feet and clutching an inhaler in one hand. She's sitting bolt upright, wide-eyed, scared, and appears to be working very hard to breathe. She says, "I can't breathe!"

You take in all of this information within the few moments it takes to actually reach her. By the time you're ready to assess her mental status, you already have a sense that she has a serious problem and is in significant distress. An experienced First Responder might communicate his or her general impression by saying, "This patient's in trouble!" or "This patient looks really sick!"

STREET NOTES

Pay attention to your "gut feeling" or intuition about how sick or injured your patient might be. It's usually correct!

CHECKING MENTAL STATUS

Another part of initial assessment is checking a patient's mental status, or **level of responsiveness**. It's a key indicator of the severity of your patient's condition. Begin by speaking to your patient. For example: "Hi, my name is Luis. I'm a First Responder with the local fire department. Looks like you may have taken a fall. Listen, if it's all right with you, I'm going to check you out to make sure you're okay." The patient's response to this introduction can give you a lot of patient information. For example, if your patient is talking, you can assume the airway is open. A reassuring touch during your introduction can serve to tell you about the condition of the patient's skin.

LEVELS OF RESPONSIVENESS

Observe your patient. An alert patient is awake and answers your questions easily with no confusion. If a patient doesn't seem to be awake, try verbal stimuli. "Hey, are you okay? Can you hear me?" If he doesn't respond, shake his arm, lightly pinch the top of his hand, or gently rub the sternum with your knuckles. Take care to prevent injury.

Even if your patient appears to be alert, watch for signs of confusion. Confusion can be caused by any illness or injury that prevents an adequate supply of oxygen from reaching the brain. Ask this patient a question or two, such as: What's your name? What day is it? What time is it? Where are you? What happened to you? Watch for behavior changes. If a patient is combative, irrational, or slow to respond, he may have a low level of responsiveness—even if he's awake. Patients like this may have significant medical problems.

Use the mnemonic **AVPU** to help you check for the four basic levels of responsiveness:

A — *Alert.* Your patient is awake and answering all questions appropriately.

V — *Verbal.* Your patient responds only when spoken to.

P — *Painful.* Your patient only responds to painful stimuli.

U — *Unresponsive.* Your patient has minimal or no response to verbal or painful stimuli.

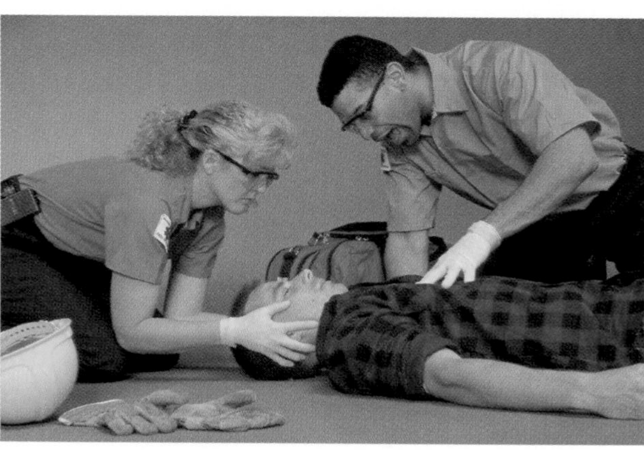

Figure 9-2
When you suspect spine injury, manually stabilize the patient's head and neck as you assess mental status.

THE UNRESPONSIVE PATIENT

If you determine that a patient is unresponsive and that the mechanism of injury suggests trauma, assume there's a spinal injury. Immediately stabilize the patient's head and neck. Then with your gloved hands bring the patient's head into a neutral, in-line position (Figure 9-2). *Neutral* means that the head shouldn't be pushed forward or pulled back. *In-line* means that the patient's nose should be in line with his or her navel. Hold that position until the patient is completely immobilized.

INFANTS AND CHILDREN

Infants and children who are less than two years of age can't respond to the usual tests of responsiveness. These patients don't speak yet and probably won't understand your questions. Assess them by observing their interaction with parents and the environment. In general, they should recognize their parents. They should be consolable, and they should be able to be distracted by interesting objects such as jingling keys or a flashing penlight. If not, this patient may have a significant problem. Be sure to ask the parents if their child is responding normally.

ASSESSING THE ABCS

After completing the AVPU check, move immediately to assess your patient's ABCs—airway, breathing, and circulation. Note that the procedures mentioned here for the treatment of life-threats will be described in detail in Chapters 10, 11, and 12.

AIRWAY

Airway management is best summarized by this First Responder: "If you don't have an airway, nothing else matters." It's the most important aspect of your First Responder practice. Without a **patent airway** (an open airway), your patient won't survive for more than a few minutes.

After forming a general impression and determining the level of responsiveness, assess your patient's airway. A responsive patient with a patent airway will be able to speak clearly and breathe without effort. If your patient is unresponsive, open the airway and clear it of vomit and other matter as needed (Figure 9-3).

> **STREET NOTES**
>
> A noisy airway is an obstructed airway. You need to clear it and open it!

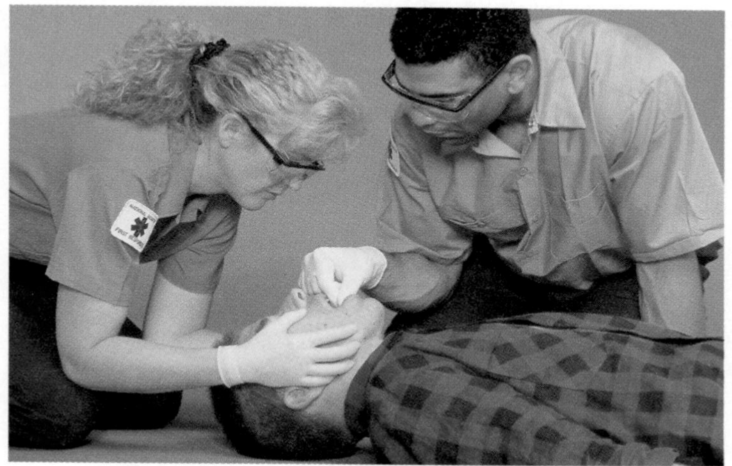

Figure 9-3
Always ensure an open airway. It's the most important aspect of First Responder practice.

BREATHING

After you ensure an open airway, assess the patient's breathing status. You don't have to count respirations at this point. During the initial assessment, just determine whether or not your patient *is* breathing and, if so, whether or not it's too fast, too slow, or labored.

Normal breathing in a responsive patient is accomplished in a relaxed manner with no obvious effort. Signs and symptoms of breathing difficulty are:

- Difficulty speaking.
- Labored breathing, with heaving of the chest and drawing in of muscles around the collarbones and base of neck *(retractions)*.
- Unusually rapid, slow, or irregular breathing.
- Air hunger (patient complains of not being able to get enough air).
- Fatigue from breathing.

To determine inadequate breathing, look for respirations that provide minimal chest rise, appear to be moving little or no air, or appear to be extremely slow. Also look for mental status changes from confusion to combativeness to unresponsiveness. **Cyanosis** is another sign, which appears as bluish, gray, or dark purple discoloration of the skin and mucous membranes.

In general, place the responsive medical patient with breathing difficulty in a sitting position. If you are equipped to provide oxygen therapy, provide high flow oxygen by mask. If your patient is unresponsive, open the airway immediately. Then look, listen, and

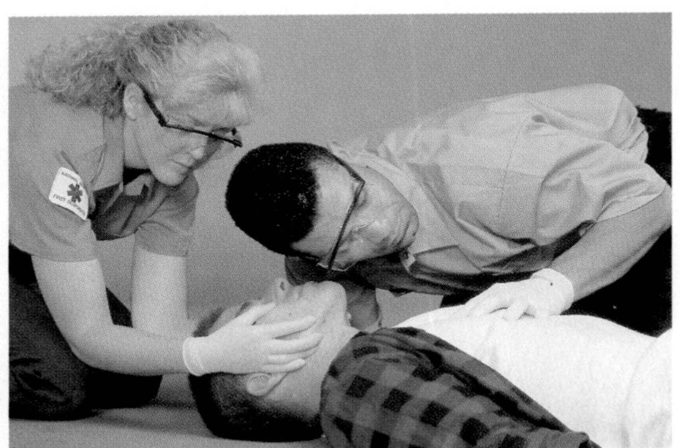

Figure 9-4
Look, listen, and feel to assess for breathing status.

feel for breathing (Figure 9-4). If there is no breathing or if breathing is inadequate, provide artificial ventilation immediately.

> **Warning** *Your patients may stop breathing if they show gasping respirations, extreme fatigue with difficulty breathing, inability to speak, or inability to maintain an upright position. Be prepared to ventilate these patients.*

CIRCULATION

Initial assessment of circulation comes after you've ensured an open airway and adequate breathing in your patient. This assessment consists of checking the patient's pulse, presence of major bleeding, and skin condition. At this stage, you must answer two questions: Does my patient have a pulse? Does my patient have signs of shock?

CHECKING PULSE

First, check to see if your patient has a pulse and get a sense of the pulse rate. If there's no pulse, start CPR immediately. If the pulse seems extremely rapid and weak or extremely slow, your patient may need to be treated for shock.

The pulse points most often used in the initial assessment are the carotid, brachial, radial, and femoral (Table 9-1).

TABLE 9-1 PULSE POINTS FOR PATIENTS

	PULSE POINT WITH RESPONSIVE PATIENT	PULSE POINT WITH UNRESPONSIVE PATIENT
Infant	Brachial	Brachial
Child	Radial or Brachial	Carotid or Femoral
Adult	Radial	Carotid

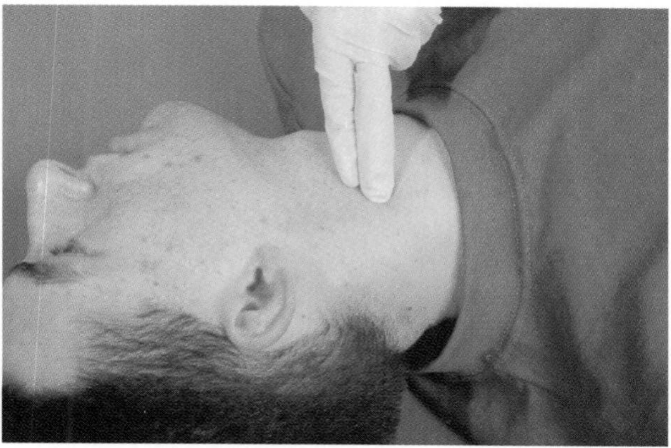

Figure 9-5
Taking a carotid pulse.

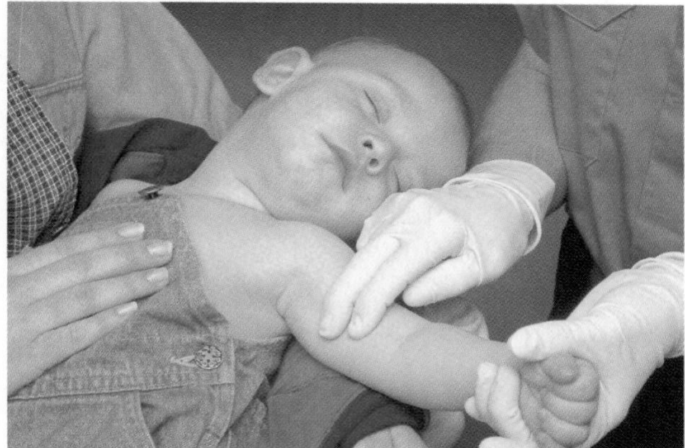

Figure 9-6
Taking a brachial pulse.

- *Carotid pulse.* The carotid pulse is usually the easiest to feel and the last pulse to be lost in a patient. To take a carotid pulse, place two gloved fingers—your index and middle fingers—on the patient's Adam's apple and then slide your fingers into the groove between it and the neck muscles (Figure 9-5).
- *Brachial pulse.* Place two or three gloved fingers into the groove between the triceps and biceps on the inside of the patient's upper arm (Figure 9-6).
- *Radial pulse.* Place two gloved fingers below the thumb on the underside of the wrist (Figure 9-7).
- *Femoral pulse.* Place the fingers of one gloved hand in the crease between the thigh and the pelvic area (Figure 9-8).

Checking for Major Bleeding

Next, perform a visual sweep of your patient. Check up and down the body and the extremities to determine if there is any major external bleeding (Figure 9-9). Run your gloved hands down the body, and slide them lightly under the sides of the patient. Look at your gloves to check for blood. Control all major bleeding immediately.

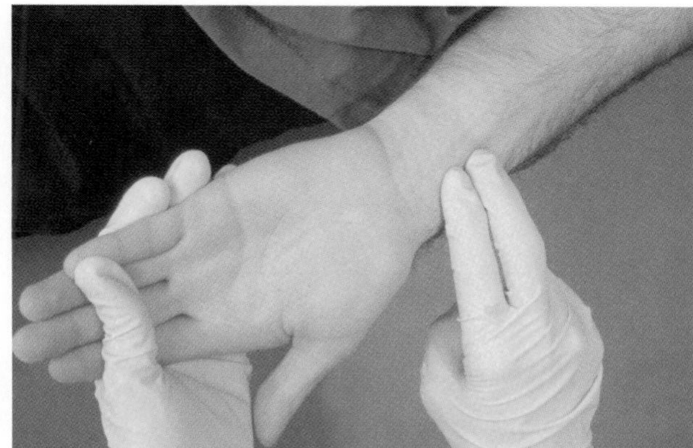

Figure 9-7
Taking a radial pulse.

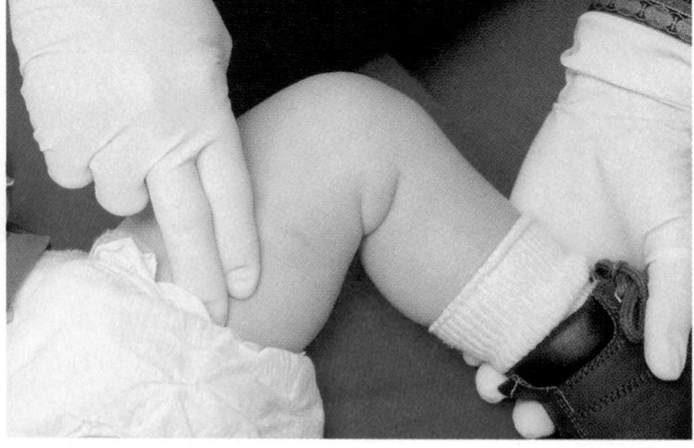

Figure 9-8
Taking a femoral pulse.

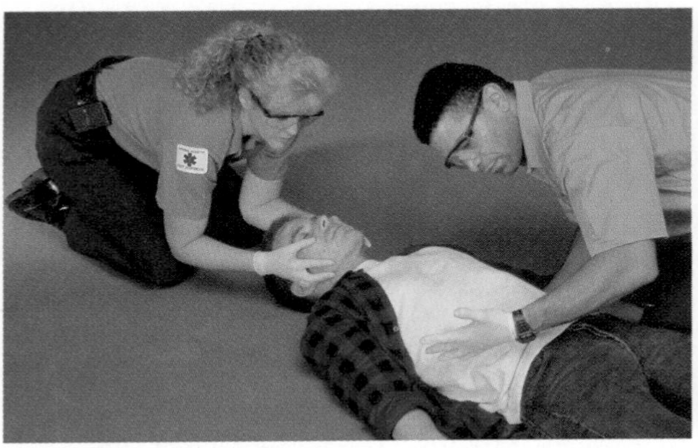

Figure 9-9
Check to see if there is any major external bleeding.

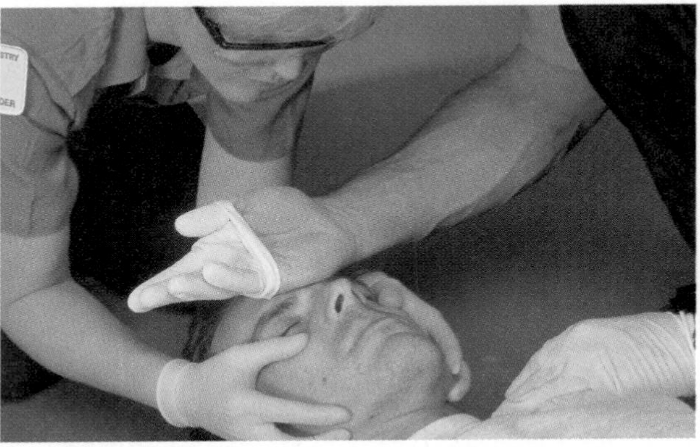

Figure 9-10
To assess body temperature, pull your glove down just a bit to feel the patient's forehead.

Checking the Skin Condition

Finally, notice your patient's skin condition. Observe the skin color. To check temperature and moisture, place the back of your hand or the inside of your forearm above the patient's brow (Figure 9-10). Normal skin usually is reported as "normal color, warm, and dry." Pale or ashy skin that is cool and wet may indicate shock in your patient. Cyanosis (blueness) can indicate the patient is not getting enough oxygen.

PRIORITIZING THE PATIENT

Now you have to prioritize the patient for transport. Any patient who has an abnormal mental status or problems with airway, breathing, or circulation, should be considered a high priority. Low priority patients have normal mental status, ABCs, and appear to be in low or moderate distress.

> **Remember** *Don't ignore your "gut feeling." If it seems to you that your patient is in a lot of distress—even with normal findings, classify him or her has a high priority.*

COMMUNICATING FINDINGS

If you have radio capability, update the responding EMS unit. Include in your report the following information about your patient:

- Sex and approximate age.
- Mechanism of injury or nature of illness.

- Chief complaint and level of distress.
- Level of responsiveness (mental status).
- Airway and breathing status.
- Circulation status.
- Priority status (high or low).

Determine from the incoming EMS unit its estimated time of arrival so you know which tasks to complete prior to its arrival. Time permitting, you should complete the physical exam and treatment prior to the hand-off of the patient.

CONCLUSION

The initial assessment takes only a minute or so, but it's the most important step in managing your patients successfully. It's designed to help you identify and treat life threats to your patient's airway, breathing, and circulation. It's also designed to help you determine if your patient is a high or low priority for transport.

The initial assessment is an integrated assessment. Though we've outlined it in a task-by-task sequence, the tasks should be completed simultaneously or very nearly so. Questions you should answer for the initial assessment include the following:

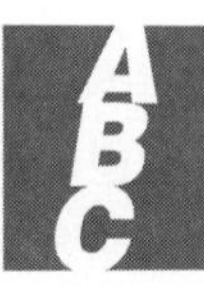

INITIAL ASSESSMENT AND TREATMENT

- Form a general impression.
  - Is my patient a trauma or medical patient? What is my evaluation of the mechanism of injury or clues to the nature of illness?
  - What is the patient's chief complaint?
  - What is the patient's sex and approximate age?
  - What is the patient's body posture?
  - What is the patient's overall level of distress?
- Check mental status.
  - What is the level of responsiveness (AVPU)?
  - Is the patient confused, combative, or otherwise behaving abnormally?

- Assess the ABCs.
  - Is there a patent airway?
  - Is there breathing? Is it adequate? Is there any difficulty?
  - Is there a pulse? Is it too weak, rapid, or slow?
  - Is there major external bleeding?
  - What is the patient's skin condition?
- Prioritize the patient and communicate findings.
  - Is my patient a low or high priority for transport?
  - Can I communicate my findings to incoming EMS personnel?

KEY TERMS

You may wish to use this list to review your understanding of key terms introduced in the chapter.

AVPU a mnemonic for the four basic levels of patient responsiveness: *alert*—awake and answering all questions appropriately; *verbal*—responds only when spoken to; *painful*—responds only to painful stimuli; *unresponsive*—has minimal or no response to stimuli.

chief complaint what the patient identifies as the problem.

cyanosis bluish, gray, or dark purple discoloration of the skin and mucous membranes due to lack of oxygen.

initial assessment and treatment part of emergency medical care designed to help rescuers find and treat life-threatening problems first; includes general impression, mental status, status of the ABCs, and transport priority.

level of responsiveness mental status.

medical patient a patient who is ill.

patent airway an open airway.

trauma patient a patient who is injured.

APPLICATION QUESTIONS

You may wish to use these questions to review your understanding of the chapter. For answers with page references, see Appendix 2.

1. Read the following example of a trauma patient being interviewed. This patient was struck on the head with flying debris

from a car crash. After reading the passage, describe how you'd interpret the patient's mental status.

"Sure I know where I am. Corner of Main and Broadway. What happened to me? No kidding, I got hit in the head? My name? It's Andy Garcia. Day of the week? Wednesday. Say could you tell me what happened? No kidding, I got hit in the old noggin? Where was I going? I'm on my lunch hour. How did I get here? Was I in an accident?"

2. You are at the scene of a patient who says she is short of breath. You observe her reclined in a chair, talking in full sentences, laughing and smiling to another First Responder who is interviewing her. The patient appears to have normal, warm, and dry skin. Her respirations seem to be a bit fast, but she's breathing without effort. You ask her what her problem is and she states, "I can't breathe." Is this a high or lower priority patient? Explain your answer.

CHAPTER 10 AIRWAY AND BREATHING MANAGEMENT

FIRST RESPONSE

Officer Tim Bradley is dispatched to a medical aid call on State Route 62 at Exit 41. There's a car at the shoulder with a four-year-old patient who has stopped breathing. He responds with lights and sirens. The dispatcher tells him that an ambulance and the fire department are en route and that rescue breathing is being attempted by the child's untrained mother.

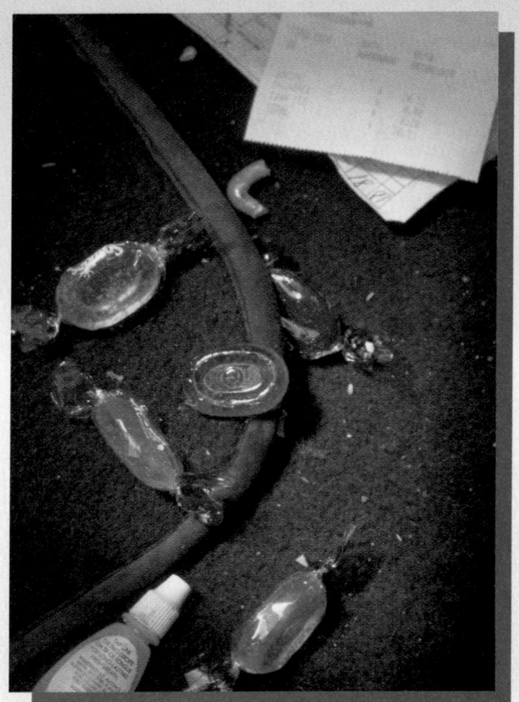

Arriving at the scene a few minutes later, Tim notes that the car is parked safely away from oncoming traffic. He quickly dons a pair of latex gloves, grabs his jump kit, and approaches the car. The child's mother is kneeling on the ground, cradling the limp body of her daughter. She's frantically trying to provide rescue breathing for the child. Tim sees a cellular phone cradled awkwardly on the mother's shoulder as she follows directions from the dispatcher.

Tim introduces himself as an officer with the highway patrol and a First Responder. "Please help my daughter!" the mother pleads. As Tim takes the child, the mother says, "I was just driving along when she began to thrash around. Before I could find a safe place to stop, she got real quiet. She isn't breathing. Please, please help her."

Tim lays the child on the ground and positions the airway. He attempts to ventilate her with a pocket face mask. He sees no chest rise. He repositions the airway and tries again. Nothing. Tim looks into the child's airway but can see nothing blocking it. He asks if there's any chance that the child ate something prior to the episode. "I don't know," the mother answers.

Tim performs five abdominal thrusts. When he checks the airway again, he sweeps away a huge piece of hard candy. The youngster immediately begins to cough, then vomits, and eventually cries for her mother. Seeing that the child is breathing on her own, Tim turns her onto her side and encourages the mother to comfort her until the ambulance arrives. Soon thereafter they hear sirens approaching.

SCENE SIZE UP

INITIAL ASSESSMENT and TREATMENT

PHYSICAL EXAM and TREATMENT

ONGOING ASSESSMENT and TREATMENT

PATIENT HAND-OFF

LEARNING OBJECTIVES

Successfully managing a patient's airway and breathing is one of the most important tasks you'll perform. As the scenario on the previous page shows, a patient's ability to breathe may be compromised at any time. Your ability to care for that patient can make the difference between life and death. In this chapter we'll walk you through the skills you need to assess a patient's airway and breathing, to treat airway and breathing problems, and to check if your interventions are actually working.

However, before you go on, you might want to review the anatomy and physiology of the respiratory system (see Chapter 4). A good way to review is to draw a rough diagram of the system and then label all its parts. Check it against the illustrations in text. Be sure to pay special attention to the differences between the airway of adults and the airway of infants and children.

By the end of the chapter, you should be able to:†

- 2-1.1 Name and label the major structures of the respiratory system on a diagram. (p. 111)
- 2-1.2 List the signs of inadequate breathing. (pp. 112-113, 122-123)
- 2-1.3 Describe the steps in the head-tilt chin-lift. (p. 114)
- 2-1.4 Relate mechanism of injury to opening the airway. (p. 114)
- 2-1.5 Describe the steps in the jaw thrust. (pp. 114-115)
- 2-1.6 State the importance of having a suction unit ready for immediate use when providing emergency medical care. (pp. 118-119)
- 2-1.7 Describe the techniques of suctioning. (pp. 118-119)
- 2-1.8 Describe how to ventilate a patient with a resuscitation mask or barrier device. (pp. 123-126)
- 2-1.9 Describe how ventilating an infant or child is different from an adult. (p. 123)
- 2-1.10 List the steps in providing mouth-to-mouth and mouth-to-stoma ventilation. (pp. 126-127)
- 2-1.11 Describe how to measure and insert an oropharyngeal (oral) airway. (pp. 119-120)

†Numbered objectives are from the 1995 U.S. DOT "First Responder: National Standard Curriculum." Asterisks indicate supplementary material.

- ■ 2-1.12 Describe how to measure and insert a nasopharyngeal (nasal) airway. (pp. 120-122)
- ■ 2-1.13 Describe how to clear a foreign body airway obstruction in a responsive adult. (pp. 136-137)
- ■ 2-1.14 Describe how to clear a foreign body airway obstruction in a responsive child with complete obstruction or partial airway obstruction and poor air exchange. (p. 138)
- ■ 2-1.15 Describe how to clear a foreign body airway obstruction in a responsive infant with complete obstruction or partial airway obstruction and poor air exchange. (pp. 140-141)
- ■ 2-1.16 Describe how to clear a foreign body airway obstruction in an unresponsive adult. (pp. 137-138)
- ■ 2-1.17 Describe how to clear a foreign body airway obstruction in an unresponsive child. (p. 138)
- ■ 2-1.18 Describe how to clear a foreign body airway obstruction in an unresponsive infant. (p. 141)
- * Describe the steps for using the bag-valve-mask to ventilate a patient. (pp. 127-130)
- * Describe the steps for using a flow-restricted oxygen-powered ventilation device. (pp. 130-132)
- * Describe the indications and steps for providing oxygen via mask. (pp. 132-135)

MANAGING THE AIRWAY

SIGNS OF BREATHING PROBLEMS

As discussed in the last chapter, a patient who is breathing normally shows no signs of respiratory distress. Normal breathing is effortless. It appears to be steady, rhythmic, and occurs with little or no noise.

Patients with labored breathing breathe more rapidly or more slowly than normal. Their breathing may be irregular, and you might see them use the muscles of the neck, ribs, or abdomen to assist with breathing. This is called accessory muscle use or breathing with retractions. Such patients may be cyanotic (bluish skin and mucous membranes, a very grave sign). They also may be quite agitated. Patients who go into **respiratory arrest** (they stop breathing) usually appear exhausted first.

Body posture will vary in patients who have difficulty breathing. In general, they sit upright with backs very straight. Patients with chronic breathing problems often will sit in the **tripod position**. That is, they sit with back straight but leaning slightly forward with hands on their knees.

Signs of breathing problems may be difficult to detect in infants and children. Look for **seesaw breathing**, where the chest and abdomen appear to move in opposite directions with each breath. Also check for **nasal flaring**, grunting sounds with breathing, and pronounced use of accessory muscles.

GENERAL GUIDELINES

Learning when to assess a patient's airway and breathing is as important as learning airway and breathing skills. So as you learn each new skill in this chapter, keep in mind the following assessment and treatment strategy:

- *Assess airway and breathing.* Does my patient have a patent airway? Is the rate and quality of breathing adequate? Do I need to support the patient's breathing with ventilations?
- *Intervene.* Open the airway, begin artificial ventilation, and so on.
- *Reassess.* Is the airway now open? Have my interventions improved the patient's breathing status? If not, what else can I do?

OPENING THE AIRWAY

After a scene size-up, perform an initial assessment of your patient. Form a general impression. Assess responsiveness. Stabilize the spine, if necessary. Then assess the patient's airway and breathing status. If your patient is not breathing or shows signs of a partially obstructed airway (such as noisy or snoring respirations), immediately open the airway.

Use either the **head-tilt/chin-lift maneuver** or the **jaw-thrust maneuver** (described below). Both can lift the tongue away from the back of the throat to allow a clear passage for air. Note that the number one cause of an obstructed airway is the tongue, especially in an unresponsive patient.

> **Remember** *Your top priority is to establish an airway. All other emergency care can wait. Remember: Airway! Airway! Airway!*

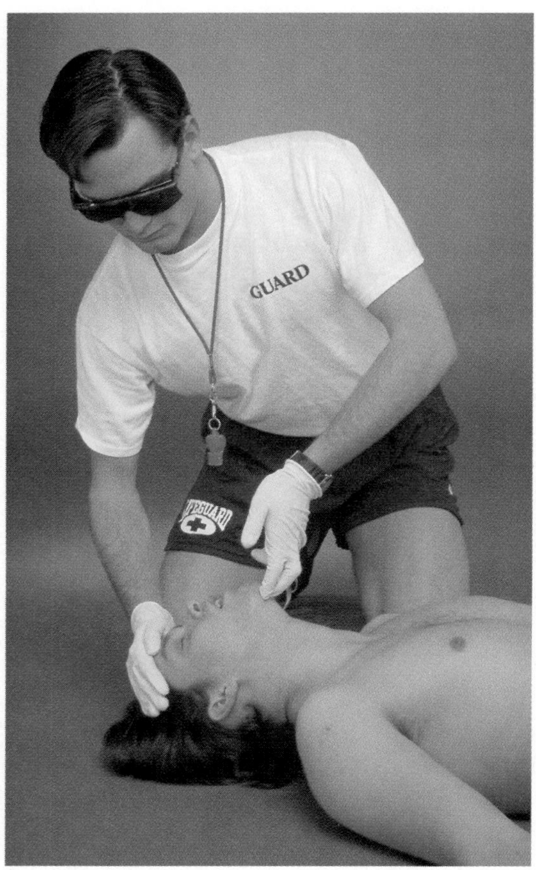

Figure 10-1
Head-tilt/chin-lift maneuver.

Head-Tilt/Chin-Lift Maneuver

Use the head-tilt/chin-lift maneuver to open the airway of uninjured, unresponsive patients. Never use it with suspected spine-injured patients. Make sure there's no mechanism of injury at the scene that suggests trauma or injury to the head or spine. Then after taking all proper BSI precautions, follow these steps (Figure 10-1):

1. Position yourself along the side of your patient's head.
2. Place one gloved hand on your patient's forehead. Then apply firm pressure to tilt the head back into a sniffing position.
3. Place the fingers of your other hand on the bony part of the patient's chin. Don't use your thumb. Then lift the chin up, while you keep the mouth open.
4. Reassess the patient. Answer these questions: Has the patient's breathing improved? Have noisy or snoring respirations cleared up? If you see no improvement, reposition the airway.

> **Caution** *To prevent further airway obstruction, keep your fingers from pressing deeply into the soft tissues of the chin.*

When you perform the head-tilt/chin-lift on an infant or child, tilt the head back only slightly. *Hyperextension*, or too much tilt backwards, can cause the windpipe to collapse. Also remember that the head in an infant or child usually is proportionately larger than the body. If you were to put this patient in a supine position, the head would tilt forwards (*hyperflexion*). A small towel beneath the patient's shoulders may help you avoid this problem.

Jaw-Thrust Maneuver

Use the jaw-thrust maneuver to open the airway of unresponsive trauma patients. Always use it when the mechanism of injury suggests a possible spine injury. Use it for patients who fell and patients with an injury to the head or neck. Use it if there's any doubt about whether you have a trauma patient or a medical patient. This maneuver keeps the patient's neck in a neutral, in-line

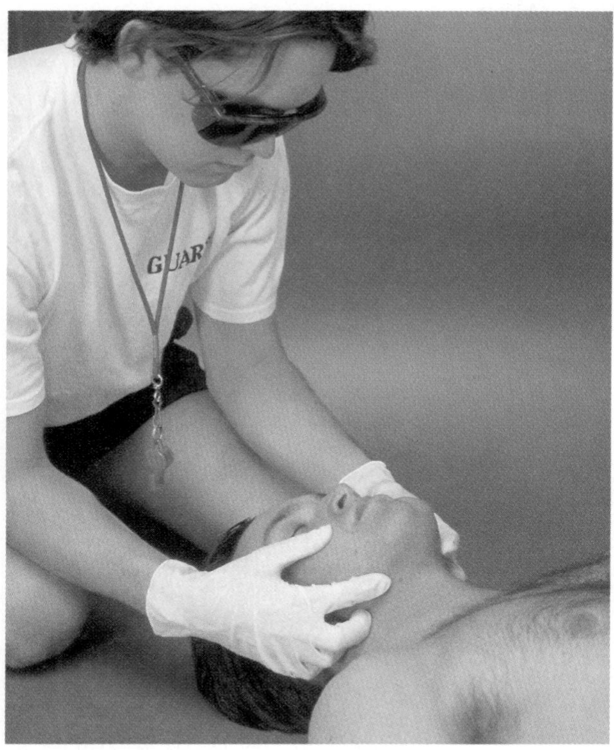

Figure 10-2
Jaw-thrust maneuver.

position while lifting the tongue off the back of the throat.

After taking all proper BSI precautions, follow these steps (Figure 10-2):

1. Position yourself above your patient's head.
2. Place your gloved hands on either side of the head. Your thumbs should be resting on the cheekbones.
3. Grasp the angles of the lower jaw with your fingers.
4. Simultaneously press down with your thumbs and up with your fingers. If the lips close, open the lower lip with your thumb.
5. Reassess the patient to ensure that the airway is now open.

Caution *Since pressure must be kept constant to keep the airway open, the jaw-thrust maneuver may be tiring. Have another rescuer relieve you.*

INSPECTING AND CLEARING THE AIRWAY

After you open the patient's airway, inspect it. Fluid and solid particles or loose dentures can block it. Altered mental status patients who cannot protect their own airways also should have their airways inspected. Using a gloved hand, open the patient's mouth and look inside. If it's blocked, clear it immediately.

There are four ways you can help to clear or maintain an open airway. They are the recovery position, the log roll, a finger sweep, and suction. They are not performed in sequence. The specific emergency situation will dictate which one is needed.

THE RECOVERY POSITION

A patient in the recovery position is on his or her side (Figure 10-3). This position uses gravity to help keep the airway open. It allows fluid to drain from the patient's mouth rather than into the airway. Unrecognized airway obstructions are less likely to occur.

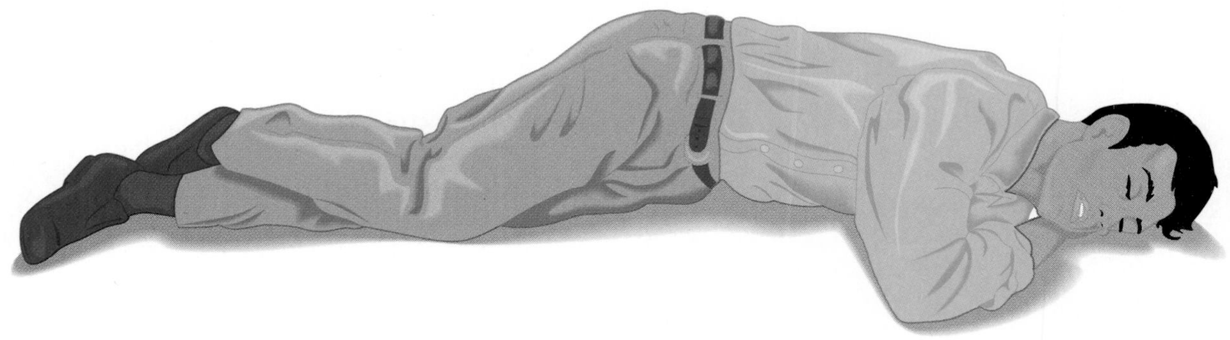

Figure 10-3
The recovery position.

Therefore, it's the best position for the uninjured, altered mental status or unresponsive patient who is breathing adequately.

After determining that the airway is open and breathing is adequate, follow these steps:

1. Lift the patient's left arm above the head. Cross the patient's right leg over the left.
2. While supporting the patient's face, grasp the right shoulder and roll the patient toward you onto his or her left side. Make sure that the head, torso, and shoulders move together without twisting.
3. Place the patient's right hand under the side of the face. The head should be as close to the midline position as possible.
4. Once in position, monitor the patient until additional EMS personnel take over care.

The Log Roll

When an unresponsive patient is prone (face down), you can't assess breathing properly and you can't provide basic life support. So you must turn the patient around to a supine (face up) position quickly and carefully. One way is to perform a log roll. It protects the suspected spine-injured patient from twisting motions that can cause injury. Though two rescuers can do it, three or more are needed to perform a log roll safely.

After taking all proper BSI precautions, follow these steps (Figure 10-4):

1. Get in position at the patient's head. Hold the patient's head and neck in neutral, in-line position.
2. The second rescuer places one of the patient's arms above the head. The patient's legs should not be crossed.

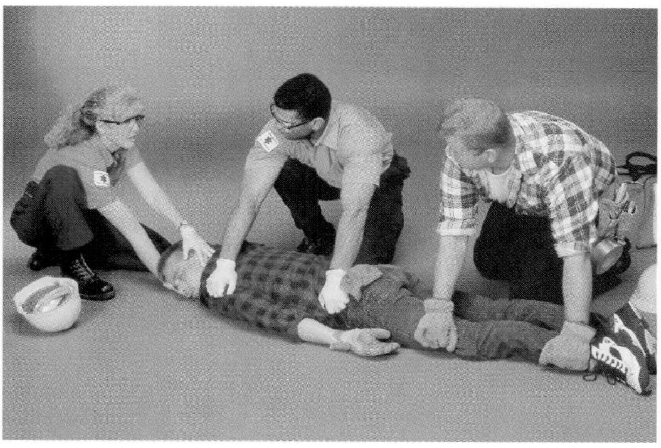

Figure 10-4
Rescuers in position to log roll a prone patient.

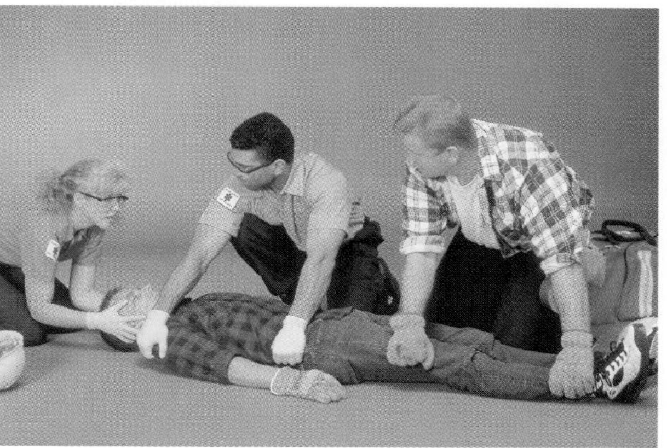

Figure 10-5
Rescuers in position to log roll a supine patient.

3. The second and third rescuers position themselves on the same side of the patient. Then they grasp the patient at the shoulders, hips, and knees. Make sure the patient's body is completely supported during the move.
4. On your signal, the second and third rescuers turn the patient as a unit in one coordinated move. Make sure that the patient's spine is kept in a neutral, in-line position throughout the move.
5. When the patient is supine, rescuers place the arms alongside the patient's body.
6. You must continue manual stabilization of the cervical spine until the patient is completely immobilized on a long backboard.

When the log roll is used to help clear an airway (Figure 10-5), the patient is rolled to his side so that vomit, blood, or other materials can drain from the patient's mouth. Be sure the patient's cervical spine is completely supported while the patient is on his or her side. When the airway is drained, the patient may be rolled back to a supine position again.

The Finger Sweep

A patient's airway can be blocked by solid objects as well as vomit or other fluids. When you use a finger sweep, you use your own gloved fingers to remove visible blockages of the airway. After taking all proper BSI precautions, follow these steps:

1. If the patient is not injured, roll him onto his side.

2. If the foreign material is visible in the mouth, remove it quickly. Wipe out liquids with your index and middle fingers covered with a cloth. Remove solid objects with a hooked index finger.

Never perform a "blind" finger sweep on an infant or child. Be sure you can see the object before trying to pluck it out with your fingers.

SUCTIONING

Suction units create negative pressure to open an airway clogged with blood, vomit, or food particles. However, suctioning doesn't usually work on solid objects like teeth or food. Portable suction units are powered either by hand or electricity (Figure 10-6). At the end of suction tubing is a catheter, which can be rigid or flexible. A rigid or tonsil-tip catheter is used to suction the mouth. A flexible catheter is used for the nose and around airway adjuncts.

STREET NOTES

Plan ahead. Keep your suction unit within arm's reach. Altered mental status and unresponsive patients may vomit without warning.

Consider suctioning your patient immediately when you hear a gurgling sound during breathing or ventilation. It's indicated if the recovery position, log roll, and finger sweeps don't help to clear the airway. To suction wear gloves and eye protection and follow these steps:

1. Place the proper catheter on the suction tubing. A rigid tonsil tip is preferred for an unresponsive patient.
2. Turn on the suction unit.
3. Insert the suction catheter to the base of the tongue without suction. If you place it any deeper, vomiting may result.
4. Begin suctioning while moving the tonsil tip from side to side and while removing it slowly from the mouth (Figure 10-7).

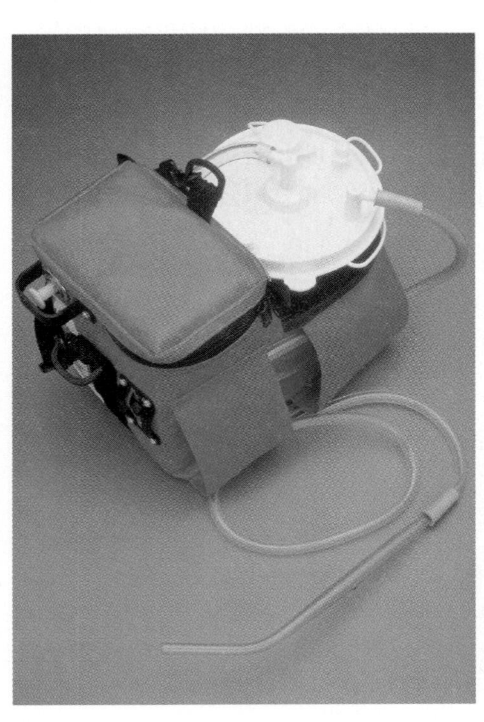

Figure 10-6a
Portable electric suction unit.

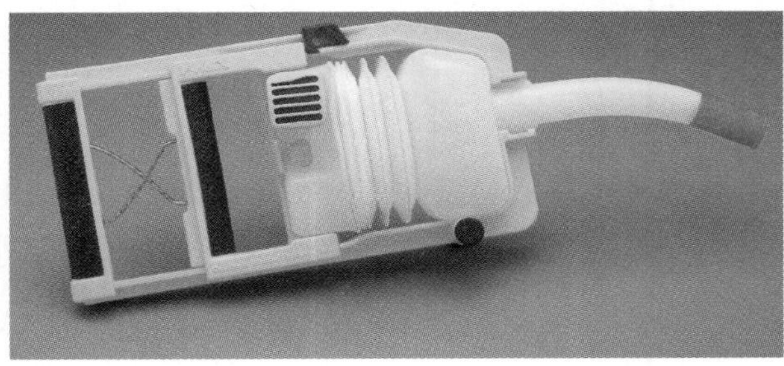

Figure 10-6b
Portable hand-operated suction unit.

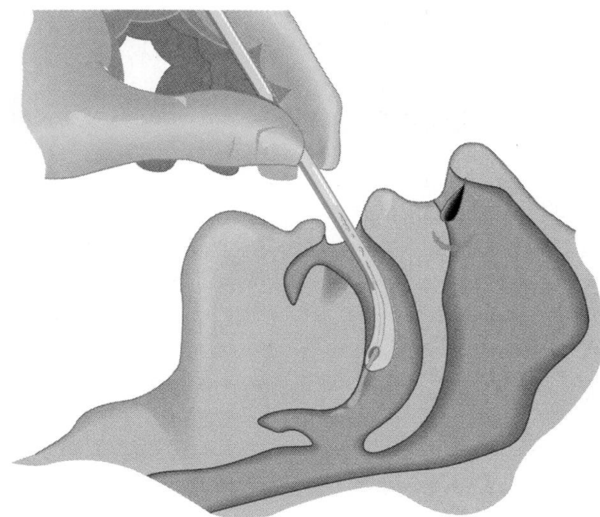

Figure 10-7
Suction by moving the tonsil tip from side to side.

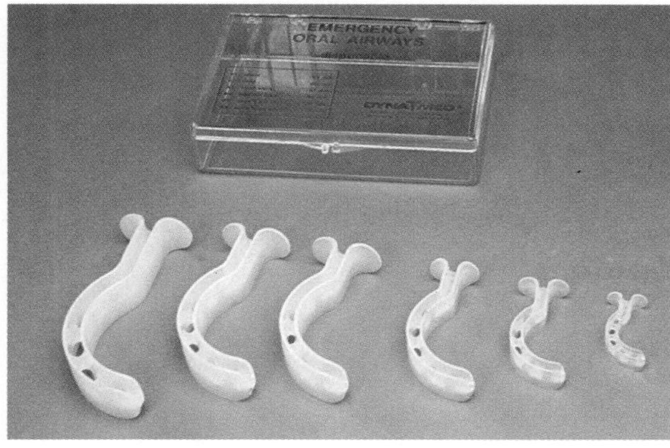

Figure 10-8
Oropharyngeal airways.

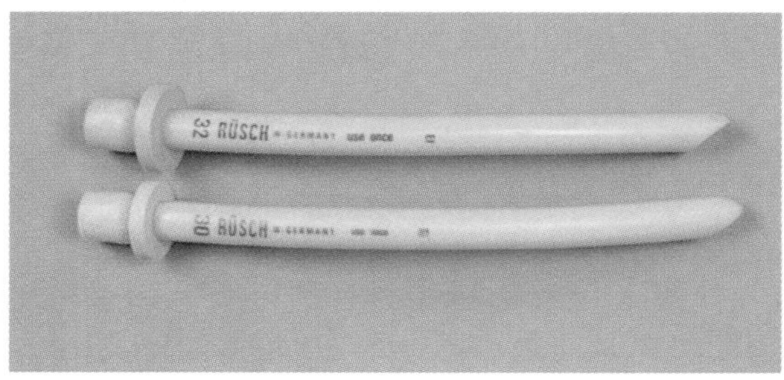

Figure 10-9
Nasopharyngeal airways.

5. Suction up to 15 seconds. If there's a lot of vomit or other fluids, suction vigorously. Then ventilate for two minutes, and suction again.
6. If the suction catheter becomes clogged, rinse it out and continue.

Because suctioning removes air, suction an infant for only five seconds and a child for only ten. If there's a decrease in an infant's heart rate, stop suctioning and ventilate. Note also that a simple bulb syringe is an excellent suction device for infants.

AIRWAY ADJUNCTS

Airway adjuncts are used to increase the effectiveness of managing the airway. Two types are the **oropharyngeal airway** (Figure 10-8) and the **nasopharyngeal airway** (Figure 10-9). Both are designed to keep the patient's airway open by keeping the tongue off the back of the throat.

> **Remember** *Unresponsive patients don't maintain their own airways!*

Oropharyngeal Airway (OPA)

The oropharyngeal airway (OPA) is used to maintain the airway of an unresponsive patient who has *no gag reflex*. To properly insert it into the patient's mouth, take all proper BSI precautions and follow these steps (Figure 10-10):

1. Determine the proper OPA size. Measure from the corner of your patient's lips to the tip of the earlobe or angle of the jaw.
2. Open the patient's mouth.
3. Insert the OPA upside down. Be sure the tip is pointed at the roof of the patient's mouth.
4. Advance the OPA gently until you feel resistance.

Inserting the Oropharyngeal Airway

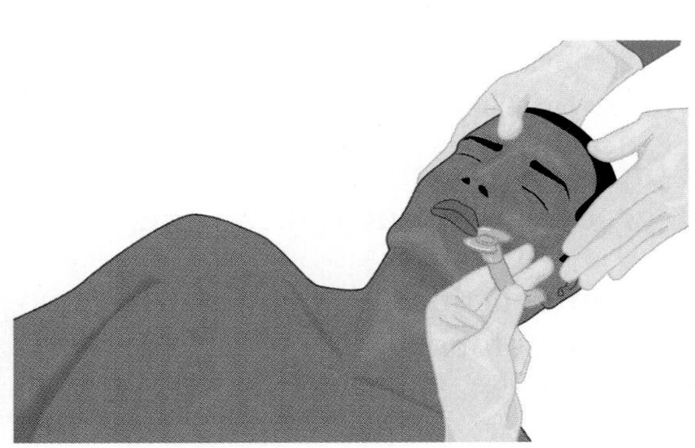

Figure 10-10a
Determine the proper airway size.

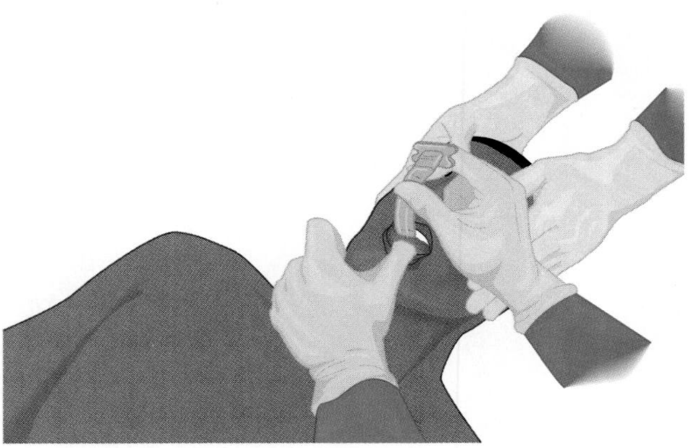

Figure 10-10b
Insert the airway upside down.

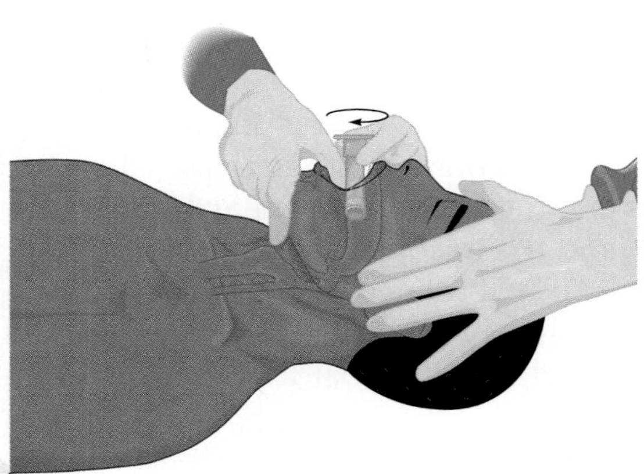

Figure 10-10c
Rotate the airway as you insert it.

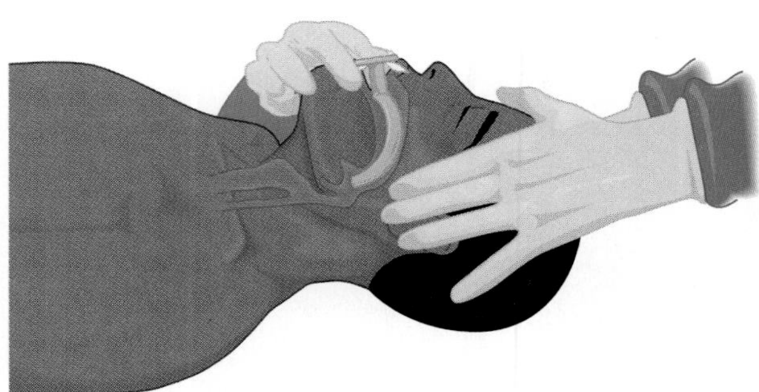

Figure 10-10d
Stop when the flange rests against the mouth.

5. Rotate the OPA 180 degrees clockwise as you continue to insert it. Stop when the flange rests against your patient's teeth.
6. Reassess the patient to ensure that the airway is open.

Modify this method for an infant or child. Don't insert the OPA upside down. Instead use a tongue depressor to press the tongue down and away. Then insert the airway right side up (Figure 10-11).

Nasopharyngeal Airway (NPA)

The nasopharyngeal airway (NPA) is a soft rubber tube with a beveled end. It's less likely to stimulate vomiting, so it's used in the altered mental status patient who still has a gag reflex. Note that this airway adjunct can be painful during insertion.

To insert the NPA into the patient's nose, take all proper BSI precautions and follow these steps (Figure 10-12):

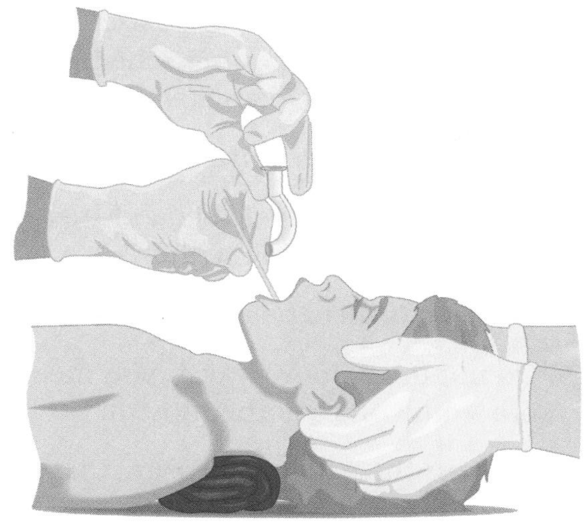

Figure 10-11
For an infant or child, insert the oropharyngeal airway right side up.

Inserting the Nasopharyngeal Airway

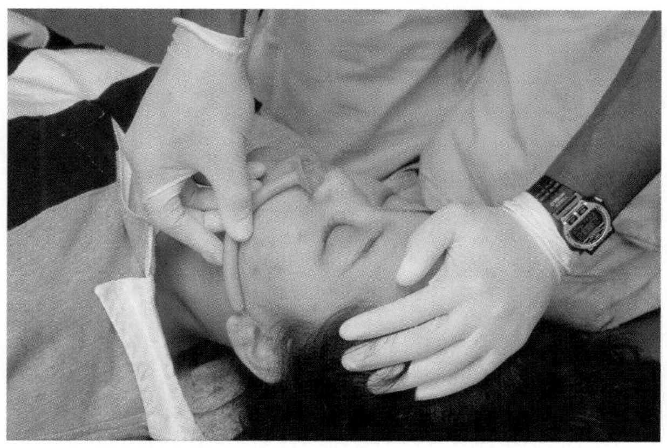

Figure 10-12a
Determine the proper size airway.

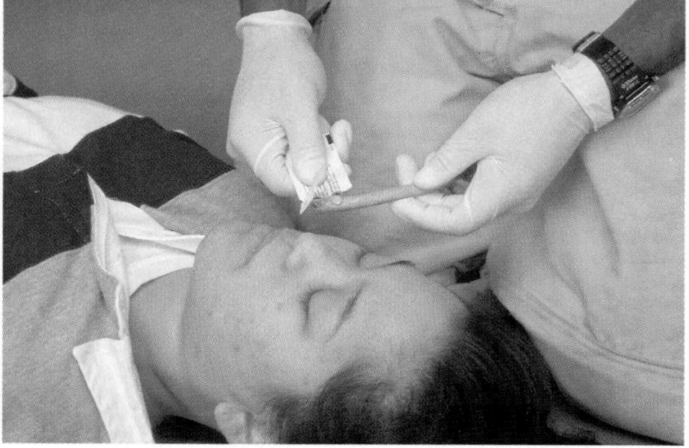

Figure 10-12b
Lubricate the airway.

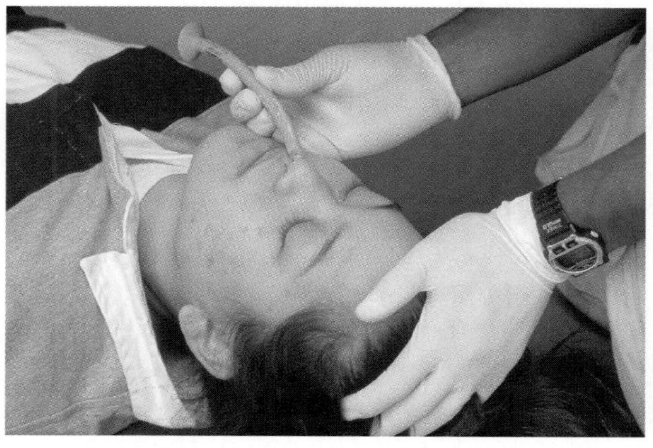

Figure 10-12c
Gently advance the airway with a rotating motion.

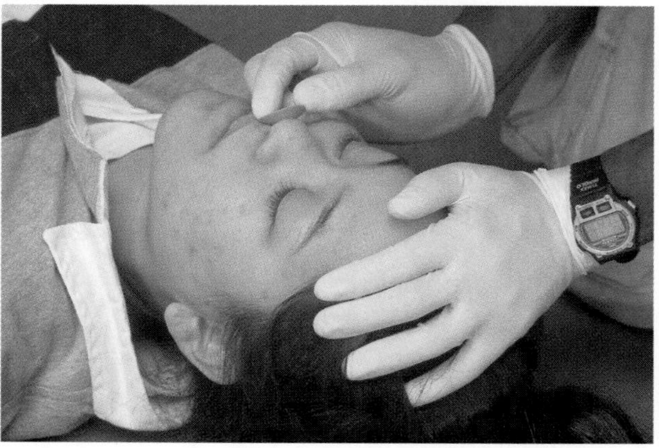

Figure 10-12d
The airway in place.

1. Determine the proper NPA size. Match the distance from the tip of the patient's nose to the tip of the ear. The tube should also fit inside the diameter of the patient's nostril.
2. Lubricate the NPA with a water-soluble lubricant.
3. Then place the beveled end of the NPA against the base of the nostril or toward the septum.
4. Gently advance the airway with a rotating motion.
5. Do not force the airway. If you meet resistance, try the same procedure on the other nostril.
6. Reassess the patient to ensure that the airway is open.

ARTIFICIAL VENTILATION

DETERMINING THE PRESENCE AND ADEQUACY OF BREATHING

Immediately after opening the patient's airway, you must check to see if the patient is breathing. At the same time, look at the effort or work of breathing. Remember normal breathing appears effortless.

When checking the breathing of a responsive patient, ask questions such as "Can you speak?" "Are you choking?" or "Are you having trouble breathing?" The ability to talk or make vocal sounds indicates that air is moving past the vocal cords. If you are assessing the breathing of an unresponsive patient, first open the airway. Then place your ear close to the patient's mouth and nose. Assess breathing as described below for three to five seconds:

- *Look* for the rise and fall of the chest.
- *Listen* for air escaping during exhalation.
- *Feel* for air entering and exiting the mouth and nose.

It's possible to see some rise and fall of the chest even when an airway obstruction is present. However, you won't hear or feel air movement. If your patient isn't breathing or breathing inadequately (Figure 10-13), you must ventilate him or her immediately. Use one of the techniques of **artificial ventilation**, or rescue breathing, described below. Whichever one you use, the rates in Table 10-1 apply.

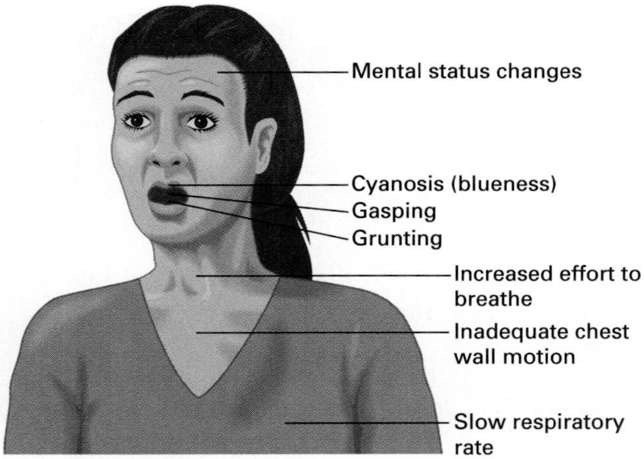

Figure 10-13
Signs of inadequate breathing.

TABLE 10-1	ARTIFICIAL VENTILATION RATES
Infant	20 breaths per minute at 1.0 to 1.5 seconds each.
Child	20 breaths per minute at 1.0 to 1.5 seconds each.
Adult	10-12 breaths per minute at 1.5 to 2.0 seconds each.

Note that just after cardiac arrest some patients have *agonal respirations* or reflex gasping (a type of muscle contraction associated with death). Don't confuse this with breathing.

MOUTH-TO-MASK VENTILATION

Mouth-to-mask ventilation is the most preferred method of artificial ventilation (Figure 10-14). Performed properly, it's very effective since it allows for a tight seal around the patient's mouth.

STREET NOTES

Dentures usually can be left in place during ventilation. However, if they become dislodged, be prepared to remove them immediately.

Be sure to use the correct mask size—infant, child, or adult. The mask should have a one-way valve that protects you from the patient's exhaled air, secretions, and vomit. It must be transparent so you can see when the patient is vomiting. Some models also have connecting ports for supplemental oxygen delivery (Figure 10-15).

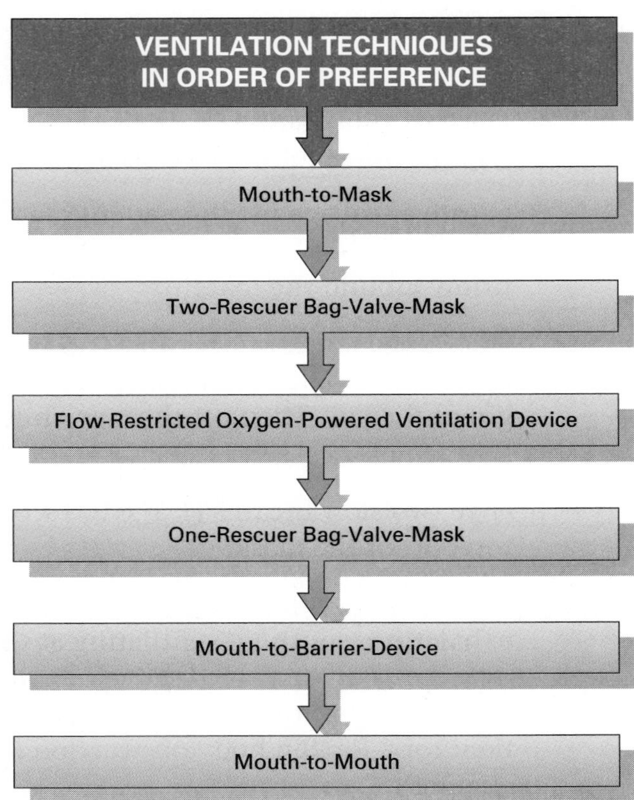

Figure 10-14
Mouth-to-mask is the preferred method of ventilation.

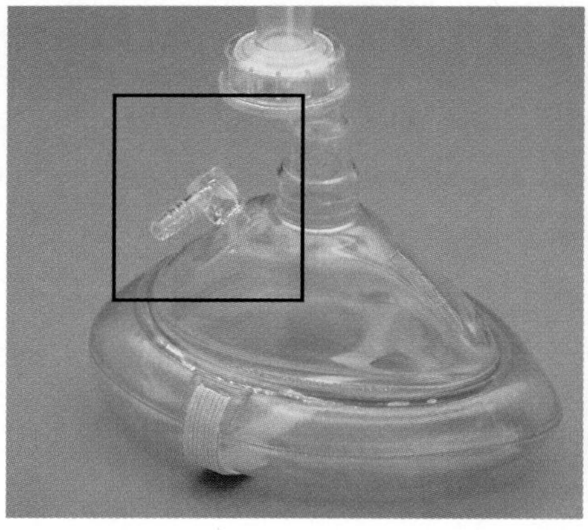

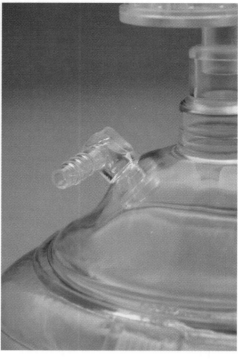

Figure 10-15
Pocket face mask with oxygen port.

After taking BSI precautions, follow these steps (Figure 10-16):

1. Open the airway with a head-tilt/chin-lift or jaw-thrust maneuver. Then check for breathing. Remember to manually stabilize the head and neck of a trauma or suspected spine-injured patient.
2. Place the mask around the nose and mouth of your patient. Use the bridge of the nose as a guide for correct position.
3. Create a seal against the patient's face. Place the heel and thumb of each hand along the border of the mask. Compress firmly around the margin.
4. Place both index fingers on the portion of the mask that covers the chin. Lock your remaining fingers along the bony margin of the jaw. Then lift the jaw while you maintain a head tilt.
5. Give two slow breaths (1.5 to 2.0 seconds each) through the top port of the mask.
6. If you see the chest rise, and hear and feel air escape during exhalation, continue ventilating at the proper rate. However, if your ventilations are inadequate, reposition the patient's airway and try again. If the second try fails, then treat the patient for a foreign body obstruction (described later in this chapter).

Providing Artificial Ventilation

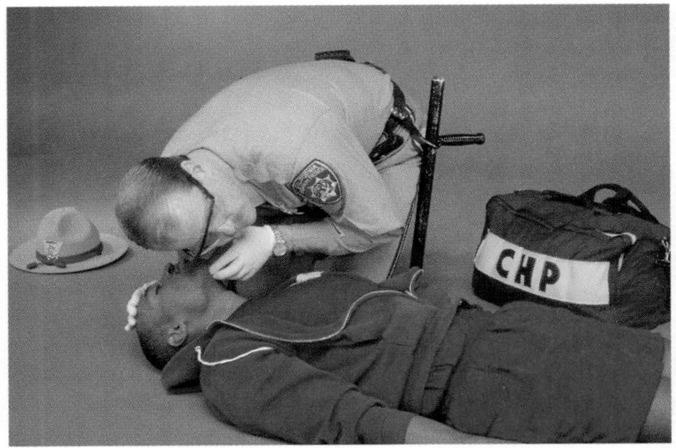

Figure 10-16a
Open the airway and check for breathing.

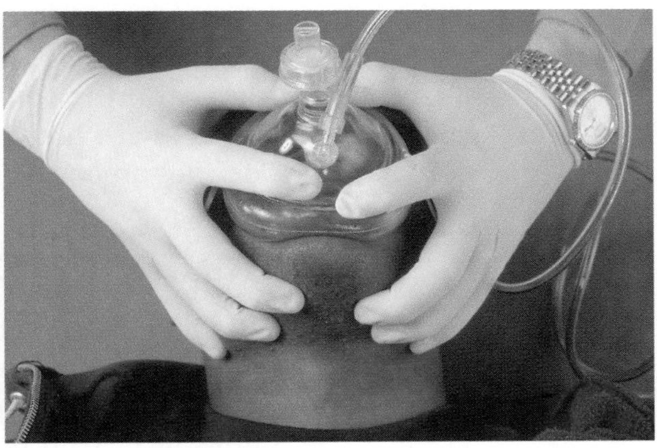

Figure 10-16b
Position the mask and create a seal.

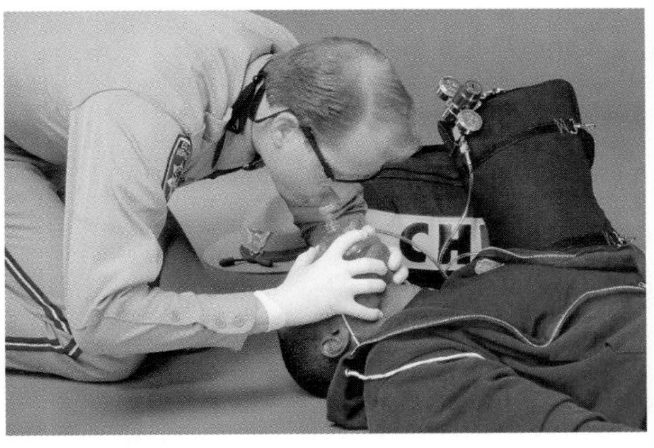

Figure 10-16c
Provide two slow breaths through the top port.

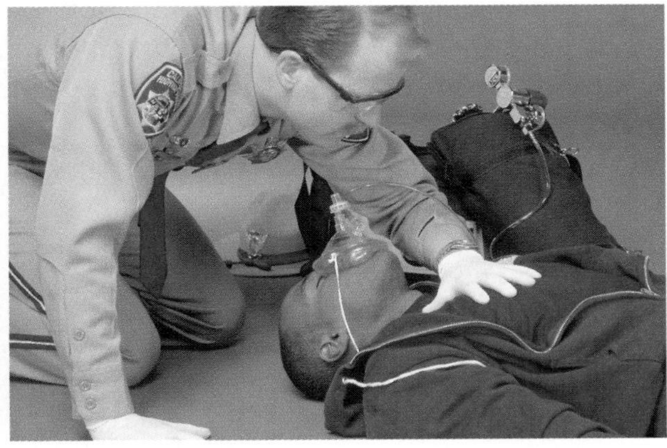

Figure 10-16d
If you see or feel the chest rise, continue ventilations at the proper rate.

Warning *Don't provide too much air or air too forcefully. If you do, air may enter the patient's stomach causing vomiting and inadequate ventilations. This problem is more common in infants and children than adults and may significantly impair your efforts.*

Whenever you provide artificial ventilation, it's absolutely critical that you assess and reassess the effectiveness of your efforts. Sending your breaths into the patient's stomach or cheeks is as effective as not ventilating at all. The key is to ask yourself constantly: Are my ventilations effective? Has my patient's color improved? Is my patient now breathing on his or her own? Is my patient's mental status improving? If your patient is not improving, you need to reassess your care: Do I need to reposition the patient's airway? Tighten the mask seal? Increase the depth or rate of ventilations?

MOUTH-TO-BARRIER DEVICE VENTILATION

When a mask isn't available, simple barrier devices may be used (Figure 10-17). Most lack one-way valves. They also commonly leak air during ventilations. However, they do protect you from contact with body fluids. Perform *mouth-to-barrier device ventilation* the same way you would perform mouth-to-mask.

MOUTH-TO-MOUTH VENTILATION

When a mask or a barrier device isn't available, *mouth-to-mouth ventilation* is your only option. This method is actually the most efficient. With it, you can create a very tight seal around the patient's mouth. You also can control the force of ventilations more easily. The downside is that it provides no protection against infection. Follow these steps:

1. Keep the airway open with a head-tilt/chin-lift or jaw-thrust maneuver. Manually stabilize the head and neck of a trauma or suspected spine-injured patient
2. Gently pinch the patient's nostrils closed with the thumb and index finger of one hand.
3. Take a deep breath. Then put your lips around the patient's mouth to create an airtight seal.
4. Give two slow breaths (1.5 to 2.0 seconds each).
5. If you see the chest rise, and hear and feel the air escape during exhalation, continue ventilations at the proper rate. However, if your ventilations are inadequate, reposition the patient's airway and try again. If the second try fails, then treat the patient for a foreign body obstruction (described later in this chapter).

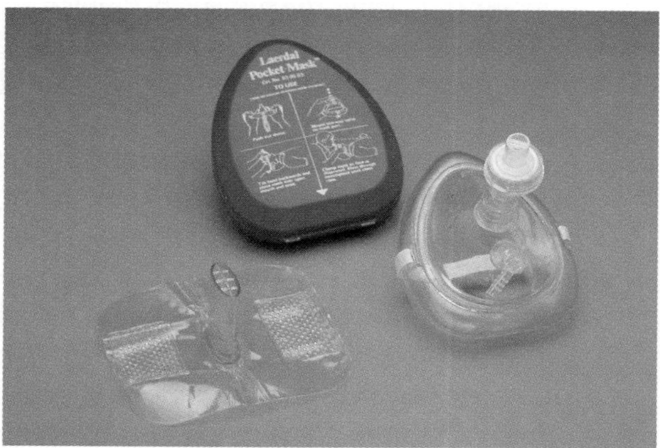

Figure 10-17
Mask and simple barrier devices.

Cover both the nose and mouth to create a seal for the infant patient. Also, adjust the volume of your ventilations to your patient's size. An infant may require only a small cheek puff of air. A larger child may require an adult-size ventilation.

MOUTH-TO-STOMA VENTILATION

In rare cases your patient may have had a *tracheostomy*. During this operation, a **stoma** (a hole) is made in the trachea and a tube commonly is inserted to create an airway. The patient may now breathe solely or only partially through the stoma.

To provide *mouth-to-stoma ventilation,* we suggest that you use a barrier device (Figure 10-18). If no barrier device is available, gently seal your lips around the tube and ventilate. If air escapes from the patient's mouth or nose, then close the mouth and pinch the nostrils while you ventilate.

BAG-VALVE-MASK VENTILATION

Bag-valve-mask ventilation is a highly effective way to provide rescue breathing to a patient. When used with supplemental oxygen, the **bag-valve-mask** (BVM) can deliver almost 100% oxygen to the patient. However, it's more difficult than other methods to master. Although one rescuer can use a BVM, it's most effective when two rescuers operate it.

The BVM is a hand-operated device (Figure 10-19). It consists of a self-inflating bag, a one-way valve, a face mask, and an oxygen reservoir. It has a volume of approximately 1600 milliliters (less than provided by way of the mouth-to-mask technique). To perform most effectively, it needs to be connected to oxygen. An oral or nasal airway may be necessary in conjunction with the BVM.

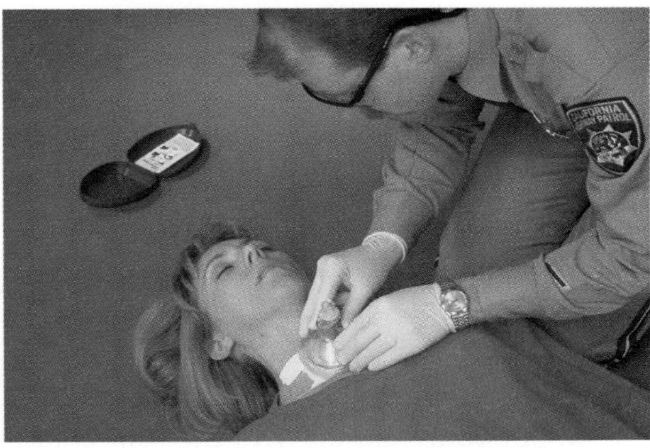

Figure 10-18
Use a barrier device to provide ventilations to a patient with a stoma.

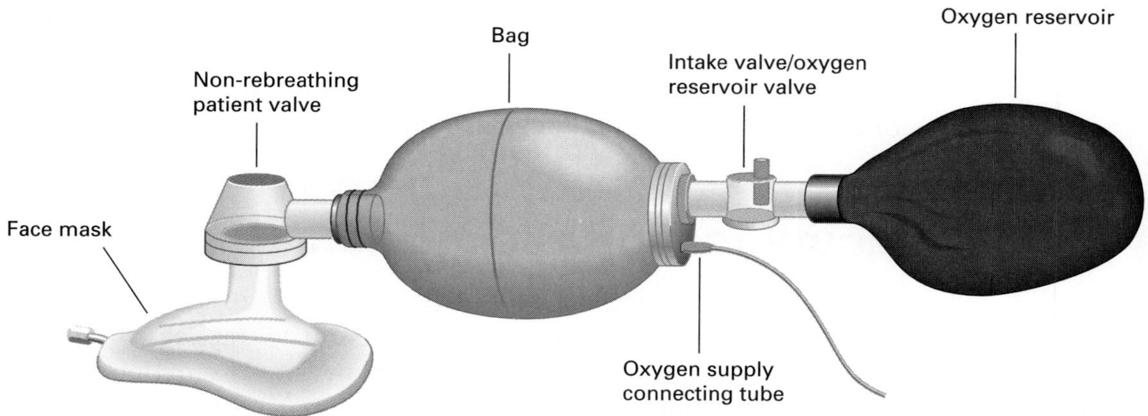

Figure 10-19
Bag-valve-mask device.

The BVM is available in infant, child, and adult sizes. Whatever the size, it should have the following features:

- A self-refilling bag that is easy to clean and sterilize.
- A non-jamming valve that allows a maximum oxygen inlet flow of 15 liters per minute (lpm).
- Either no pop-off valve or a pop-off valve that can be disabled. Failure to disable a pop-off valve may result in inadequate ventilations.
- Standardized 15/22 mm fittings.
- An oxygen inlet and reservoir to allow for a high concentration of oxygen.
- A true one-way valve.
- Can perform in all environmental conditions and temperature extremes.

BVM Ventilation—Medical Patient

For the medical patient (no suspected trauma), take all proper BSI precautions and follow these steps for two-rescuer BVM ventilation (Figure 10-20):

1. Select the correct size BVM for the patient.
2. Both you and your partner should be in position at the patient's head. Keep the airway open with a head-tilt/chin-lift.
3. Put your thumbs over the top half of the mask with index and middle fingers over the bottom half. Then place the narrow

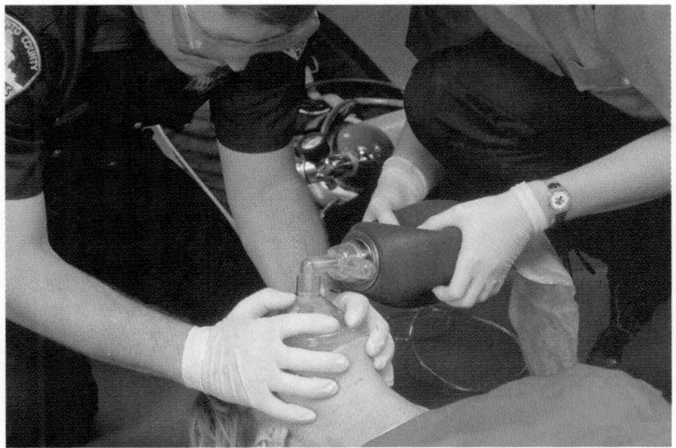

Figure 10-20
Two-rescuer BVM method.

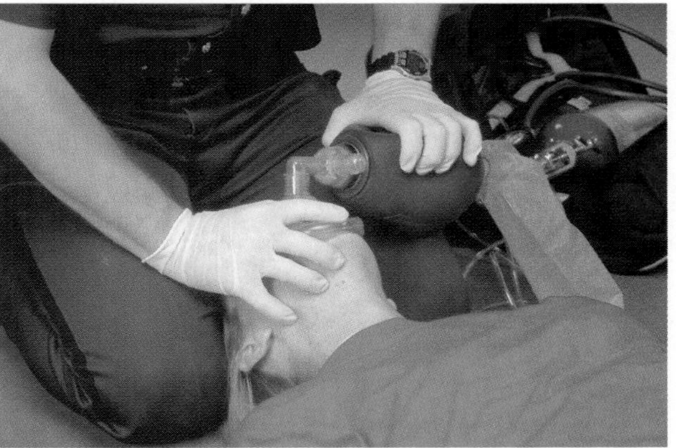

Figure 10-21
One-rescuer BVM method.

end (apex) of the mask over the bridge of the patient's nose. Lower the mask over the mouth and upper chin. If the mask has a large round cuff around the ventilation port, center the port over the patient's mouth.

4. Use your ring and little fingers to bring the patient's jaw up to the mask. The mask can be connected to the bag now if you haven't already done so.

5. Then your partner can squeeze the bag with both hands until the patient's chest rises.

If you're alone, form a "C" around the ventilation port with your thumb and index finger. Use your middle, ring, and little fingers under the patient's jaw to maintain the correct chin lift and complete the seal. Compress the bag against your thigh (Figure 10-21).

If the patient's chest doesn't rise and fall, reevaluate the patient to make sure there is no airway obstruction. If the chest doesn't rise, reposition the patient's head. If air is escaping around the mask, reposition your fingers and check placement of the mask. If the patient's chest still does not rise and fall, switch to another ventilation method, such as mouth-to-mask. If necessary, consider the use of an oropharyngeal or nasopharyngeal airway.

BVM Ventilation—Trauma Patient

To ventilate the trauma patient with a BVM, take all proper BSI precautions and follow these steps:

1. Select the correct size BVM for the patient.

2. Both you and your partner should be in position at the patient's head. Keep the airway open with a jaw-thrust.

3. Immobilize the patient's head and neck. One way is to hold the patient's head immobile with your knees. Another way is to have your partner manually stabilize the head and neck while you perform one-rescuer BVM ventilation.
4. Put your thumbs over the top half of the mask with index and middle fingers over the bottom half. Then place the narrow end (apex) of the mask over the bridge of the patient's nose. Lower the mask over the mouth and upper chin. If the mask has a large round cuff around the ventilation port, center the port over the patient's mouth.
5. Use your ring and little fingers to bring the patient's jaw up to the mask without tilting the head or neck. At this point the mask should be connected to the bag if you haven't already done so.
6. Then your partner can squeeze the bag with both hands until the patient's chest rises.

If the patient's chest doesn't rise and fall, reevaluate the patient to make sure there is no airway obstruction. If the patient's abdomen rises, reposition the jaw. If air is escaping from under the mask, reposition your fingers and check placement of the mask. If the patient's chest still does not rise and fall, switch to another ventilation method. If necessary, consider the use of an oropharyngeal or nasopharyngeal airway.

BVM-to-Stoma Ventilation

To ventilate a patient with a stoma, attach an infant or child-size BVM to the endotracheal tube. Then ventilate as you would any other patient, with one exception. The patient doesn't need a head-tilt/chin-lift or jaw-thrust to open the airway. Also, be careful not to dislodge the endotracheal tube while attempting to ventilate the patient.

FLOW-RESTRICTED OXYGEN-POWERED VENTILATION DEVICE (FROPVD)

The flow-restricted oxygen-powered ventilation device (FROPVD) is used only in adults (Figure 10-22). It provides a peak flow rate of 100% oxygen at up to 40 liters per minute (lpm). This device has a pressure relief valve that opens at about 60 centimeters of water, and vents into the atmosphere. If it can't vent, gas flow should stop. An alarm sounds whenever the relief valve pressure is exceeded. It also should have a trigger that is positioned so that both hands of the rescuer can remain on the mask. The

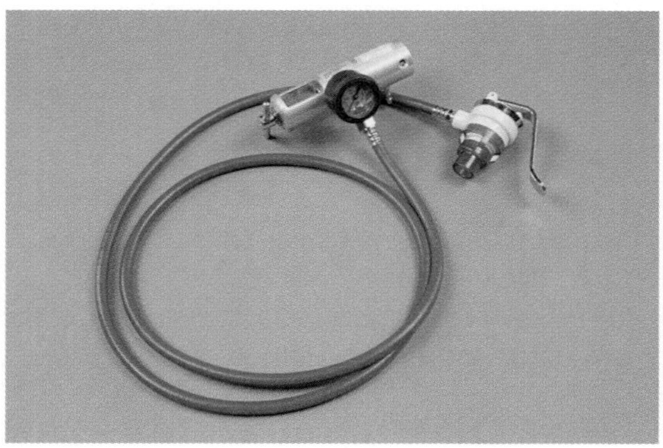

Figure 10-22a
Manually triggered flow-restricted oxygen-powered ventilation device (FROPVD).

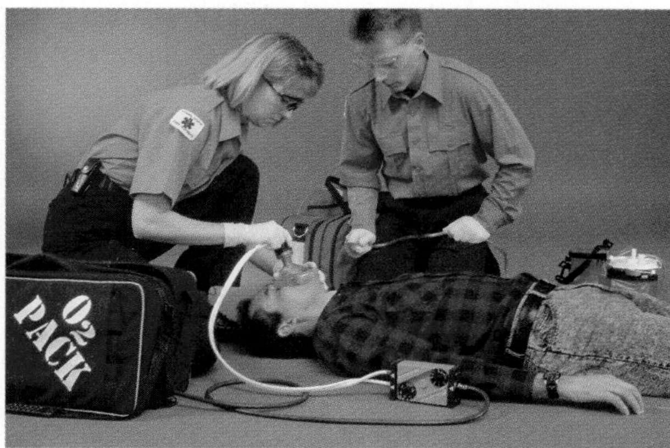

Figure 10-22b
Automatic FROPVD on the patient.

FROPVD should operate well under ordinary environmental conditions as well as in extremes of temperature.

FROPVD

To ventilate a patient with a FROPVD, take all proper BSI precautions and follow these steps:

1. After you open the patient's airway with a head-tilt/chin-lift or a jaw-thrust, insert an oral or nasal airway. Attach an adult-size mask to the FROPVD. If you have to immobilize the patient's head and neck, use your knees or have a second rescuer hold the patient's head and neck manually.
2. Place the mask on the patient. First, position your thumbs over the top half of the mask and your index and middle fingers over the bottom half. Then place the apex (narrow end) over the bridge of the patient's nose. Lower it over the mouth and upper chin. Use your ring and little fingers to lift the patient's jaw up to the mask without tilting the head or neck.
3. Connect the FROPVD to the mask if it hasn't already been done.
4. Trigger the FROPVD until you see the patient's chest rise. Repeat every 5 seconds. For an automatic FROPVD, set the desired volume and rate. Follow local protocols.

If the chest doesn't rise with each ventilation, reposition the patient's jaw. If air escapes around the mask, reposition your fingers and check the placement of the mask. If the patient's chest still doesn't rise, switch to another ventilation method. Make sure the patient doesn't have an airway obstruction.

OXYGEN THERAPY

Oxygen (O_2) is a colorless, odorless, tasteless gas that humans need to survive. Remember, the human body can do without oxygen only for a few minutes before brain cells start to die. Patients who benefit from oxygen therapy include:

- Patients with airway, breathing, and circulation problems.
- Patients complaining of chest pain.
- Patients who are cyanotic, cool, clammy, or short of breath.
- Patients with any degree of altered mental status.

Note that concerns about giving too much oxygen to an infant, child, or a patient with chronic obstructive pulmonary disease (COPD) aren't valid in the out-of-hospital setting. If an infant, child, or patient with COPD needs oxygen, they should receive high concentrations.

OXYGEN CYLINDERS

Oxygen cylinders, or tanks, are available in several different sizes. For example, D cylinders (350 liters) and E cylinders (625 liters) are small enough to be used in portable oxygen kits (Figure 10-23). Those commonly found in ambulances include the M (3000

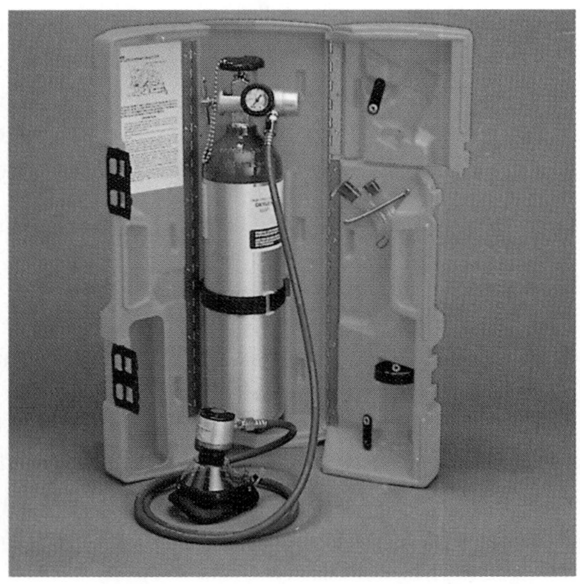

Figure 10-23
A basic oxygen cylinder kit.

liters), G (5300 liters), and H (6900 liters) cylinders. The gas in oxygen tanks is under pressure, usually at about 2000 pounds per square inch. So they need to be handled very carefully. Protect the valve-gauge assembly from blows. Be sure to place a tank on its side to prevent a fall, and secure an upright tank in an approved stand. Secure all oxygen tanks during transport.

Humidifiers are available to attach to oxygen cylinders. However, since dry oxygen is not harmful to a patient for short-term use, humidified oxygen generally isn't used in the field.

OPERATING PROCEDURES

To administer oxygen to a patient, follow these steps (Figure 10-24):

1. Remove the protective seal from the tank.
2. Quickly open and then shut the valve. This will clean away any debris.
3. Attach the regulator-flowmeter to the top of the tank. Make sure there is an approved gasket between the tank and the regulator.
4. After the regulator is hand-tight, open the valve by making a one-quarter turn. Attach the proper delivery device to the flowmeter.
5. Open the flowmeter to the desired setting. Then administer oxygen to the patient.
6. When you remove the device from the patient, turn off the valve and bleed off all pressure from the regulator.

OXYGEN DELIVERY EQUIPMENT

Oxygen delivery devices get the oxygen from the regulator to the breathing patient. Typically made from soft plastic or rubber, they are connected to the regulator by a thin piece of flexible tubing. Such devices include the **nonrebreather mask** and **nasal cannula**.

Providing up to 90% oxygen to the patient, the nonrebreather is the preferred method of administration (Figure 10-25). Be sure to select the correct mask size. After it's on the patient, adjust flow rate to keep the reservoir bag inflated when the patient takes a breath. For the adult patient, this will be approximately 15 liters per minute (lpm).

The nasal cannula provides lower concentrations of oxygen (a maximum of six liters per minute). The oxygen is delivered

Administering Oxygen

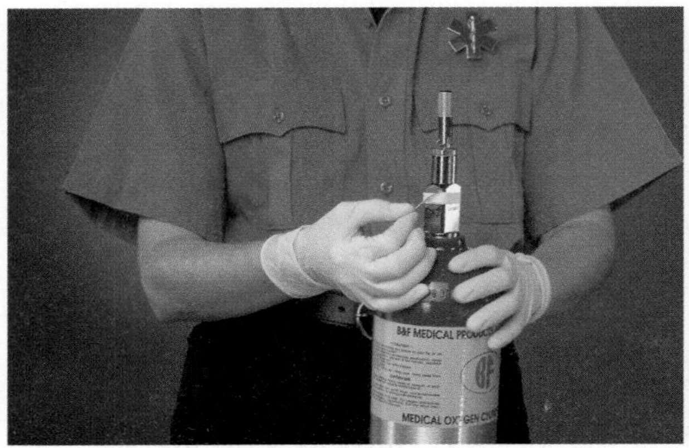

Figure 10-24a
Remove the protective seal.

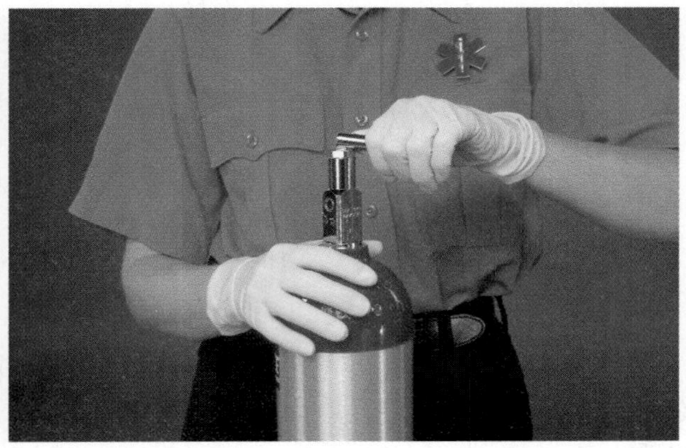

Figure 10-24b
Quickly open and then shut the valve.

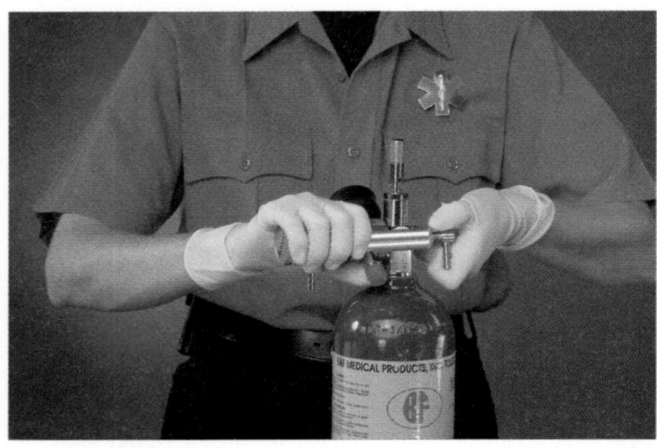

Figure 10-24c
Attach the regulator-flowmeter to the top of the tank.

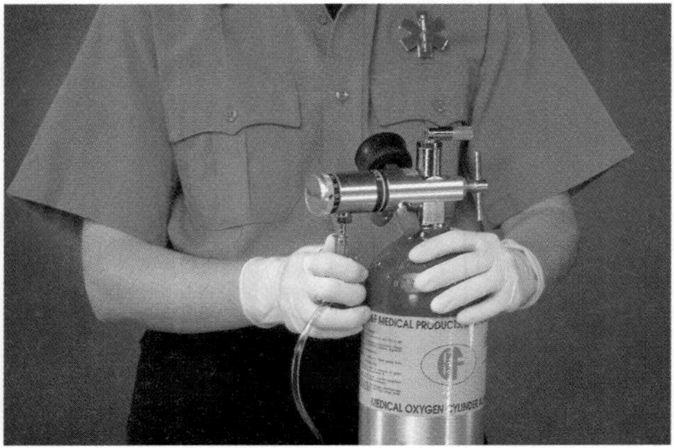

Figure 10-24d
Attach the proper delivery device to the flowmeter.

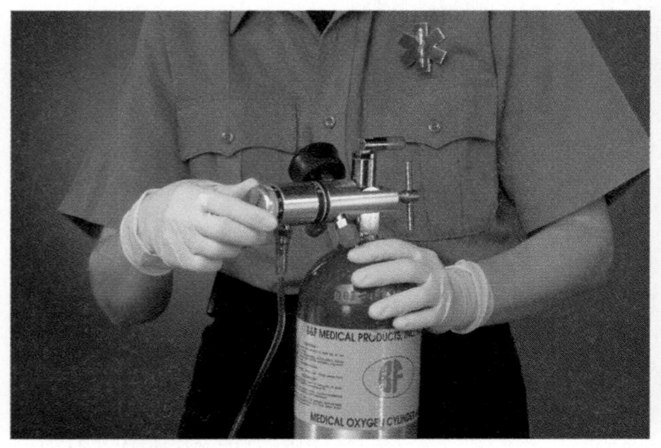

Figure 10-24e
Open the flowmeter to the desired setting.

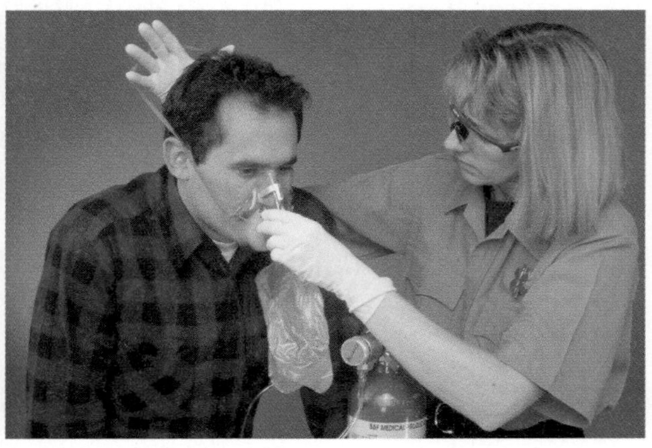

Figure 10-24f
Administer oxygen to the patient.

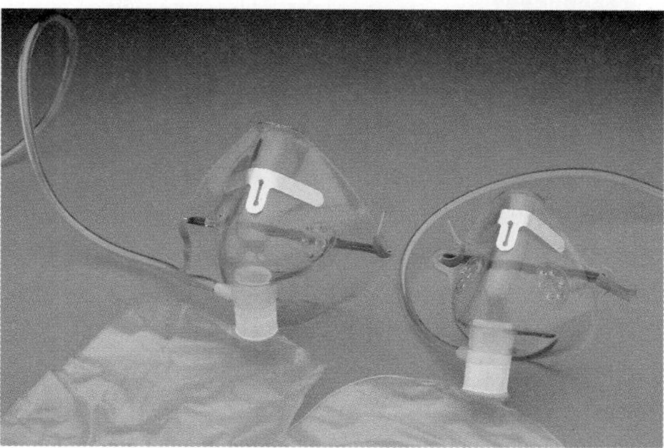
Figure 10-25a
Nonrebreather.

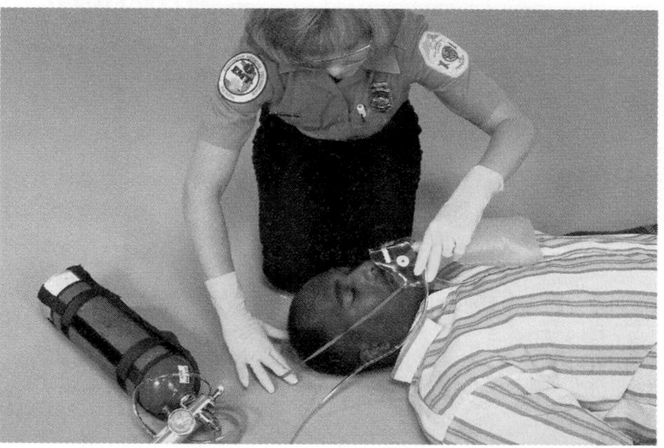
Figure 10-25b
Nonrebreather on the patient.

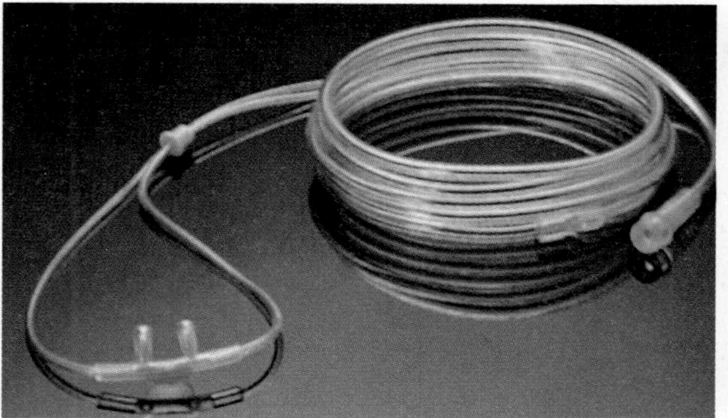
Figure 10-26a
Nasal cannula.

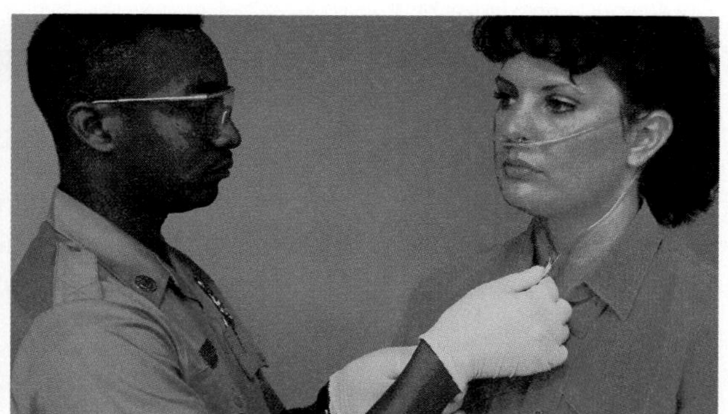
Figure 10-26b
Nasal cannula on the patient.

through two prongs that fit into a patient's nostrils (Figure 10-26). Use it only when patients won't tolerate a nonrebreather.

FOREIGN BODY AIRWAY OBSTRUCTION (FBAO)

Choking emergencies are quite common. Most choking episodes clear up by themselves. However, if a blocked airway isn't cleared, the patient can die in minutes.

All patients—adults, children, and infants—with a partial airway obstruction are still able to breathe. They can talk a bit, cough, and wheeze. They'll also work to relieve the airway problem. Let them! Keep them calm, and tell them that EMS is responding. Don't try to perform any maneuvers (like slapping

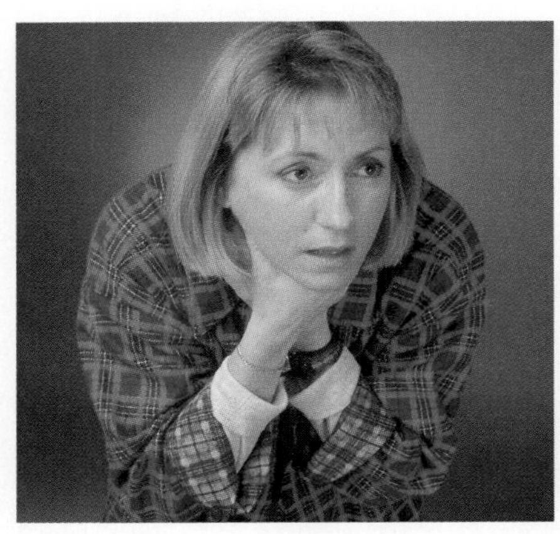

on the back). You could cause a partial obstruction to turn into a complete one.

Partial airway obstructions may cause patients to have poor air exchange and an ineffective cough. They'll appear to be in a great deal of distress and cyanotic. These patients may be getting some air but not enough to sustain them. Treat them in the same way you'd treat a patient with a complete airway obstruction.

A complete airway obstruction occurs when patients cannot breathe at all. Unable to speak or cough, they'll clutch at the neck in the universal signal for choking (Figure 10-27). They'll be extremely agitated and panicky. Don't try to reason with them. Your job is to relieve the blocked airway as soon as possible. These patients require immediate emergency care.

Figure 10-27
The universal sign of choking.

AIRWAY OBSTRUCTIONS IN ADULTS

FBAO IN THE RESPONSIVE ADULT

The *Heimlich maneuver* is recommended for relieving foreign-body airway obstructions. Perform it on the responsive adult by following these steps (Figure 10-28):

> **STREET NOTES**
>
> Whenever you hear "Heimlich maneuver," think "abdominal thrusts" and vice versa.

1. Determine if there is an airway obstruction. Find out if the patient can speak or cough. Ask, "Are you choking?" If the patient indicates "yes" or uses the universal sign for choking, then proceed with the abdominal thrusts.

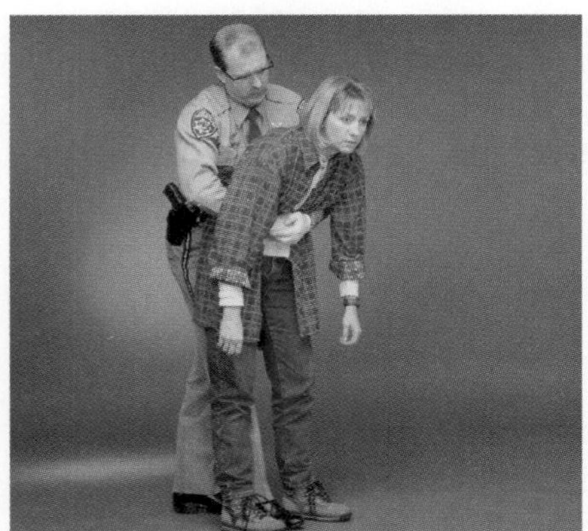

Figure 10-28
Performing abdominal thrusts on an adult.

2. Stand behind the patient. To help keep your balance if the patient becomes unresponsive, place one of your legs between the patient's legs.
3. Wrap your arms around the patient's waist.
4. Make a fist with one hand. Then place the thumb side against the patient's abdomen halfway between the navel and sternum (breastbone).
5. Grab your fist with your free hand. Press into the patient's abdomen with a quick inward and upward thrust.
6. Repeat the thrusts until the obstruction is relieved or until the patient becomes unresponsive.
7. When the patient resumes effective breathing, place him or her in the recovery position or position of comfort.

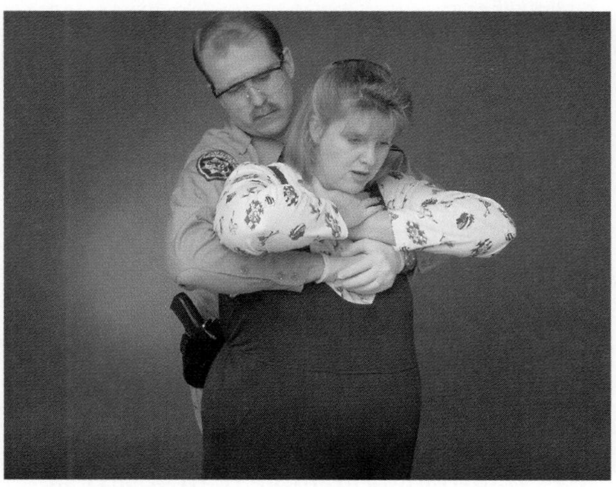

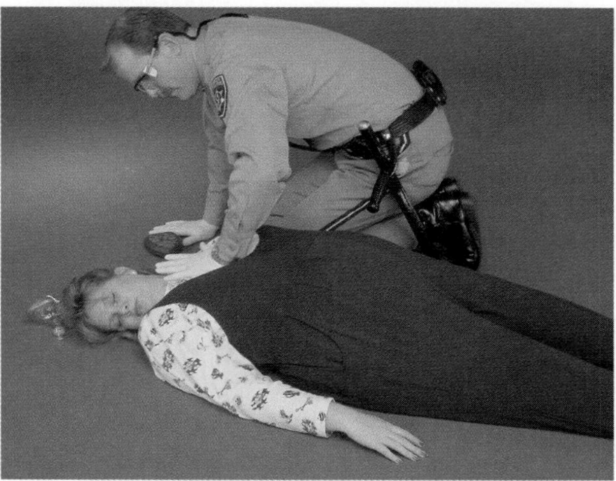

Figure 10-29
Perform chest thrusts on standing or supine pregnant and obese patients.

If you can't wrap your arms around a large patient, or if your patient is pregnant, perform chest thrusts instead of abdominal thrusts (Figure 10-29). The procedure is the same, with this exception: place your arms under the patient's armpits and around the chest, with your hands at the middle of the patient's sternum. All other steps are identical.

You also can perform the Heimlich maneuver on yourself. If you're choking, press your upper abdomen quickly over any firm surface, such as the back of a chair, side of a table, or porch railing. Several thrusts may be needed to clear the airway.

FBAO IN THE UNRESPONSIVE ADULT

Your patient may become unresponsive as you work to relieve an obstruction. You also may be called to the scene of an unresponsive patient with an FBAO. In either case, establish unresponsiveness, activate EMS, and proceed with the following (Figure 10-30):

1. Open the patient's airway with a head-tilt/chin-lift or jaw-thrust. Ventilate. If the airway is obstructed, reposition the head and try to ventilate again.
2. If there's still no breathing, kneel astride the patient's thighs. Place the heel of one hand on the patient's abdomen, midline slightly above the navel and well below the sternum. Place your other hand on top of the first. Then press into the abdomen up to five quick upward and inward thrusts.
3. Perform a **tongue-jaw lift** (open the mouth by grasping the tongue and lower jaw between thumb and fingers). Then perform a finger sweep to remove the obstruction.

FBAO in the Unresponsive Adult

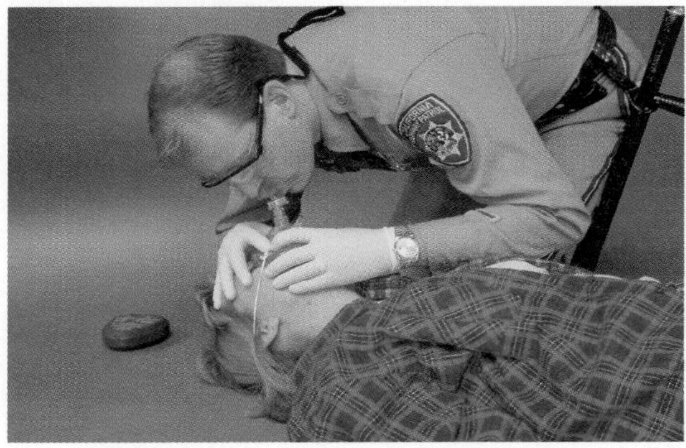

Figure 10-30a
Open the airway and provide ventilations.

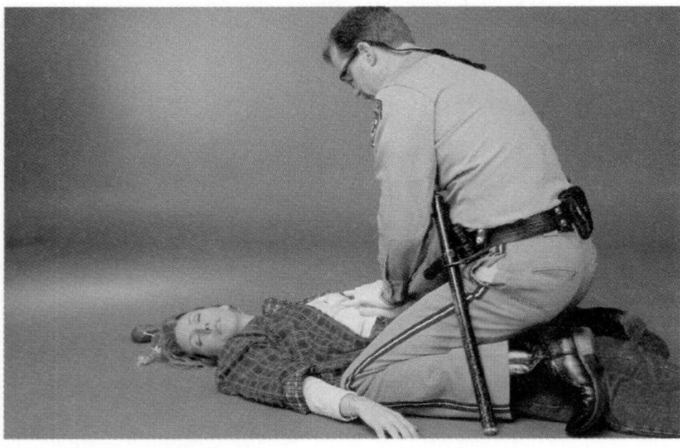

Figure 10-30-b
If no breathing, kneel astride the patient and position your hands. Provide five abdominal thrusts.

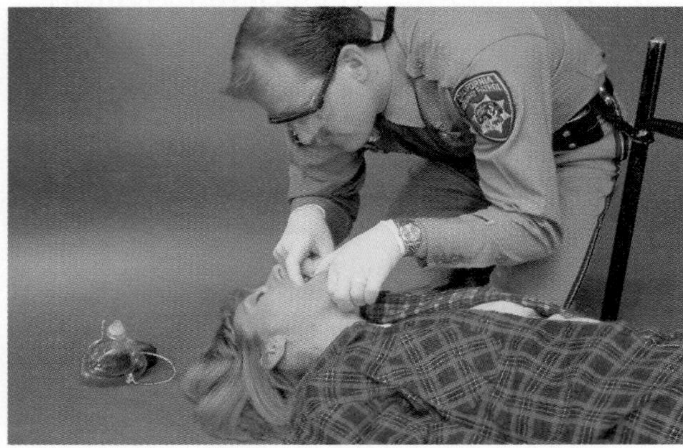

Figure 10-30c
Perform a finger sweep to remove the obstruction.

4. Repeat steps 1 through 3 in rapid sequence until the airway is clear or until you're relieved by other EMS personnel.

5. When the patient resumes effective breathing, place him or her in the recovery position.

AIRWAY OBSTRUCTIONS IN INFANTS AND CHILDREN

According to the U.S. Department of Transportation, more than 90% of all deaths from foreign body obstruction occur in children younger than five. About 65% of all choking victims are infants. Anything that can fit into an infant's or child's mouth is potentially lethal. Such objects include toys, balloons, hot dogs, hard candy, nuts, and grapes. Infection also can be the cause of obstruction. Suspect an airway obstruction with any infant or child who develops sudden respiratory distress with coughing, **stridor** (a high-pitched noise when the patient inhales), wheezing, or gagging.

Remember *Never perform blind finger sweeps in an infant or child.*

FBAO IN THE RESPONSIVE CHILD

Care for a choking child in much the same way as you'd care for a choking adult (Figure 10-31). However, do not perform blind finger sweeps. Instead, perform the tongue-jaw lift, look down into the airway, and use your finger to pluck out the foreign body only if you actually see it.

FBAO IN THE UNRESPONSIVE CHILD

This technique is performed very much like the technique used for unresponsive adults (Figure 10-32). Don't perform blind finger sweeps. If the airway obstruction is not relieved after one minute of care, activate the EMS system.

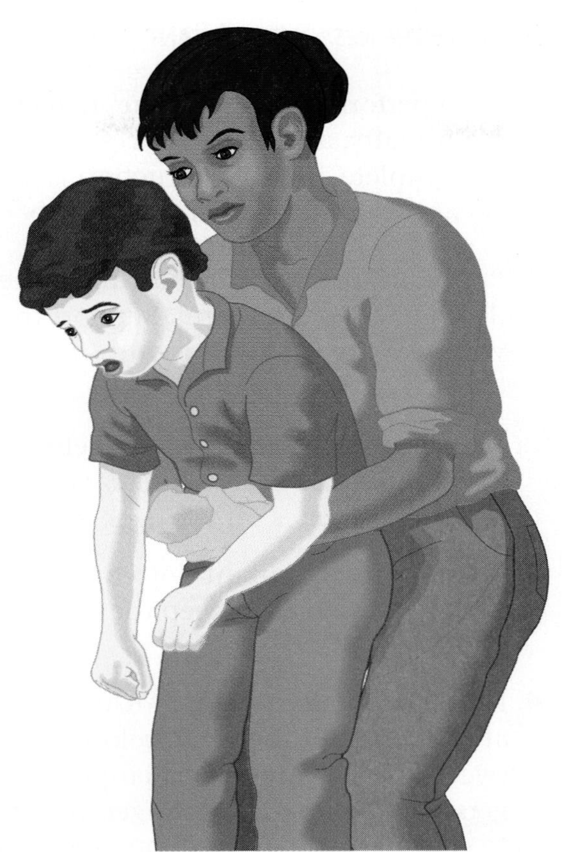

Figure 10-31
Abdominal thrusts in a responsive child.

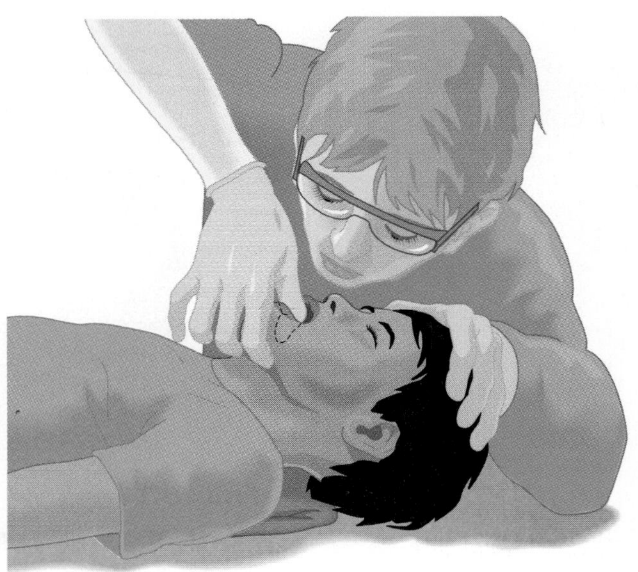

Figure 10-32
Performing the tongue-jaw lift in an unresponsive child.

FBAO in the Responsive Infant

To perform this procedure, first check for serious breathing difficulty, an ineffective cough, and weak or absent cry. Once complete airway obstruction is confirmed, deliver back blows and chest thrusts as described below (Figure 10-33):

1. Rest your forearm on your thigh. Then place the infant face down over your forearm. Support the face and head, while you keep the nose and mouth free. Keep the infant's head lower than the rest of the body.
2. Deliver up to five back blows between the infant's shoulder blades with the heel of one hand. Raise your hand approximately six inches off the back for each blow.
3. Then rotate the infant onto his or her back. Support the head and neck as you do. Keep the head lower than the rest of the body.
4. Deliver up to five chest thrusts. First, place your index finger at the center of the chest below an imaginary line drawn between the two nipples. Then place your middle and ring fingers next to your index finger. Use the middle and ring fingers to compress the sternum one-half to one inch.

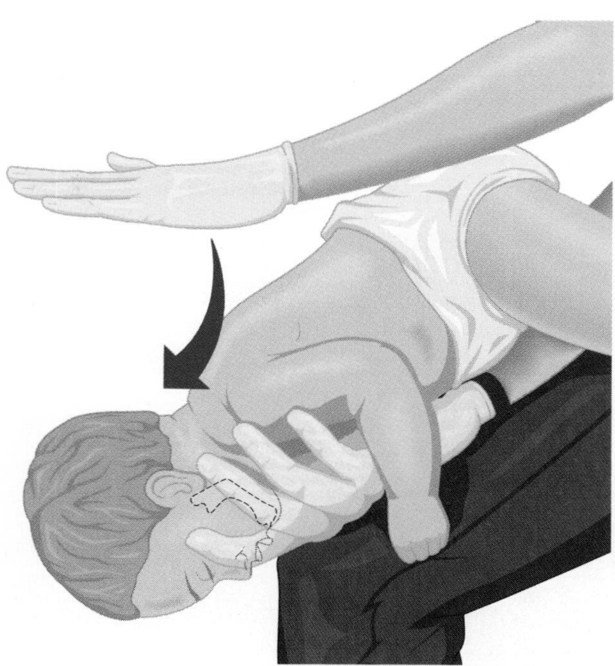

Figure 10-33a
Back blows for an infant with an FBAO.

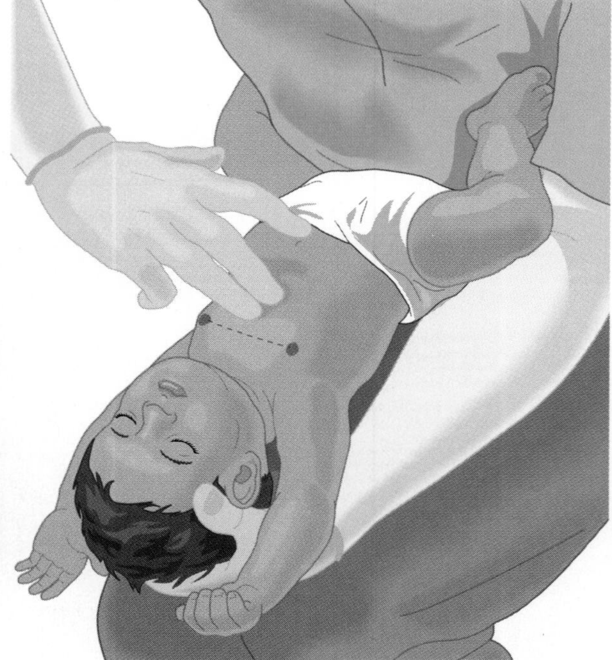

Figure 10-33b
Chest thrusts for an infant with an FBAO.

5. Repeat steps 2-4 until the foreign object is expelled or the infant becomes unresponsive.
6. When the infant resumes effective breathing, place him or her in the recovery position.

FBAO IN THE UNRESPONSIVE INFANT

If the choking infant becomes unresponsive or if you find the infant unresponsive, follow these steps:

1. Determine unresponsiveness by tapping or gently shaking the infant's foot. If you're alone, call out "Help!" If someone comes, have him or her activate the EMS system.
2. Open the airway and try to ventilate. If the airway is still obstructed, reposition the head and try to ventilate again.
3. Give up to five back blows and five chest thrusts.
4. Perform a tongue-jaw lift. If you see the foreign object, pluck it out with a finger.
5. Repeat steps 2 through 4 until the airway is clear or until you are relieved by other EMS personnel.
6. If you are alone and your efforts are unsuccessful, activate the EMS system after one minute of care.
7. When the infant resumes effective breathing, place him or her in the recovery position.

CONCLUSION

Most of your patients won't require any airway or breathing care. However, those who do will have a much better chance of survival because of your training. Remember the key strategy for successful airway and breathing management:

- *Assess airway and breathing.* Does my patient have a patent airway? Is the rate and quality of breathing adequate? Do I need to support the patient's breathing with ventilations?
- *Intervene.* Open the airway, begin artificial ventilation, and so on.
- *Reassess.* Is the airway now open? Have my interventions improved the patient's breathing status? If not, what else can I do?

More than any other skill, airway and ventilation skills can dramatically increase the possibility that your patient will survive critical injuries and illness. Be aggressive!

KEY TERMS

You may wish to use this list to review your understanding of key terms introduced in the chapter.

artificial ventilation method of forcing air into the lungs of a patient who is not breathing or breathing inadequately. *Also called* pulmonary resuscitation, positive pressure ventilation, rescue breathing.

bag-valve-mask (BVM) device a hand-operated device used to provide artificial ventilation to a patient; consists of a bag reservoir, a one-way flow valve, and a face mask. *Also called* bag-valve-mask resuscitator.

FBAO abbreviation for foreign body airway obstruction.

head-tilt/chin-lift maneuver a technique for opening the airway of an unresponsive medical patient (a patient who is not suspected of trauma).

jaw-thrust maneuver a technique for opening the airway of an unresponsive trauma patient.

log roll a move used to place a suspected spine-injured patient who is prone in a supine position; also a move to turn a suspected spine-injured patient onto his or her side for the purpose of draining the airway.

nasal cannula an oxygen delivery device made of two prongs that fit into a patient's nostrils.

nasal flaring occurs when patients (usually infants or children) spread the nostrils to help them increase air flow to the lungs.

nasopharyngeal airway (NPA) a flexible tube that is inserted into the nose of an unresponsive patient to maintain an open airway. *Also called* nasal airway.

nonrebreather mask an oxygen delivery device made of a reservoir bag and a one-way valve.

oropharyngeal airway (OPA) a firm tube that is inserted into the mouth of an unresponsive patient to maintain an open airway. *Also called* oral airway.

recovery position the patient is lying on his or her side, to allow for drainage from the mouth and to keep the tongue from blocking the airway.

respiratory arrest breathing has stopped.

seesaw breathing the chest and abdomen appears to move in opposite directions with each breath. *Also called* paradoxical breathing.

stoma a small opening in the trachea that is created artificially.

stridor a high-pitched noise made when inhaling.

tongue-jaw lift a technique used to open an unresponsive patient's mouth.

tripod position sitting position in which patient has a straight back but is leaning slightly forward with hands on the knees.

APPLICATION QUESTIONS

You may wish to use these questions to review your understanding of the chapter. For answers with page references, see Appendix 2.

1. As the First Responder at the county fairgrounds, you can get plenty busy when rock concerts get rowdy. Tonight is no different. At the request of security, you approach an adult male lying on the ground under the bleachers. You observe that he is making loud snoring sounds as he breathes. He is unresponsive. How would you manage this patient?

2. While on bicycle patrol, you are dispatched to find an unresponsive young adult female with multiple head wounds. Bystanders tell you that her bicycle crashed, and she struck her head on the ground. She was not wearing a helmet and has been unresponsive for about five minutes. She is breathing very slowly, and her face and throat are blue. How would you manage this patient?

3. Your neighbor is screaming and pounding on your front door. When you open it, she shoves her unresponsive 13-month-old baby into your arms. She says the baby is choking and can't breathe. You see that the baby is awake, appears calm, and there's good skin color. However you can hear some whistling sounds when the baby breathes in. How would you manage this patient?

CHAPTER 11 CIRCULATION AND CPR

FIRST RESPONSE

Keiko is the assistant manager of a large food outlet. As of a few weeks ago, she's also the safety team coordinator. "I really hope I don't have to use this training," she told one of her First Responder classmates. "Performing CPR on mannequins is one thing, but doing it for real? I'd just rather not." Keiko spoke too soon.

It's a busy Thursday afternoon. Keiko looks through her office window down to the floor of the supermarket. One of the checkers is frantically trying to rouse an elderly woman who has collapsed on the floor. Almost without thinking, Keiko grabs her jump kit and runs to the stricken customer. "I don't think she's breathing," says the worried checker.

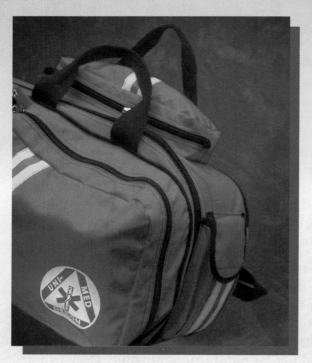

"Call 9-1-1," Keiko says and kneels beside the patient. The woman appears to be unresponsive and turning blue. Keiko quickly pulls on a pair of latex gloves. "Stay calm" she says to herself. "Do it just like in class." She shakes the patient's shoulder gently and says loudly, "Miss, are you okay?" There's no response. Keiko opens the patient's airway, bends down to her face, and finds that there's no breathing. Grabbing her pocket face mask from the jump kit, Keiko ventilates the patient, confirms pulselessness, and begins chest compressions. As curious people look on, Keiko performs CPR as if she's done it a thousand times before. She stays focused and in control. When the patient begins to vomit, Keiko quickly turns her onto her side without missing a beat.

After a while, the local fire crew arrives and takes over care. When the Paramedics arrive, they place a breathing tube into the patient's windpipe, administer several drugs, and ready the patient for transport to the hospital. "We've got a pulse," one of them says. Before they leave, a Paramedic tells Keiko, "She's got you to thank for starting CPR."

"Thank you," she says and smiles to herself as she helps the checkers get things back to normal.

SCENE SIZE UP

INITIAL ASSESSMENT and TREATMENT

PHYSICAL EXAM and TREATMENT

ONGOING ASSESSMENT and TREATMENT

PATIENT HAND-OFF

LEARNING OBJECTIVES

CPR is truly a life-saving intervention. Without it, most cardiac arrest patients would die in the first few minutes. In the scenario at the beginning of the chapter, Keiko's CPR gave the patient a very valuable gift—time. CPR supplied the patient's brain and heart with oxygen until the EMT-Paramedics could respond with other life-saving techniques and interventions.

Before you go on with this chapter, you may want to go back to Chapter 4 to review the circulatory system.

By the end of the chapter, you should be able to:[†]

- 4-1.1 List the reasons for the heart to stop beating. (p. 146)
- 4-1.2 Define the components of cardiopulmonary resuscitation. (pp. 147-148)
- 4-1.3 Describe each link in the chain of survival and how it relates to the EMS system. (pp. 146-147)
- 4-1.4 List the steps of one-rescuer adult CPR. (p. 152)
- 4-1.5 Describe the technique of external chest compressions on an adult patient. (pp. 148, 150)
- 4-1.6 Describe the technique of external chest compressions on an infant. (p. 150)
- 4-1.7 Describe the technique of external chest compressions on a child. (p. 150)
- 4-1.8 Explain when the First Responder is able to stop CPR. (p. 156)
- 4-1.9 List the steps of two-rescuer adult CPR. (p. 152)
- 4-1.10 List the steps of infant CPR. (pp. 155-156)
- 4-1.11 List the steps of child CPR. (pp. 154-155)

[†]Numbered objectives are from the 1995 U.S. DOT "First Responder: National Standard Curriculum." Note also that content presented in this chapter is in accordance with the 1992 American Heart Association, "Guidelines for Cardiopulmonary Resuscitation and Emergency Cardiac Care," published in the *Journal of the American Medical Association (JAMA)*, October 28, 1992.

CPR AND CARDIAC ARREST

When in **cardiac arrest**, a patient's heart stops beating. Blood stops flowing through the patient's body. In four to six minutes, brain cells begin to die. In eight to 10 minutes, brain damage becomes irreversible. External chest compressions combined with artificial ventilation help to circulate blood and oxygen to vital organs, especially the brain. These combined actions are called **cardiopulmonary resuscitation**, or **CPR** for short.

There are many reasons why cardiac arrest occurs. Respiratory arrest is the main reason for infants and children. Heart disease is the main reason for adults. Stroke, allergic reactions, and poisoning are common causes. So are drowning, suffocation, and trauma (Table 11-1). No matter what the cause, emergency care of cardiac arrest is CPR.

CPR only works for a short period, and it becomes less effective over time. Even with the best CPR, blood flow in the patient's body is only about 30% of normal. So start CPR as early as possible. Restoring a patient's pulse is a hollow victory if the patient has no brain function.

THE CHAIN OF SURVIVAL

The most important factors in the survival of a cardiac arrest patient are illustrated by the "chain of survival" (Figure 11-1). The chain includes: early access, early CPR, early **defibrillation**, and early **advanced cardiac life support** (ACLS). If there are any weak or missing links in the chain, the patient's chances of surviving are greatly reduced.

TABLE 11-1 GENERAL REASONS FOR THE HEART TO STOP BEATING
Sudden death and heart disease.
Respiratory arrest, especially in infants and children.
Medical emergencies including stroke, epilepsy, diabetes, and allergic reactions.
Electrical shock.
Poisoning.
Drowning, suffocation.
Congenital abnormalities.
Trauma and bleeding.

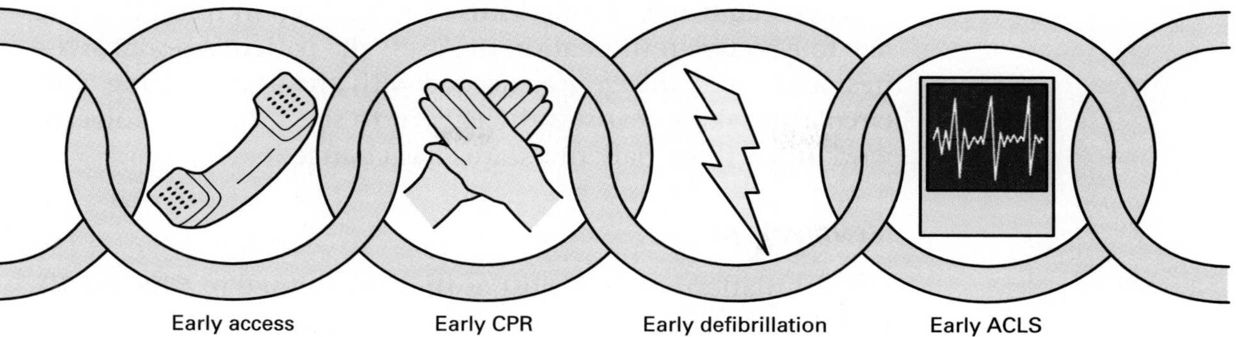

Figure 11-1
Chain of survival.

- *Early access* means the cardiac arrest should be recognized as soon as it occurs. The EMS system should be activated before CPR is provided. The EMS dispatcher should provide CPR instructions as needed. Time is the biggest killer in cardiac emergencies. Early access tends to be the weakest link in the chain.
- *Early CPR* is critical if a patient in cardiac arrest is to survive. Families with members who have heart disease should all be trained in CPR. Bystander CPR also is essential because they can provide CPR before EMS arrives.
- *Early defibrillation* can help up to 90% of all cardiac arrest patients. It's a method of applying electric shocks to restore a patient's normal heart rhythm. Because it must be started within the first few minutes after cardiac arrest, many First Responders are taught this EMT-Basic skill (see Appendix 1).
- *Early advanced cardiac life support (ACLS)* is the next link in the chain. It begins with the arrival of the EMT-Intermediates and EMT-Paramedics. They continue CPR, administer medications, and use specialized airways for more efficient and effective ventilation.

Though traditionally not included in the "chain of survival," early **definitive care** is the last essential factor necessary to the survival of a cardiac patient. It means that patients should be transported rapidly to an emergency department for additional advanced care. Later in the treatment of the patient, definitive care also may include rehabilitation.

MAJOR COMPONENTS OF CPR

CPR is not a single skill. It's actually a combination of two—external chest compressions and artificial ventilations. Performed in exact preset ratios, these two skills provide the maximum oxygen and blood flow possible.

As you continue through this chapter, keep in mind that the key to effective resuscitation is: *Assess* the patient's responsiveness and ABCs. *Intervene* as needed with airway, breathing, and circulation skills. *Reassess* the patient to see if interventions are working or if the patient's status has changed

VENTILATIONS

Use ventilation methods just as they're outlined in Chapter 10. Patients in cardiac arrest benefit from supplemental oxygen. So use oxygen with a BVM or pocket face mask if you're equipped to do so. Remember that CPR must circulate blood with enough oxygen in it to keep the patient's brain alive.

EXTERNAL CHEST COMPRESSIONS

External chest compressions press the heart between the sternum and the spine and increase pressure in the chest cavity. This causes blood to circulate in the body. To properly perform chest compressions, the patient must be supine (face up) on a hard flat surface and his or her head should be on the same level as the heart. See Figure 11-2 for the "landmarks" related to the correct CPR compression site.

External Chest Compressions—Adult Take BSI precautions, and then follow these steps (Figure 11-3):

1. Kneel alongside the patient. Locate the lower margin of the patient's ribs on the same side.

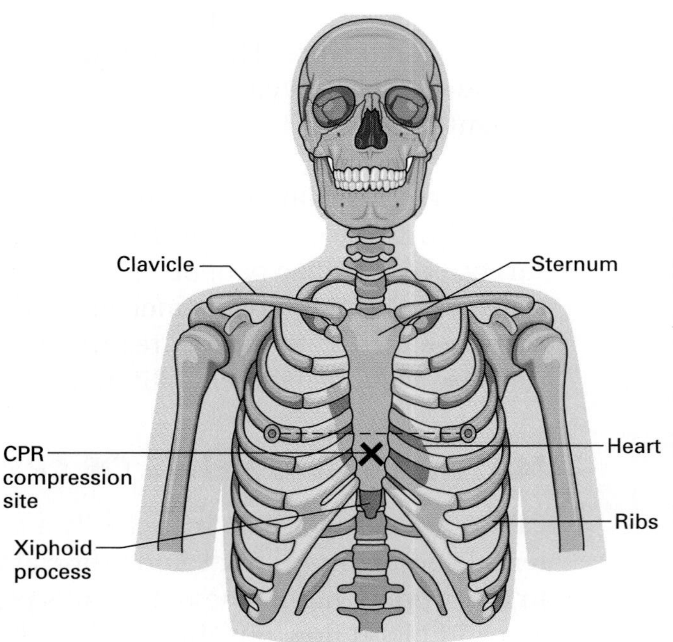

Figure 11-2
CPR compression site and related structures.

Positioning for Chest Compressions

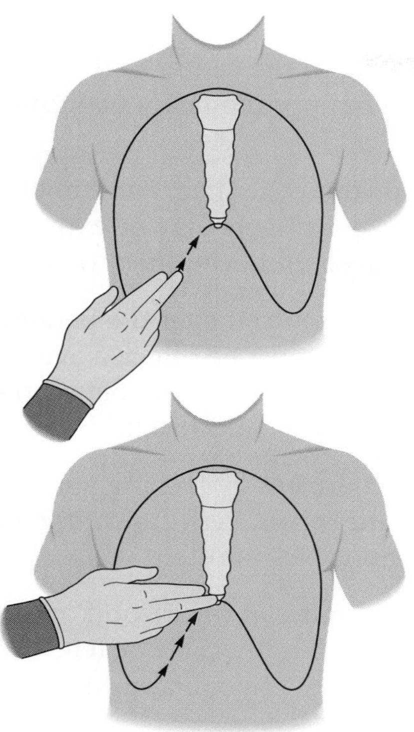

Figure 11-3a
Locate the lower margin and run your fingers up the rib margin until you reach the xiphoid process.

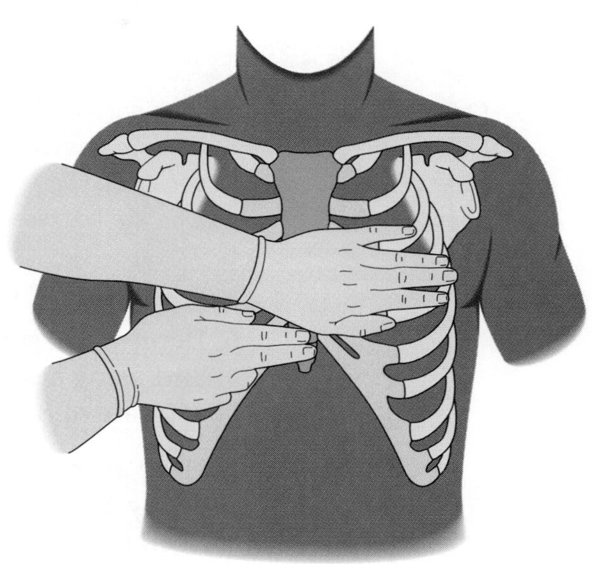

Figure 11-3b
Place the heel of one hand on the lower sternum about two finger-widths above the notch.

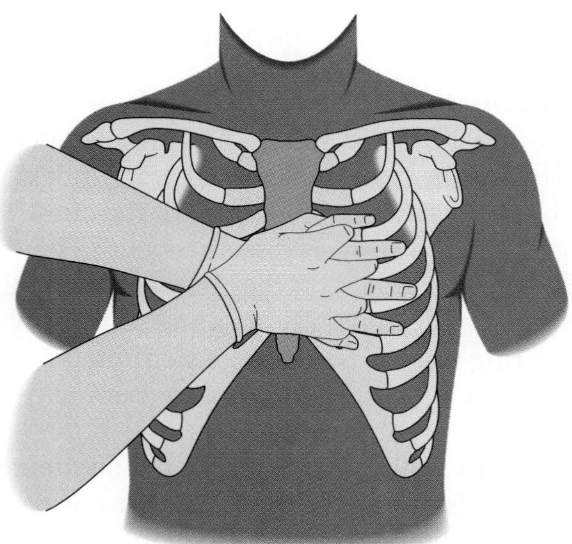

Figure 11-3c
Place your other hand on top. Keep your fingers off the chest.

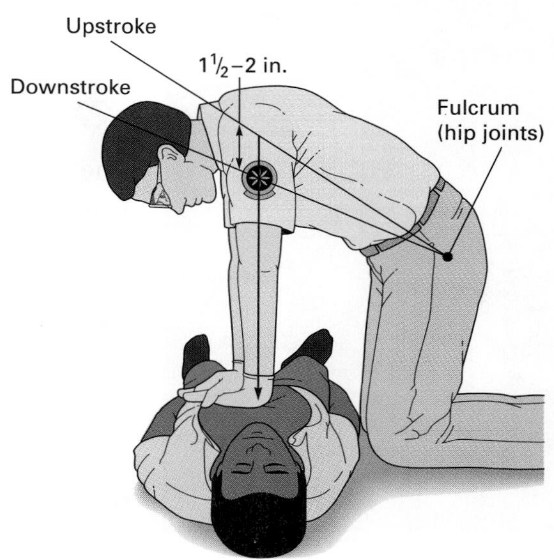

Figure 11-3d
Position yourself over the patient, and depress the sternum using a straight downward thrust.

2. Run the fingers of one gloved hand up the rib margin until you reach the xiphoid process (the notch where the ribs join the lower sternum).

3. Place the heel of your free hand in the center of the chest on the lower sternum. It should be approximately two finger-widths above the notch.

> **STREET NOTES**
>
> Correct hand position during chest compressions is important. Be sure to stay clear of the xiphoid process. It can be snapped off if compressions are too close to it.

4. Place your other hand on top of the first. Your fingers may be extended or interlaced, but keep them off the chest.

5. Position yourself over the patient. Your shoulders must be directly over an imaginary line running between the patient's nose and naval.

6. Depress the sternum 1.5 to 2.0 inches by locking your arms and using a straight downward thrust. Perform compressions at a rate of 80-100 compressions per minute.

7. Have another rescuer feel for a pulse at the carotid or femoral artery after each compression. If a pulse can't be felt, you may need to increase the depth or force of your compressions.

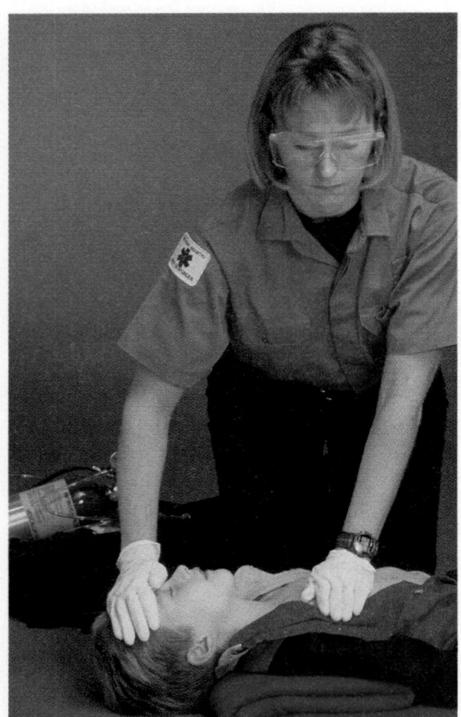

Figure 11-4
Depending on the child's size, use one or two hands to compress the chest wall.

External Chest Compressions—Child The correct hand position on a child is one finger-width above the notch where the ribs and sternum meet. Chest compressions are 1.0 to 1.5 inches deep. Depending on the child's size, use one or two hands to compress the chest wall (Figure 11-4). Compression rate for a child is 100 compressions per minute.

External Chest Compressions—Infant To position your hand on an infant, find an imaginary line that lies between the two nipples. Place your index finger directly below that line at the center of the chest. Place your ring and middle fingers directly over the sternum, and raise the index finger off the chest wall (Figure 11-5). Chest compressions generally are done using only your middle and ring fingers. Depress the sternum 0.5 to 1.0 inch at a rate of at least 100 compressions per minute.

Just like an adult and child, an infant should be supine on a hard flat surface for most effective CPR. However, you can deliver chest compressions to an infant who is lying supine on your forearm. Be sure your palm supports the infant's back. This position will allow the infant's head to tilt back slightly, allowing the airway to stay open.

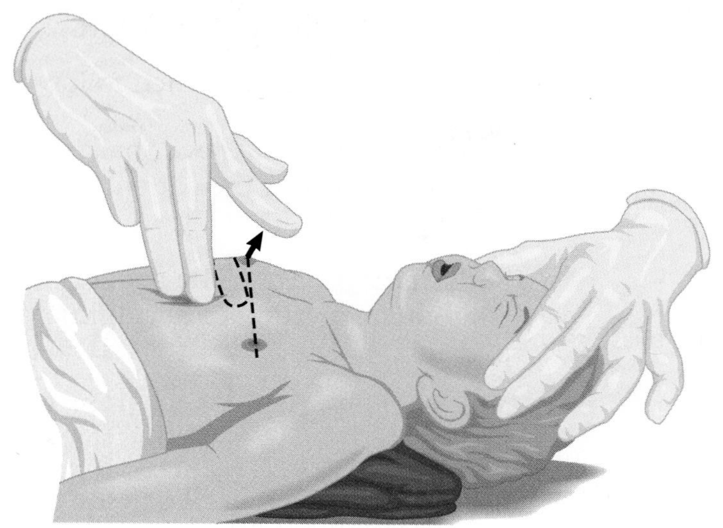

Figure 11-5
Correct hand position for delivering chest compressions to an infant.

PERFORMING CPR

For the purposes of CPR an infant is less than one year of age and a child is between the ages of one and eight. The following text lists the steps for performing CPR on an infant, child, and adult. Refer to Table 11-2 for a summary of all three techniques.

STREET NOTES

During CPR the patient is very likely to vomit. Typically the airway gets very messy. So make sure you've got your suction unit within arm's reach.

TABLE 11-2 SUMMARY OF CPR TECHNIQUES

	INFANT	CHILD	ADULT
RATIO (compressions to breaths)	5:1	5:1	15:2 (one-rescuer CPR) 5:1 (two-rescuer CPR)
COMPRESSION RATE	At least 100 per minute	100 per minute	80-100 per minute
COMPRESSION DEPTH	0.5 to 1.0 inch	1.0 to 1.5 inches	1.5 to 2 inches
BREATH RATE	20 per minute	20 per minute	10-12 per minute
BREATH LENGTH	1.0 to 1.5 seconds each	1.0 to 1.5 seconds each	1.5 to 2.0 seconds each
HAND POSITION	Two fingers on lower third of sternum	One hand on lower half of sternum	Two hands on lower half of sternum

ADULT CPR—ONE RESCUER

Take BSI precautions, and then follow these steps (Figure 11-6):

1. *Establish unresponsiveness.* Shake the patient gently, or shout "Are you okay?" If the patient is unresponsive, activate the EMS system.

2. *Position the patient.* If the patient is prone (face down), use the appropriate method to turn him or her to a supine (face up) position.

3. *Open the airway.* Use the head-tilt/chin-lift or jaw-thrust maneuver as appropriate.

4. *Establish breathlessness.* Look, listen, and feel for breathing. If your patient is breathing and there's no evidence of trauma, place him or her in the recovery position. If the patient is not breathing, proceed to the next step.

5. *Provide two slow breaths.* If the first attempt is unsuccessful, reposition the airway and try again. If still unsuccessful, perform the foreign body airway obstruction (FBAO) sequence.

6. *Establish pulselessness.* Check the patient's carotid pulse for at least five seconds. If there's a pulse, continue artificial ventilation. Recheck the pulse every minute. If there's no pulse, proceed to the next step.

7. *Perform CPR.* Perform one cycle of 15 chest compressions at 80-100 per minute followed by two slow breaths. Repeat this cycle three more times. Then check the carotid pulse. If there's still no pulse, continue CPR. Check the pulse after every four cycles.

8. *When the pulse returns, check for breathing.* If there's breathing, place the patient in the recovery position and monitor breathing and pulse. If there's no breathing, provide artificial ventilation and monitor the pulse.

ADULT CPR—TWO RESCUERS

To perform two-rescuer CPR on an adult, ventilate the patient while another rescuer provides chest compressions (Figure 11-7). The sequence is the same as for one-rescuer CPR, except the ratio changes from 15:2 to 5:1 (five compressions to one ventilation). Once pulselessness is confirmed, one rescuer performs five chest compressions at a rate of 80-100 per minute. This is followed by one full ventilation by the second rescuer. Check the patient's pulse every minute. When either of the rescuers tires, they can switch positions.

One-Rescuer Adult CPR

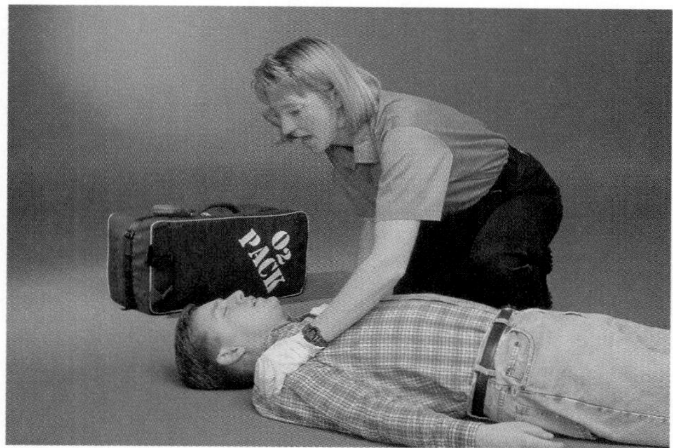

Figure 11-6a
Establish unresponsiveness, and activate the EMS system.

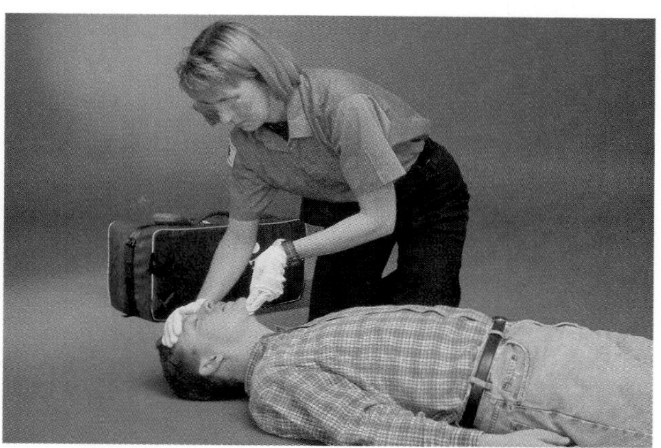

Figure 11-6b
Position and patient, and open the airway.

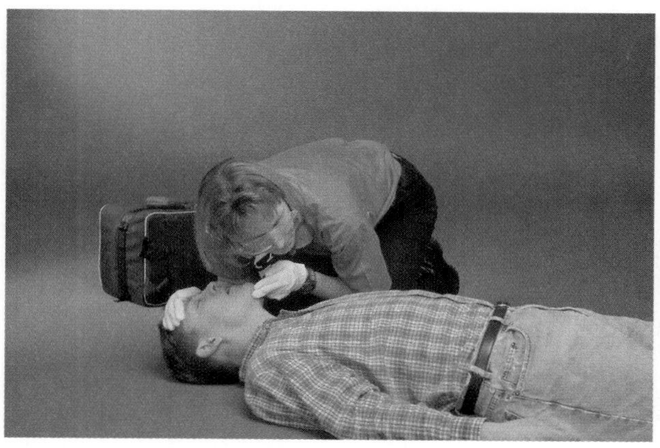

Figure 11-6c
Establish breathlessness.

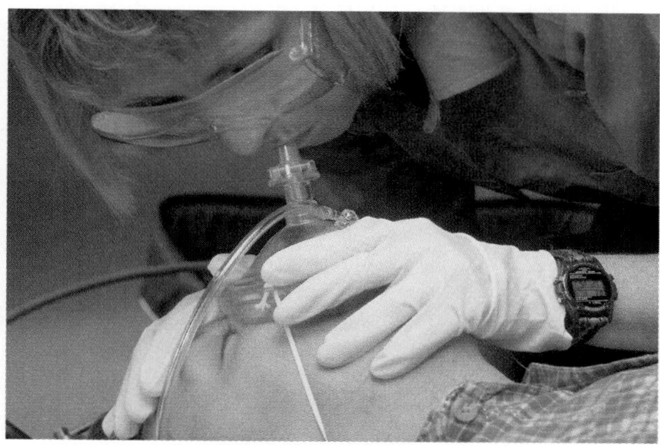

Figure 11-6d
Provide two slow breaths.

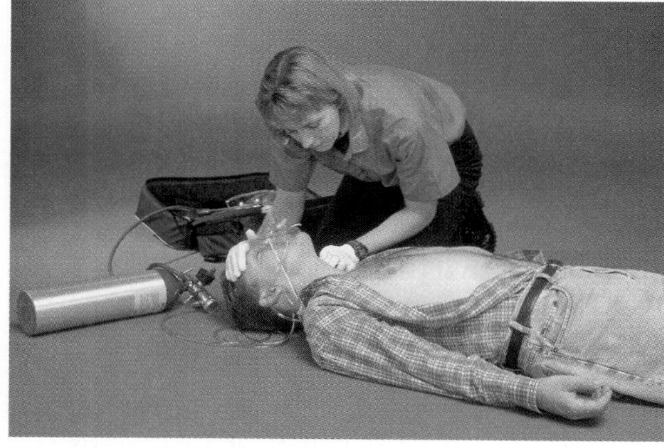

Figure 11-6e
Determine pulselessness

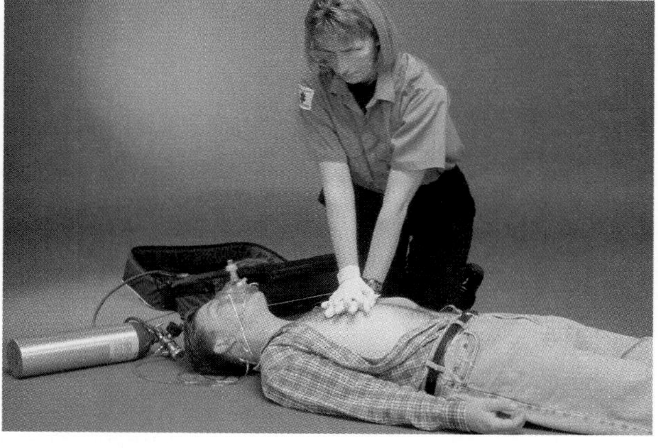

Figure 11-6f
Perform CPR.

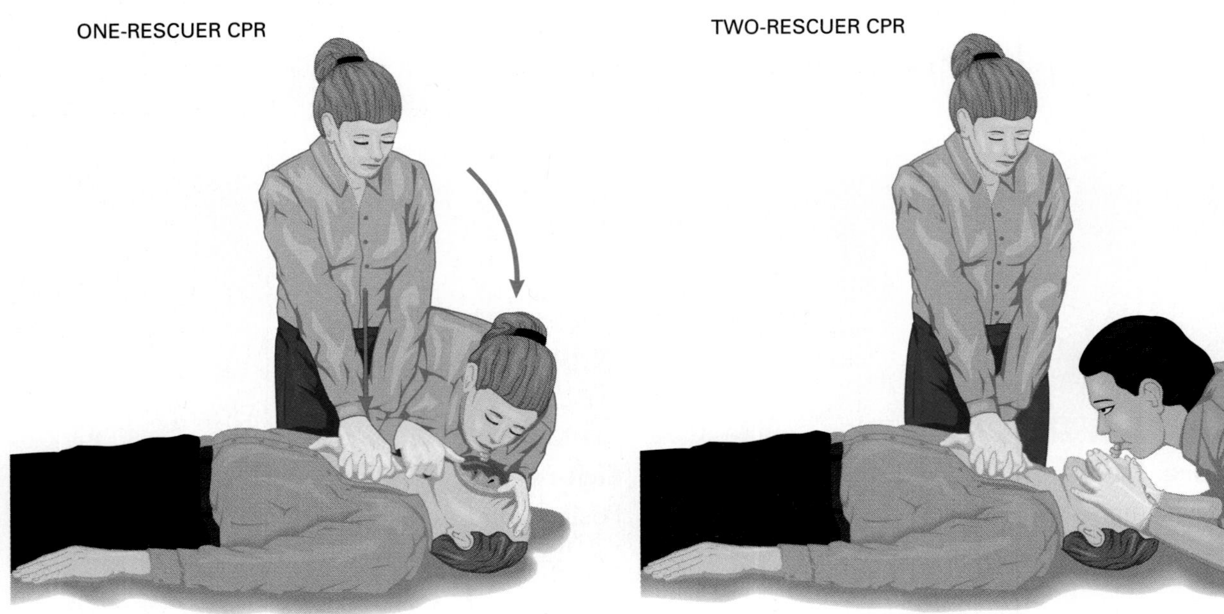

Figure 11-7
One-rescuer CPR vs. two-rescuer CPR.

CHILD CPR

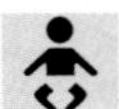 Take BSI precautions, and then follow these steps:

1. *Establish unresponsiveness*. Shake the patient gently, or shout "Are you okay?" If the patient is unresponsive and you're alone, call out "Help!" If others are present, have one of them activate EMS.

2. *Position the patient*. If the patient is prone (face down), use the appropriate method to turn him or her to a supine (face up) position.

3. *Open the airway*. Use the head-tilt/chin-lift or jaw-thrust maneuver as appropriate. Be sure to avoid overextending the neck since this could cause the airway to collapse.

4. *Establish breathlessness*. Look, listen, and feel for breathing. If the child is breathing and there's no evidence of trauma, place him or her in the recovery position. If the patient is not breathing, proceed to the next step.

5. *Provide two slow breaths*. If the first attempt is unsuccessful, reposition the airway and try again. If still unsuccessful, perform the foreign body airway obstruction (FBAO) sequence.

6. *Establish pulselessness*. Check the patient's carotid pulse for at least five seconds. If there's a pulse, continue artificial ventilation and recheck the pulse every minute. If there's no pulse, proceed to the next step.

7. *Provide one minute of CPR.* Provide five chest compressions at 100 per minute followed by one slow breath. Then check the carotid pulse. If there's no pulse, repeat the cycle about 20 times or for about one minute. Then, if you're alone, activate the EMS system.

8. *Check pulse. If absent, continue CPR.* Be sure to check pulse every few minutes.

9. *When pulse returns, check for breathing.* If there's breathing, place the child in the recovery position and monitor breathing and pulse. If there's no breathing, provide artificial ventilation and monitor the pulse.

If a second rescuer is qualified in basic life support and you're tired, have him check the patient's pulse. If no pulse, he can proceed with chest compressions and ventilations. Monitor the procedure. Watch for the patient's chest to rise and fall during artificial ventilation and feel for a pulse during chest compressions.

INFANT CPR

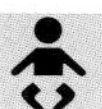 Take BSI precautions, and then follow these steps:

1. *Establish unresponsiveness.* Shake the patient gently. If the patient is unresponsive and you're alone, call out "Help!" If others are present, have one of them activate EMS.

2. *Position the patient.* If the patient is prone (face down), use the appropriate method to turn him or her to a supine (face up) position.

3. *Open the airway.* Use the head-tilt/chin-lift or jaw-thrust maneuver as appropriate. Be sure to avoid overextending the neck since this could cause the airway to collapse.

4. *Establish breathlessness.* Look, listen, and feel for breathing. If the infant is breathing and there's no evidence of trauma, place him or her in the recovery position. If the patient isn't breathing, proceed to the next step.

5. *Provide two slow breaths.* If the first attempt is unsuccessful, reposition the airway and try again. If still unsuccessful, perform the foreign body airway obstruction (FBAO) sequence.

6. *Establish pulselessness.* Check the patient's brachial pulse for at least five seconds. If there's a pulse, continue artificial ventilation and recheck the pulse every minute. If there's no pulse, proceed to the next step.

7. *Provide one minute of CPR.* Provide five chest compressions at a rate of at least 100 per minute followed by one slow breath. Then check the brachial pulse. If there's no pulse, repeat the cycle about 20 times or for about one minute. Then, if you're alone, activate the EMS system.
8. *Check pulse and continue CPR.* Be sure to check pulse every few minutes.
9. *When the pulse returns, check for breathing.* If there's breathing, place the infant in the recovery position and monitor breathing and pulse. If there's no breathing, provide artificial ventilation and monitor the pulse.

WHEN TO STOP CPR

You may stop CPR under the following conditions:

- Circulation and breathing are restored.
- Emergency care is transferred to qualified EMS workers.
- Emergency care is transferred to a physician who determines resuscitation efforts should stop.
- The resuscitation team is too exhausted to continue.
- Environmental hazards place the rescuers in danger.
- Valid Do Not Resuscitate (DNR) orders are presented to the rescue team.

CONCLUSION

CPR supplies the brain and the heart with oxygenated blood, which buys more time for the EMS system to respond with additional resources. It's truly a life-saving intervention. Without it, cardiac arrest patients will not survive. In order for CPR to work, it must begin within the first few minutes after cardiac arrest and it must be done correctly. Your job as a First Responder is to recognize a cardiac emergency, begin effective CPR, and activate the EMS system. Remember the key to effective resuscitation:

- *Assess* the patient's responsiveness, airway, breathing, and circulation.
- *Intervene* as appropriate with airway, breathing, and circulation skills.

- *Reassess* the patient to see if your interventions are working or if the patient's status has changed.

KEY TERMS

You may wish to use this list to review your understanding of key terms introduced in the chapter.

advanced cardiac life support (ACLS) patient care provided by EMT-Intermediates and EMT-Paramedics and hospital emergency department personnel.

cardiac arrest the heartbeat has stopped.

cardiopulmonary resuscitation (CPR) method of forcing oxygenated blood to circulate to the vital organs of a cardiac arrest victim by way of external chest compressions and artificial ventilation.

defibrillation a method of applying electrical shocks to restore a patient's normal heart rhythm.

definitive care the highest level of care possible; generally refers to hospital care.

APPLICATION QUESTIONS

You may wish to use these questions to review your understanding of the chapter. For answers with page references, see Appendix 2.

1. You are called to a day care center where CPR is being performed on a small child. The director tells you they all thought the child was just napping. When they tried to wake her, they noticed blood coming from her nose. There was no breathing and no pulse, so they started CPR. What should your first action be when they hand over care of the child to you?

2. You arrive at the scene where another First Responder is performing artificial ventilation on a patient. He seems flustered and unsure when he says to you, "I think this guy has a pulse, but he's not breathing." You note the patient appears to be very blue. What action should you take?

CHAPTER 12 SHOCK AND BLEEDING CONTROL

FIRST RESPONSE

Chen hears the factory alarm, shuts down his forklift, and sprints across the cement floor, dodging equipment and other workers. He slides through a tight knot of workers and stops abruptly. The scene in front of him hits him like a sucker punch, and for a moment all he can do is stare.

Edward, another forklift operator, must have been loading crates onto a pallet when he slipped and caught his thigh on a sharp metal hook. Now he's sprawled on the concrete floor, propped up against one of his coworkers, ashen, sweaty, and anxious. Blood is spurting from a seven-inch gash in his right thigh. A large pool of blood is collecting on the cement.

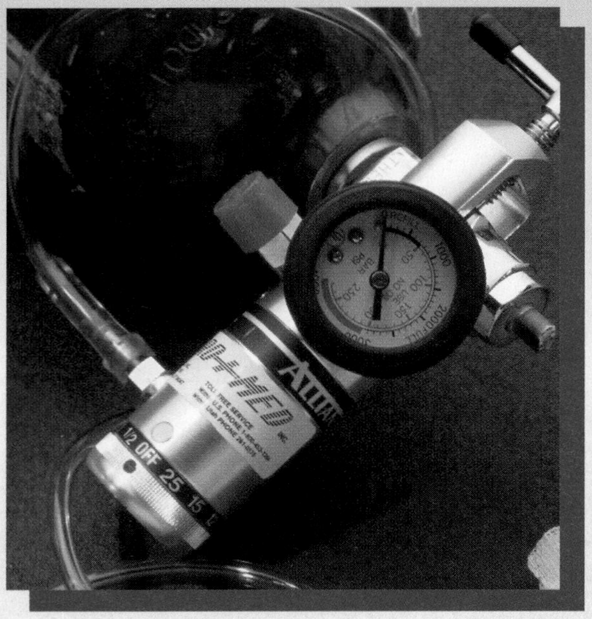

Chen knows he has to work fast. He turns to one of his coworkers: "Call 9-1-1. Hurry." Chen grabs some gloves and large dressings from a first aid station, where he also pushes the plant alarm. Then he gloves up and applies direct pressure to the wound site. "Let's have Edward lie down," he says. They elevate the leg. After 30 seconds or so, Chen sees that bleeding hasn't slowed. So with his free hand, Chen applies pressure to the femoral artery in Edward's groin. Just then two other trained First Responders show up.

"We heard the alarm. What can we do?" they ask.

"We need to get him on oxygen. I think he's in shock," Chen answers. They run to get a tank from the first aid station in the main office. In less than a minute they've applied high flow oxygen via nonrebreather.

The bleeding to Edward's leg is slowing when EMT-Paramedics arrive from the fire department and take over care. Chen gives them his report, and later helps to package the patient for transport. As the ambulance is about to leave, one of the EMTs points to the pool of drying blood and tells Chen, "Good thing you stopped the bleeding. We could have lost this guy if you hadn't. Thanks." As the factory workers go back to their jobs, they thank Chen too.

SCENE SIZE UP

INITIAL ASSESSMENT and TREATMENT

PHYSICAL EXAM and TREATMENT

ONGOING ASSESSMENT and TREATMENT

PATIENT HAND-OFF

LEARNING OBJECTIVES

Managing shock and bleeding is the last step in the initial assessment and treatment of life threats. Patients in shock aren't getting enough oxygen in their bodies. Shock kills. Bleeding, or hemorrhage, is one of the most common causes of shock.

***By the end of the chapter, you should be able to:*†**

- 5-2.1 Differentiate between arterial, venous, and capillary bleeding. (p. 160)
- 5-2.2 State the emergency medical care for external bleeding. (pp. 160-163)
- 5-2.3 Establish the relationship between body substance isolation and bleeding. (p. 159)
- 5-2.4 List the signs of internal bleeding. (p. 163)
- 5-2.5 List the steps in the emergency medical care of the patient with signs and symptoms of internal bleeding. (p. 163)

* Describe what shock is and how it presents in patients. (pp. 164-165)
* List the steps in the emergency medical care of the patient with signs and symptoms of shock. (pp. 165-166)

BLEEDING CONTROL

Normally when bleeding occurs, the body works to control it. Blood vessels contract, and clots develop at the bleeding site. Eventually, bleeding stops. Serious injury can cause the body's bleeding control mechanisms to fail. Uncontrolled bleeding can lead to severe blood loss, shock, and death.

To manage life-threatening bleeding you've got to recognize it early and treat it aggressively. External bleeding is easy to see. As one First Responder puts it, "It's more red stuff on the outside than on the inside." Internal bleeding is not so easy. Recognizing it often depends on noticing signs and symptoms, like changes in skin condition, mental status, and pulse rate and quality.

> **Remember** *Patients with life-threatening bleeding can be a threat to your life, too. Keep in mind that blood and body fluids can transmit infectious diseases. Always take all appropriate BSI precautions before approaching the patient!*

†Numbered objectives are from the 1995 U.S. DOT "First Responder: National Standard Curriculum." Asterisks indicate supplemental material.

EXTERNAL BLEEDING

In recent reports, an office worker stepped out of a transit bus and slipped, opening a huge gash in her upper leg. Bystanders stood and watched as the woman went down on the sidewalk, bleeding profusely. By the time the EMT-Paramedics arrived she already had gone into shock. She died from blood loss. If someone had applied the few simple procedures described in this chapter, she may have survived.

External bleeding may be caused by injury to an artery, vein, or capillary. Each type of bleeding may be recognized by the following characteristics (Figure 12-1):

- In **arterial bleeding** bright, oxygen-rich red blood spurts from a wound because it's under high pressure. This makes it most difficult to manage. As blood pressure drops, spurting may become less.
- In **venous bleeding** dark, oxygen-poor blood flows from a wound in a steady stream. It's under much less pressure than blood in the arteries, so it's easier to manage. Venous bleeding also is more common than arterial bleeding, because veins generally are closer to the surface of the skin.
- In **capillary bleeding** dark red blood tends to ooze from a wound because it's under very low pressure. This type of bleeding tends to be easy to control and, in fact, tends to clot spontaneously.

External Bleeding Control

Life-threatening bleeding should be treated during the initial assessment, after you've assessed and treated any airway and breathing problems. In some cases when there's someone who

Figure 12-1
Three types of bleeding.

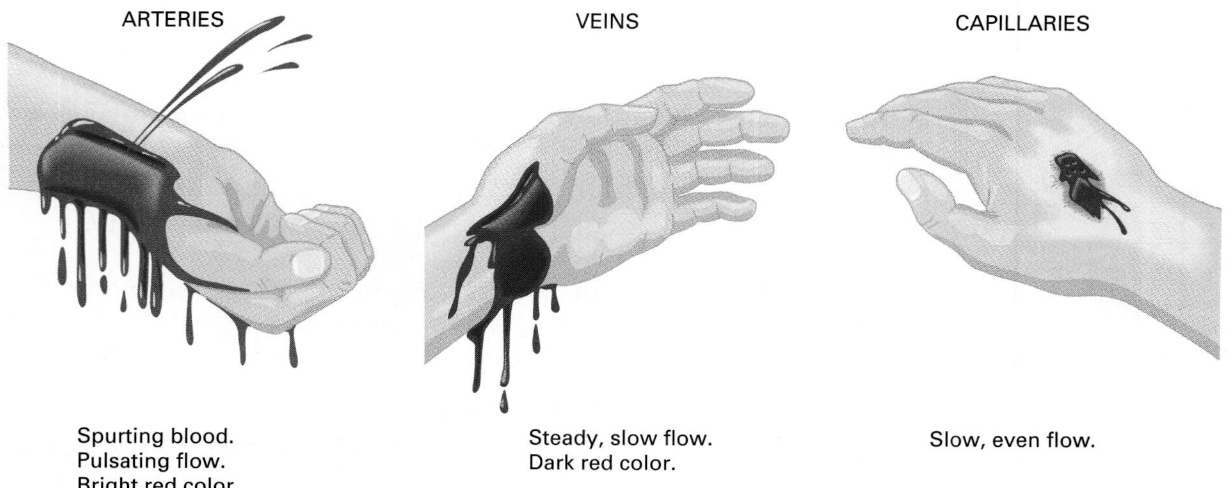

can help you, the ABCs may be managed simultaneously. Minor external bleeding can wait until after you've completed a more in-depth physical exam.

Ways to control external bleeding include **direct pressure**, **elevation**, and the use of **pressure points**. To proceed take BSI precautions and follow these steps (Figure 12-2):

1. *Apply direct pressure*. Use the flat part of your fingertips to apply direct pressure to the point of bleeding. If the wound is large and gaping and fingertip pressure isn't controlling bleeding, you may need to use sterile gauze and direct hand pressure.

Controlling External Bleeding

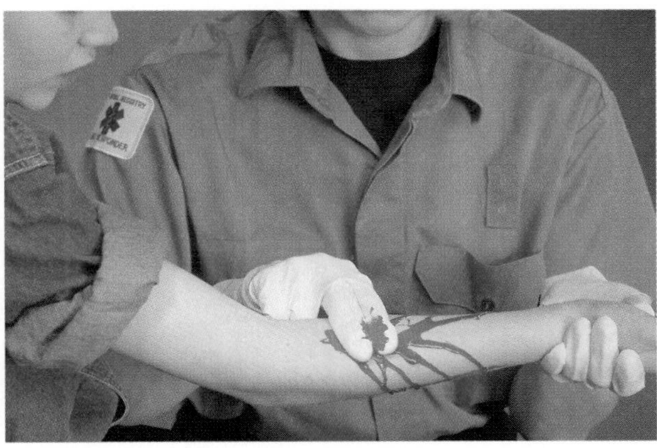

Figure 12-2a
Apply direct pressure with the fingertips.

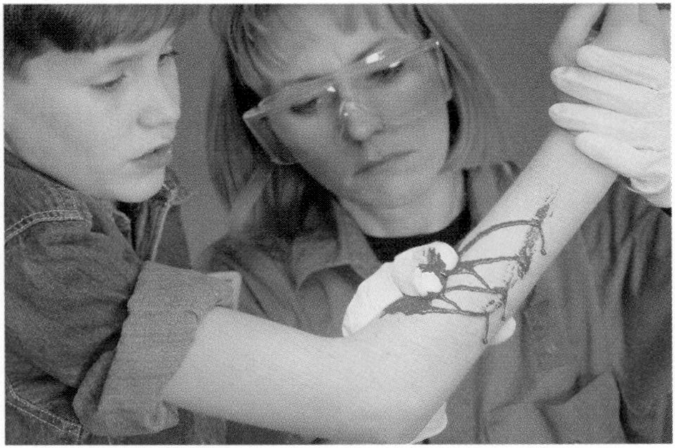

Figure 12-2b
Elevate an extremity.

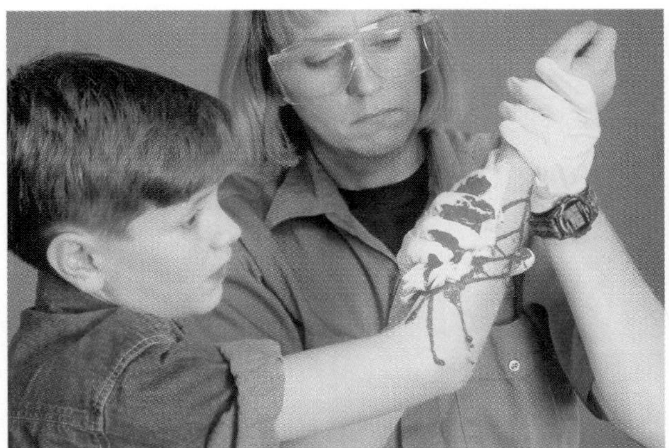

Figure 12-2c
If bleeding hasn't stopped, apply direct hand pressure.

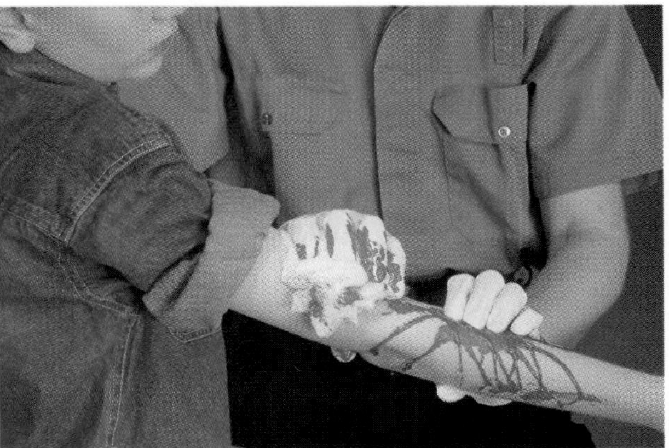

Figure 12-2d
If bleeding hasn't stopped, reassess the wound and apply additional pressure.

STREET NOTES

Almost all external bleeding can be managed using direct pressure and elevation. Be persistent. It may be necessary to apply them for several minutes.

2. *Elevate the extremity*. However, do so only if there's no major injury to the underlying muscle or bone. Continue to apply direct pressure at the same time.
3. *Reassess the wound if bleeding doesn't stop*. Remove any dressing to inspect the wound. If there's more than one bleeding site, apply additional pressure as needed.
4. *Use pressure points for bleeding in the upper and lower extremities* (Figure 12-3). If bleeding in the extremities doesn't stop with direct pressure and elevation, use a pressure point (the place where an artery lies over a bone close to the surface of the body). For the arm, compress the brachial artery. For the leg, compress the femoral artery. Use the flat part of your fingers or the palm of your hand. Do this while you maintain direct pressure and elevation of the wound site.

Note that the care for external bleeding described above is controversial. *Follow your local protocols*. In some EMS systems First

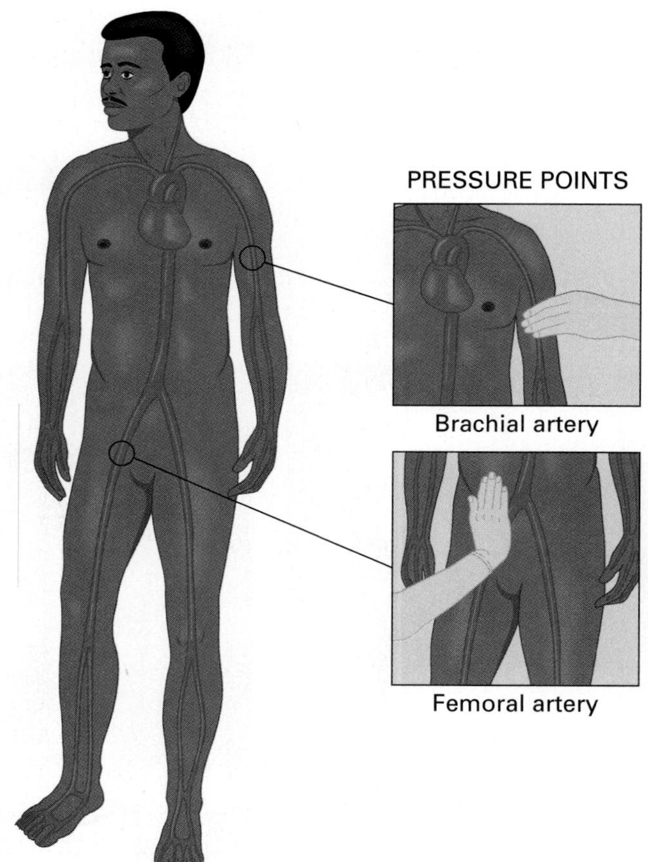

Figure 12-3
Location of pressure points for bleeding in the arms and legs.

Responders are told to use a dressing to apply direct fingertip pressure to the site of bleeding. The dressing is kept on the wound so that a clot won't get dislodged. If this dressing becomes soaked, First Responders are told to put more dressings on top of it.

Caution *If you are responsible for using this method of controlling external bleeding, then don't apply too many layers of dressings to the wound. They'd make it too difficult to apply direct pressure properly. They'd also make it too difficult to monitor bleeding properly.*

The key process to effective management of external bleeding is: *Assess* the wound and bleeding point. *Intervene* by using direct pressure, elevation, and pressure points. *Reassess* the bleeding to determine if your bleeding control methods are effective.

INTERNAL BLEEDING

When the internal organs of the body are injured or damaged, internal bleeding may occur. Painful, swollen, deformed extremities also may lead to serious internal blood loss. Whatever the cause, internal bleeding often is hidden. Take an injured 27-year-old male, for example. Someone has beat him in the chest and abdomen with a steel pipe. Your exam may show that his abdomen is tender and rigid. Though you see no obvious signs of bleeding, it's there, "hiding" in both the chest and the abdomen. If it's not managed quickly enough, the patient will go into shock.

The signs and symptoms of internal bleeding are as follows:

- Discolored, tender, swollen, or hard tissues.
- Increased pulse and respiration rates.
- Pale, cool skin.
- Nausea and vomiting.
- Thirst.
- Mental status changes.

The treatment for major internal bleeding is the same as the treatment for shock (see page 164). Recognize the signs and symptoms early and treat them aggressively. Start during the initial assessment. Be sure to take all proper BSI precautions, and arrange for immediate transport.

SHOCK

Shock is also called **hypoperfusion** (*hypo* means "less than" and *perfusion* refers to the oxygen supply to tissues). Shock is the result of too little oxygen being delivered by way of the blood to the body's tissues. This can occur when there are problems with the heart, the blood supply, or the blood vessels. For example:

Shock from heart failure: A 47-year-old male suffers a massive heart attack. Much of the heart muscle dies and can no longer work to deliver oxygenated blood to the body. This leads to shock.

Shock from a blood supply problem: A 15-year-old girl is hit by a car while crossing the street. She suffers massive internal injuries and loses two liters of blood. Now there's not enough blood in this patient's body to adequately deliver oxygen to the tissues. This patient also slips into shock.

Shock from a problem with the blood vessels: A 23-year-old woman is stung by a bee. She has a severe allergic reaction, which causes her blood vessels to **dilate** (expand). As a result, her blood doesn't fill the enlarged vessels and transport of oxygen to the body's tissues can't occur. This patient becomes shocky.

In all three cases, the end result is that too little oxygen is reaching the body's tissues. If these conditions are allowed to occur, all three patients would die even if they get to the hospital alive. If vital organs aren't *perfused* (supplied with adequate oxygen) for any significant period of time, the patients will die.

SIGNS AND SYMPTOMS OF SHOCK

Many of the signs and symptoms of shock actually are the body's attempt to compensate for problems with the heart, blood supply, or blood vessels. For example, when a patient's tissues don't receive enough oxygen due to blood loss, the body responds by increasing respiration and pulse rate. It also shunts blood from the patient's extremities and skin to where it's needed most: the brain, heart, liver, kidneys, and other vital organs.

Note that the brain is very sensitive to any decrease in its oxygen supply. Too little oxygen can cause a person's mental status to range from slightly confused to completely unresponsive. Most patients become unresponsive after losing 35% to 40% of their blood supply.

Signs and symptoms of shock include (Figure 12-4):

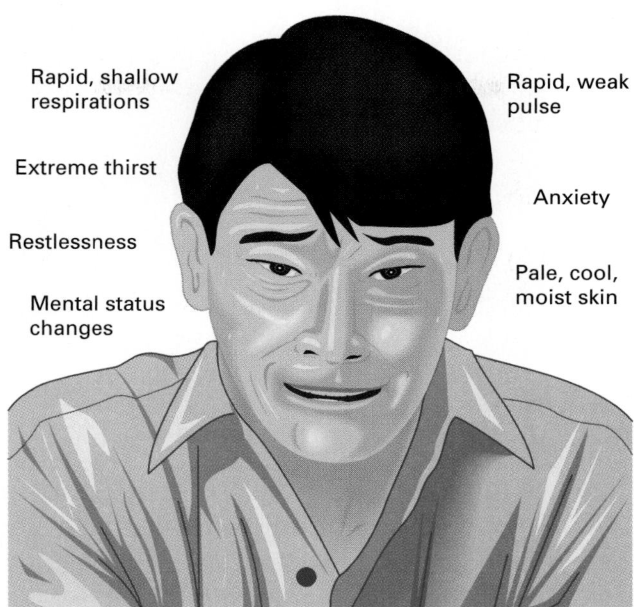

Figure 12-4
Signs and symptoms of shock.

- Extreme thirst.
- Restlessness.
- Anxiety.
- Mental status changes.
- Rapid, shallow respirations.
- Rapid, weak pulse.
- Pale, cool, moist skin.

TREATMENT OF SHOCK

After completing a scene size-up, conduct an initial assessment. Begin to treat your patient for shock at this time. Be sure to take all appropriate BSI precautions, and arrange for immediate transport. The most critical factor in the survival of a shock patient is time. The longer patients remain in shock, the greater the likelihood that they'll die.

Treat for shock as follows:

1. Maintain the patient's airway and breathing. Provide high flow oxygen via nonrebreather mask if you are equipped and trained to do so.

STREET NOTES

A patient who shows signs and symptoms of shock is a high priority patient. Call dispatch and arrange for transport immediately!

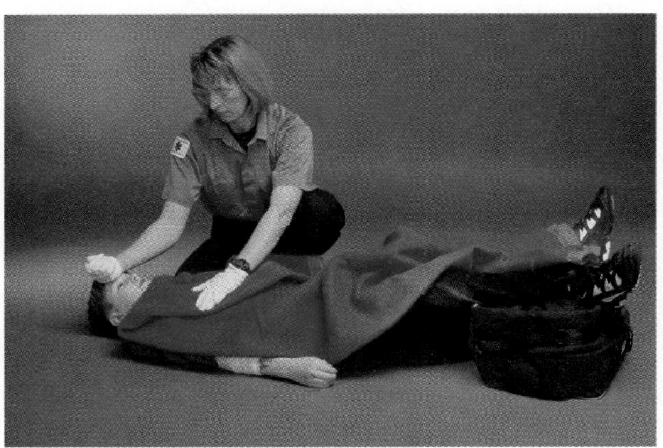

Figure 12-5
The shock position.

2. Prevent any further blood loss.
3. Place the patient in the **shock position** (Figure 12-5). That is, have the patient lie down and elevate the lower extremities about eight to 12 inches. If the patient has serious injuries to the pelvis, lower extremities, head, chest, abdomen, neck, or spine, keep the patient supine. *Follow local protocols.*
4. Cover the patient with a blanket to help prevent the loss of body heat.
5. Withhold all food and drink (patients in shock often vomit).
6. Provide care for specific injuries as needed.
7. Comfort, calm, and reassure your patient while waiting for transport.

If you're allowed to transport patients, memorize this "time rule": If the intervention is not essential for keeping a shock patient alive, do it en route to the hospital. Time is too important to stay on scene.

CONCLUSION

Treating shock and bleeding is the last step in initial assessment and treatment. Remember that shock kills and that bleeding is one of its most common causes. The key process to effective management of external bleeding is:

- *Assess* the wound and bleeding point.
- *Intervene* by using direct pressure, elevation, and pressure points.
- *Reassess* the bleeding to determine if your bleeding control methods are effective.

Signs and symptoms of internal bleeding and shock must be recognized and treated early and aggressively. Constantly reassess the ABCs. Shock is never "cured" in the field. So no matter what the cause, shock in a patient requires rapid transport to a medical facility.

KEY TERMS

You may wish to use this list to review your understanding of key terms introduced in the chapter.

arterial bleeding bleeding characterized by bright, oxygen-rich red blood that spurts from a wound.

capillary bleeding bleeding characterized by dark red blood that tends to ooze from a wound.

dilate expand, enlarge.

direct pressure force applied to a wound site by the fingertips or whole hand to control bleeding.

elevation lifting a wounded arm or leg to allow the effects of gravity help control bleeding.

hypoperfusion the insufficient supply of oxygen to the body's tissues which results from inadequate circulation of the blood. *Also called* shock.

pressure point the point where an artery lies over a bone close to the surface of the body; by compressing the brachial or femoral pressure point, arterial bleeding may be controlled in an extremity.

shock position the patient usually is supine with lower extremities elevated about eight to 12 inches.

venous bleeding bleeding characterized by dark, oxygen-poor blood flowing from a wound in a steady stream.

APPLICATION QUESTIONS

You may wish to use these questions to review your understanding of the chapter. For answers with page references, see Appendix 2.

1. You're observing another First Responder manage a shock patient. The patient has an altered mental status and is breathing rapidly. No oxygen is being administered, though the First Responder is trained and equipped to do so. The reason? "My patient is getting enough oxygen." Do you agree or disagree? Explain your answer.

2. Why is the "time rule" so important when treating patients in shock?

CHAPTER 13 THE PHYSICAL EXAM

FIRST RESPONSE

Jenny McPherson is one of several First Responders at a rock concert when she gets a call for a 19-year-old male involved in an assault on the bleachers. She and her partner Dwayne respond. "We're not sure what's going on with this guy," one of the security guards tells them. "He got hit, and he smells like he's drunk. Who knows what else. We can't find the assailant, so my partner and I'll stay here with you. Two more men are on the way to hold back the crowd."

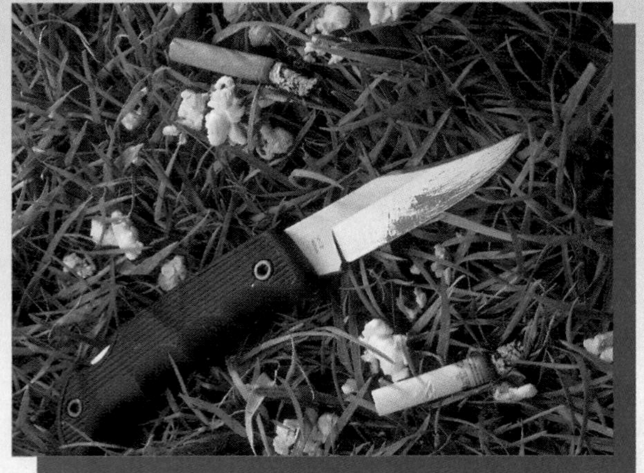

Jenny gloves up as she listens and asks, "Any weapons involved?" The guard says none that they can find. Jenny sizes up the scene and begins an initial assessment of the patient. He's lying across one of the benches. "Hey there," she calls out to the patient. He turns to her without answering, looking very pale, sweaty, and scared. Jenny says to one of the guards, "He looks pretty bad. Have you called EMS dispatch?" The guard nods and tells her to expect them any minute. She continues her assessment and finds that the patient has labored, rapid breathing and a weak, rapid pulse. With Dwayne's help she puts the patient in the shock position and applies high-flow oxygen via mask. Again she turns to the guard, "Any witnesses?"

"No witnesses. I've got a man below the bleachers checking to see if the assailant dropped anything. So far, nothing," he answers. He listens to his radio for a moment. "Paramedics just arrived at the entrance. They'll be here in about two minutes."

Jenny sees that the patient appears more agitated and short of breath. "He's getting worse," she says and begins a head-to-toe exam. When she opens his jacket and shirt, she sees a small stream of blood coming from a slit below the right nipple. "This guy's been stabbed," she says to Dwayne. She sees the blood bubble with each exhalation. "Dwayne, I need an airtight dressing now." Dwayne responds immediately. Jenny seals the wound. The patient's agitation seems to ease up almost immediately, just in time for the Paramedics who take over care.

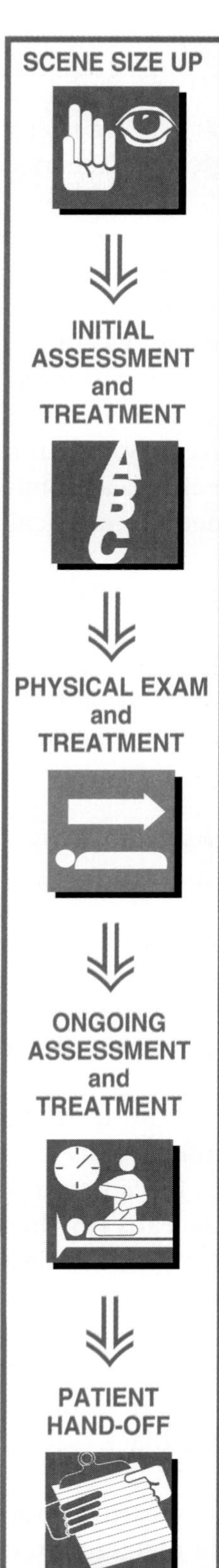

LEARNING OBJECTIVES

This chapter will introduce you to the First Responder physical exam and treatment. This step in the patient care plan is performed after the scene size-up and initial assessment and treatment. It's designed to give you more in-depth patient information from which you can make good patient care decisions.

By the end of the chapter, you should be able to:†

- 3-1.16 Discuss the components of the physical exam. (p. 169)
- 3-1.17 State the areas of the body that are evaluated during the physical exam. (pp. 174-176)
- 3-1.18 Explain what additional questioning may be asked during the physical exam. (p. 170)
- 3-1.19 Explain the components of the SAMPLE history. (pp. 171-174)

* Discuss how history-taking is modified based on your patient's chief complaint. (p. 170)

* Describe the methods for obtaining patient vital signs. (pp. 177-182)

AN OVERVIEW OF THE PHYSICAL EXAM

The physical exam is performed after scene size-up and initial assessment and treatment. It includes gathering a patient's medical history, performing a head-to-toe exam, and taking vital signs. However, in certain cases you may find that you never reach this step.

The need to care for a patient's life-threats—a blocked airway, for example—always takes priority and may keep you busy until the EMTs arrive. In another case you may gather a history and perform the head-to-toe exam, both at the same time. For trauma and altered mental status patients, you may want to do a head-to-toe exam before you gather a history. Whatever the situation, remember treatment of life-threats always takes priority.

The physical exam described in this chapter is a very general one. It applies to all patients. Physical exams and treatments specifically "tailored" to patients with different conditions are included in Section 3 of this book.

†Numbered objectives are from the 1995 U.S. DOT "First Responder: National Standard Curriculum." Asterisks indicate supplemental material.

GATHERING A PATIENT HISTORY

A patient history is the story behind the events leading up to the current illness or injury. It also includes background facts necessary to understand the patient's problem.

Gathering a patient's history can be a Pandora's box. If you ask too many questions, you'll get too much data. For example, asking about knee surgery that occurred seven years ago won't help you to understand the patient's shortness of breath today. To get an effective patient history, you must be organized and aimed at solving the patient's immediate medical problem.

> **STREET NOTES**
>
> Keep your questions relevant to the patient's chief complaint. Begin your questioning with open-ended questions and move to yes-or-no ones as necessary.

Gathering an accurate history can be a challenge. Patients may leave out information by mistake or on purpose. If you can't speak the patient's language, you may have to ask questions by way of a translator or not at all. Patients in pain or with altered mental status may not be able to give you accurate information.

> **Caution** *Gathering a poor patient history can lead to delivering poor patient care.*

So, one of the best ways to focus your efforts is to begin by asking open-ended questions. For example, instead of asking "Are you having chest pain?" you might ask "What's bothering you today?" This type of question encourages the patient to describe his or her own problem.

Questions that require only yes-or-no answers can lead your patient into agreeing with a complaint that isn't actually occurring. They also can force you into a guessing game that leads nowhere. This type of question isn't useless however. Use them with patients who are vague or unsure or with patients who have a communication problem. They're also helpful when you need specific information, such as "Did you black out?" or "Does your knee hurt when you move it?"

> **STREET NOTES**
>
> Use all "historians" on the scene as necessary. Family, friends, or even bystanders can provide valuable insights into the problem.

Obtaining a good patient history really begins during your scene size-up. When you scan the scene for the mechanism of injury or nature of illness, you're looking for the answer to the question, "What's going on?"

THE *SAMPLE* HISTORY

One way to make sure you get all the information you need in a patient history is to use the acronym SAMPLE as a guide. Each letter of the acronym stands for a topic of questioning:

S—Signs and symptoms

A—Allergies

M—Medications

P—Pertinent past history

L—Last oral intake

E—Events leading to the injury or illness

S—Signs and Symptoms

This section of the SAMPLE history helps you to identify your patient's chief complaint and related signs or symptoms. The term **sign** refers to any medical or trauma condition that you can observe in the patient. Signs include hearing the sounds of respiratory distress, seeing bleeding, or feeling a patient's cool skin. A **symptom** is a condition that only the patient can be aware of, such as headache, pain, and so on. Questions that will get this information include:

- Why did you call EMS today?
- How are you feeling? What's wrong?
- Are you having any pain? If so, where?
- Are you having any other complaints today?

It can be difficult for patients to describe their pain. A mnemonic that can help you to get an accurate description is **PQRST**. It prompts the following questions:

P—Provocation. What were you doing when the pain started?

Q—Quality. Is the pain dull, sharp, a pressure?

R—Region and radiation. Where is the pain? Does it move or spread?

S—Severity. On a scale of one to ten, how bad is your pain?

T—Time. How long have you had this pain?

Your patient may give you specific answers to these questions. If not, feel free to follow up with questions that require yes-or-no answers. For example, if your patient says "My chest doesn't feel quite right," follow up with "Are you having chest pain? Discomfort? Pressure?"

A—ALLERGIES

Find out if your patient has allergies to any medications, foods, or factors in the environment. The patient's emergency may be related to an allergic reaction. This information also will be helpful to EMTs and emergency department personnel if they have to administer medicine to the patient. Questions that will get this information include:

- Are you allergic to anything? What?
- Do you have any allergies to medications?
- Do you have any food allergies or allergies to pollen or dust?

M—MEDICATIONS

The medications your patient is taking can provide other EMS workers with critical information about the emergency. Do a good job of finding them.

Find out what current prescription and nonprescription drugs the patient is taking. Also find out what he or she was taking in the recent past. For example, if your patient has abdominal pain, knowing that she took antibiotics last month for a bladder infection could be important. Changes in a patient's prescriptions also can cause problems. This is very common for patients who take insulin for diabetes or medications to control high blood pressure.

Questions that will get this information include:

- Do you take any prescription or nonprescription drugs?
- Have you recently stopped taking a prescription or nonprescription drug?
- Have there been any recent changes in your medications?

P—PERTINENT PAST HISTORY

A medical history can give valuable clues to a patient's current medical problem. Try to be accurate. It isn't enough to report that Mrs. Jones has had a heart attack or two. When did Mrs. Jones have a heart attack? Did the doctors perform any related surgery? Use your common sense. A patient with shortness of breath shouldn't take ten minutes to tell you about oral surgery done 20 years ago. Gathering details about a patient's childbirth history also isn't going to help you manage her injured ankle.

Questions that will get pertinent information include:

- Are you seeing a doctor for any medical problems?
- Have you ever been admitted to the hospital for injuries, illness, or surgery?
- Have you recently been ill or injured?

STREET NOTES

When conducting a patient history, try to guide the patient into giving you pertinent information.

If your patient gives vague answers to open-ended questions, use the patient's chief complaint and related signs and symptoms to help you develop specific questions. For example: Do you have any chronic heart or lung problems or conditions? Are you a diabetic? Have you ever suffered a stroke or heart attack? Do you have epilepsy? Have you ever had a convulsion?

L—Last Oral Intake

Last oral intake refers to the last time your patient had anything to eat or drink. This information is especially important for infant, child, and diabetic patients, and if the patient has to go to surgery.

Questions that will get this information include:

- When was the last time you had anything to eat or drink?
- How much did you have to eat or drink?

E—Events Leading to the Injury or Illness

This is the patient's story of what led to the emergency. If your patient was injured, this information should give you a better understanding of the mechanism of injury. If your patient has a medical problem, find out what the patient was doing when the complaint began. Questions that will get this information include:

- How long have you been sick?
- What has been the course of your sickness? That is, have you gotten sicker and sicker as time goes by or have you stayed the same?

- Has anything made your illness better or worse?
- Can you describe the events of your illness?

THE HEAD-TO-TOE EXAM

The head-to-toe exam is designed to guide treatment of the patient. So it should be both patient and injury specific. For example, if your patient is complaining of a cut finger and the mechanism of injury suggests no other trauma, there's really no need to examine the head or chest.

Conduct the physical exam in a logical manner. In general start at the head and continue to the neck, chest, abdomen, pelvis, and extremities. Use the acronym **DOTS** to help you remember to look and feel for signs of illness or injury:

D—Deformities.

O—Open injuries.

T—Tenderness.

S—Swelling.

Infants and children often are extremely wary of a head-to-toe exam. Sometimes it helps to begin at the patient's toes and work up to the head. This will give him or her a chance to get used to your touch. If your patient is a crying infant, complete as much of your exam as you can simply by inspecting your patient's body visually.

THE HEAD

Look and feel for DOTS to the face and scalp (Figure 13-1). Note any blood or fluids draining from the ears, nose, and mouth. Examine your patient's mouth for broken teeth, blood, loose dentures, or other foreign objects that could obstruct the airway.

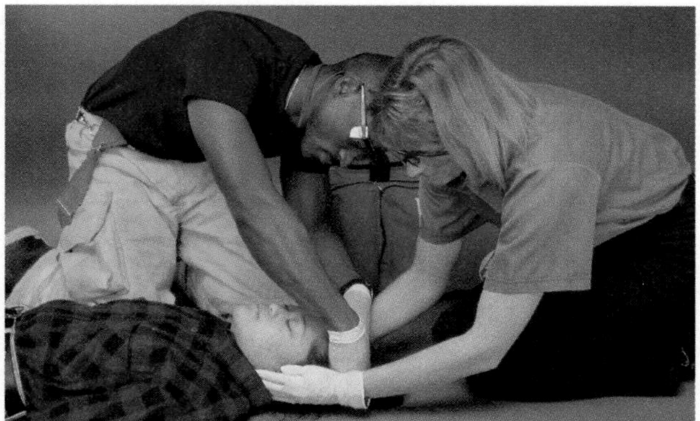

Figure 13-1
Examine the head and scalp.

THE NECK

Look at the neck for DOTS (Figure 13-2). Look to see if the patient is using accessory muscles to breathe. You'll see the muscles at the base of the neck between the collarbones draw in when the patient inhales. If so, he or she is in respiratory distress. Also, be on the lookout for a Medic Alert medallion around the patient's neck.

If you suspect spine injury in your patient, don't **palpate** (feel) your patient's neck to look for pain or tenderness. It could worsen a spinal injury. Tell possible spine-injured patients to keep very still. Then manually stabilize the head and neck in neutral alignment until the patient can be completely immobilized.

THE CHEST

Look for DOTS to the chest (Figure 13-3). Also look for bruising or major scars that could indicate previous heart surgery. Look for the use of accessory muscles (the muscles between the ribs and between the ribs and abdomen) during breathing. If the patient is sitting or on his or her side, palpate (feel) the chest by gently pressing on the sternum and back simultaneously. Then gently squeeze the rib cage from side to side. Since the sternum and ribs form a circle, this front-to-back and side-to-side palpation causes increased pain if there's any injury to any part of the rib cage.

Don't forget to check the patient's back. While this often is done at the end of the exam, the back is really the back side of the chest. If you suspect spinal injury in your patient, minimize movement. Don't palpate the spinal column to look for pain or tenderness.

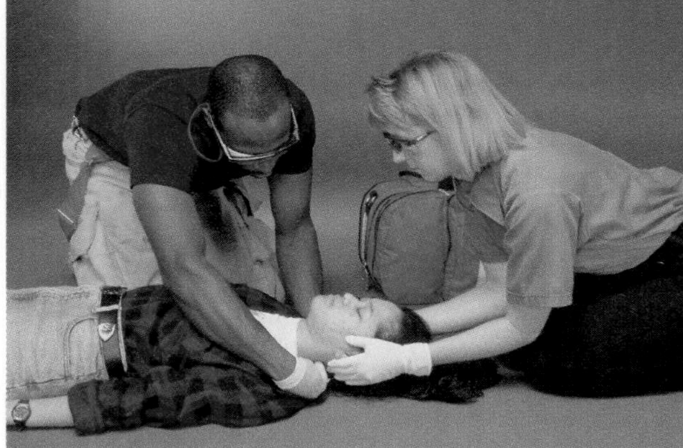

Figure 13-2
Examine the neck.

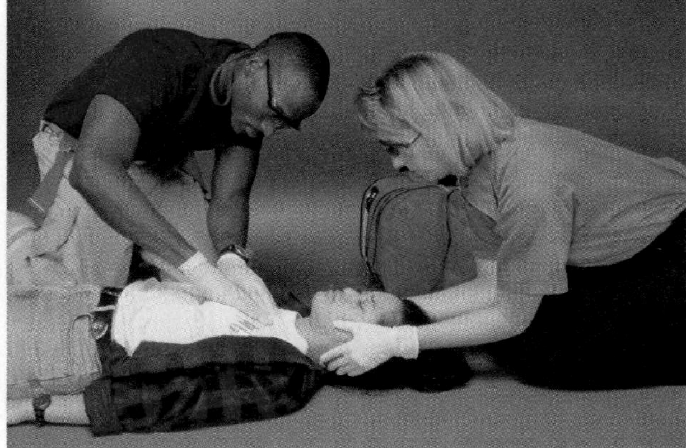

Figure 13-3
Examine the chest.

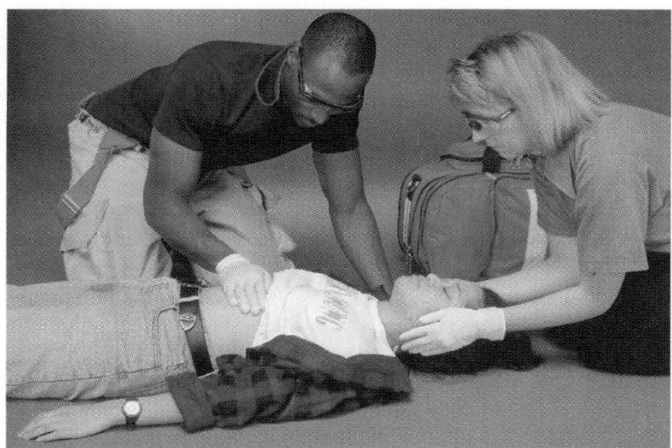

Figure 13-4
Examine the abdomen.

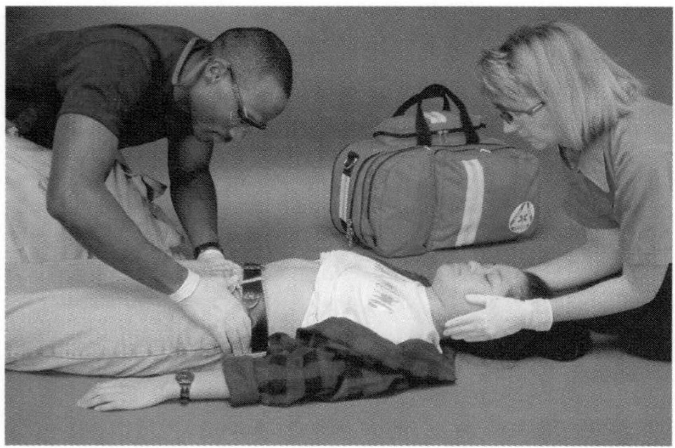

Figure 13-5
Examine the pelvis.

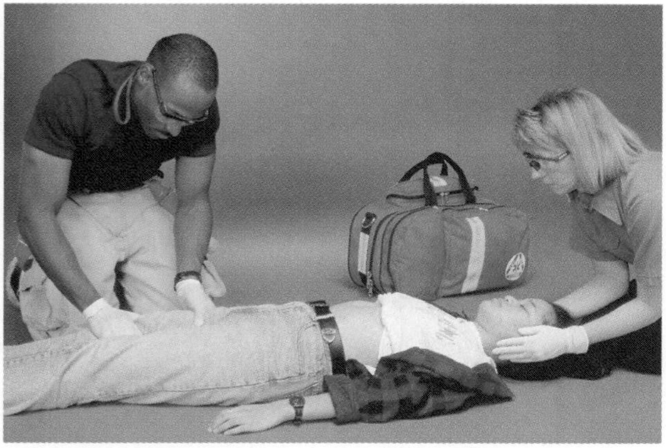

Figure 13-6
Examine the extremities.

It's especially important in infants and children for you to look for the use of accessory muscles in breathing. Also look for "seesaw" breathing.

THE ABDOMEN

Look for DOTS to the abdomen (Figure 13-4). However, change the "D" from *deformity* to *distention*. Also look for bruising and surgical scars. Injuries can cause the abdomen to become distended, rigid or hard, and tender. To palpate it, use a flat hand and press gently. If your patient says you're hurting him or her, stop. Absolutely never palpate deeply into the abdomen.

THE PELVIS

Look for DOTS to the pelvis (Figure 13-5). Since the pelvis forms a circle, palpate it from side-to-side to discover any tenderness. Also check for urine or feces to see if the patient lost control of the bladder or bowels. This could mean the patient lost consciousness at some point.

THE EXTREMITIES

Look for DOTS to all four extremities (Figure 13-6). Patients who can move their arms and legs probably have no serious extremity injuries. Be alert for any reduction of motion. Paralysis or reduced movement of the arm and leg on one side of the patient's body could indicate stroke. If the patient can't move the legs, or legs and arms, he or she may have a spinal injury. If you have any doubt about a patient's ability to move the extremities, ask the patient to lift or move each one. Keep a lookout for a Medic Alert bracelet.

VITAL SIGNS

After the head-to-toe exam of the patient, take a complete set of **vital signs**. They're key indicators of the patient's airway, breathing, and circulation status. You already checked them during the initial assessment when you determined the patient's mental status and assessed breathing, pulse, and skin condition. Now take the time to record them more completely and accurately. Organize them as you would during an initial assessment:

- Level of responsiveness
- Airway
- Breathing
- Pulse
- Skin
- Blood pressure (optional)

In general, vital signs should be assessed and recorded at least every 15 minutes in a stable patient and every five minutes in an unstable patient. You also should assess vital signs after any medical intervention. Recheck a patient's ABCs every time you observe a significant change in the patient's condition.

Remember *Vital signs can tell you if the patient is getting worse, staying the same, or improving. Ask yourself: Are your patient's vital signs changing? Are respiratory rates and pulse rates really high, really low, or somewhere in between where you want them to be?*

LEVEL OF RESPONSIVENESS

In the initial assessment you used the AVPU scale to help determine the patient's level of responsiveness. Now take the time to measure more thoroughly. Confirm that your patient is truly alert by asking the following questions:

- What's your name?
- What day is it?
- What time is it?

- Where are you?
- What's happened to you?

Patients with head injuries or any problem that causes less oxygen to reach the brain may only seem to be alert. In fact they may be confused about where they are and what happened to them. Pay attention to any unusual behavior in your patient. Look for signs of combativeness, odd or irrational thinking, or slowness. These signs may indicate a serious condition.

If the patient is alert, determine if there's any change from your previous assessment. Remember that a patient's level of responsiveness is one of the most sensitive indicators of status change.

AIRWAY

Reconfirm your patient's airway status.

BREATHING

To assess breathing properly, assess both rate and quality (Figure 13-7). Begin by observing the rise and fall of your patient's chest. Then count the patient's respirations for 30 seconds. (An inhale plus an exhale equals one respiration.) Then multiply by 2 to get the respiratory rate.

The quality of breathing may be determined at the same time you assess the rate. See if it fits into one of four categories—normal, shallow, labored, or noisy:

- *Normal* — Observe average chest wall motion. There is no use of accessory muscles during normal breathing.
- *Shallow* — Observe very slight chest or abdominal wall motion during shallow breathing.

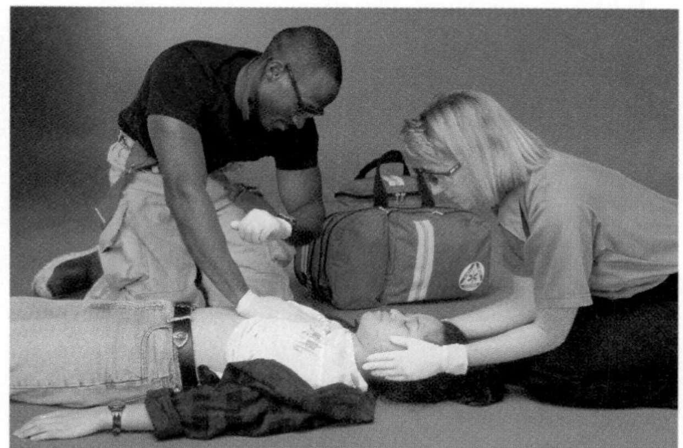

Figure 13-7
Measure the rate and quality of breathing.

- *Labored* — There is an increase in the effort of breathing, characterized by the use of accessory muscles. You may hear grunting and stridor, and sometimes gasping. There also may be nasal flaring.
- *Noisy* — Notice an increase in the sounds of breathing, which may include snoring, wheezing, gurgling, and crowing.

Recheck the effectiveness of your patient's respirations and his or her response to any breathing interventions.

PULSE

During the initial assessment you checked to see if your patient has a pulse, its approximate speed (too fast or too slow), and its strength (weak or strong). Now take the time to count the pulse accurately.

Generally the radial pulse is assessed in all patients at one year of age and older. In patients less than one year, take a brachial pulse. Whichever pulse is taken, count the beats for 30 seconds and multiply by 2 to get the rate. Then verify the strength or quality of the pulse. Generally it's characterized as strong, weak, regular, or irregular.

If the radial pulse can't be felt in an adult, assess the carotid pulse. Remember that you should never attempt to assess a carotid pulse on both sides of the neck at the same time.

 If the brachial pulse can't be felt in an infant, take a pulse at the femoral pulse point.

SKIN

When you assess a patient's skin, you are determining the adequacy of *perfusion*. (Perfusion results from the adequate circulation of blood through the body.) Examine skin color, temperature, and general condition. Be sure to note any changes from the observations you made during the initial assessment.

Assess skin color by looking at the nail beds and the mucous membranes of the mouth and inner eyelids. Pink is the normal healthy color of these parts. Abnormal skin colors include pale, cyanotic, flushed, and jaundiced:

- *Pale* may indicate impaired blood flow.
- *Cyanotic* (bluish, gray, or dark purple) may indicate a lack of oxygen.
- *Flushed* (red) may indicate exposure to heat or carbon monoxide poisoning.

- *Jaundiced* (yellow) may indicate a liver abnormality.

Check skin color in infants and children by looking at the palms of the hands and soles of the feet. These too should be pink.

Assess a patient's skin temperature by placing the back of your hand on the patient's skin. Normal skin temperature is warm. Abnormal skin temperatures include hot, cool, and cold:

- *Hot* may indicate fever or heat exposure.
- *Cool* may indicate impaired blood flow or exposure to cold.
- *Cold* may indicate extreme exposure to cold.

A patient's skin condition is normally dry. Wet or moist skin may indicate shock or heat exposure. Skin that is abnormally dry could indicate a spinal injury or severe dehydration.

In infants and children under six years old, you can also assess **capillary refill**. Press on the patient's skin or nail bed (Figure 13-8). Then measure the time it takes for the skin to return to its original color. Normal capillary refill in infants and children is less than two seconds. Abnormal capillary refill is more than two seconds.

BLOOD PRESSURE

In the out-of-hospital setting, blood pressure is the least important of all the vital signs. It's also a poor indicator of shock. Level of responsiveness, skin condition, and pulse are much more sensitive indicators. They'll show signs of shock in its earliest stages while blood pressure drops only when shock becomes severe. Many First Responders aren't equipped or trained to measure

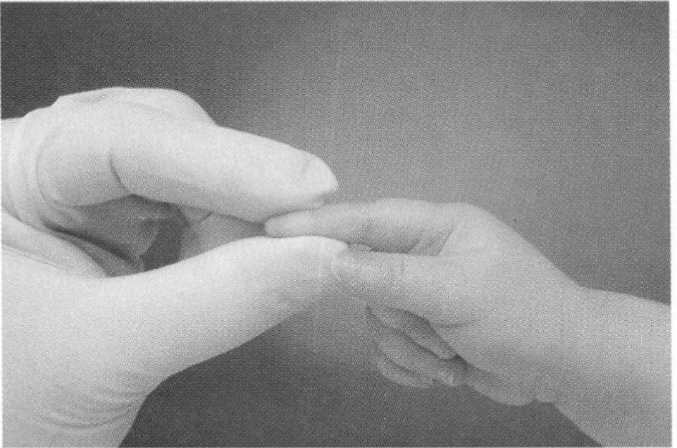

Figure 13-8
Capillary refill in infants and children under six.

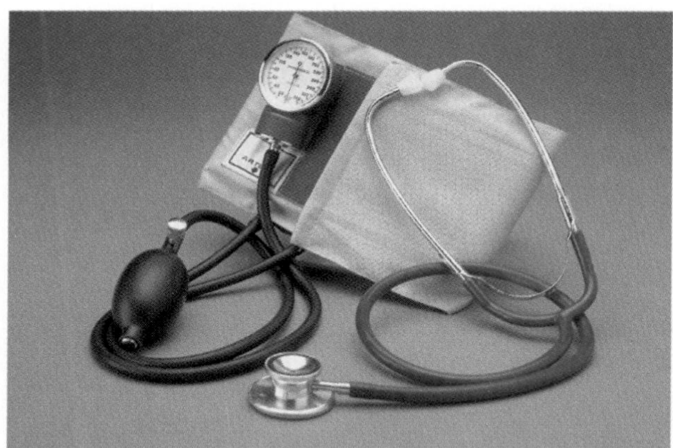

Figure 13-9
A blood pressure cuff and a stethoscope.

blood pressure. Others are required to take it. Follow your local protocols.

A patient's blood pressure reading includes two measurements—the **systolic blood pressure** and the **diastolic blood pressure**. They are indications of the pressure being exerted in the arteries during contraction (systole) and relaxation (diastole) of the heart. A patient's systolic pressure always will be greater than the diastolic, because the pressure inside the arteries always will be greater during contraction.

Blood pressure fluctuates constantly. It rises during work and physical exertion. It drops during rest. Average blood pressure for adults is anywhere from 90/60 to 140/90. Note that the systolic pressure always is written above the diastolic.

There are two methods used to measure blood pressure—**auscultated blood pressure** and **palpated blood pressure**. With either one you need a *sphygmomanometer*, or blood pressure cuff with gauge and bulb (Figure 13-9).

Assessing Blood Pressure by Auscultation

An auscultated blood pressure is measured using a blood pressure cuff and stethoscope. In this case you'll listen for both the systolic and diastolic sounds. To assess blood pressure by auscultation, take all proper BSI precautions and follow these steps (Figure 13-10):

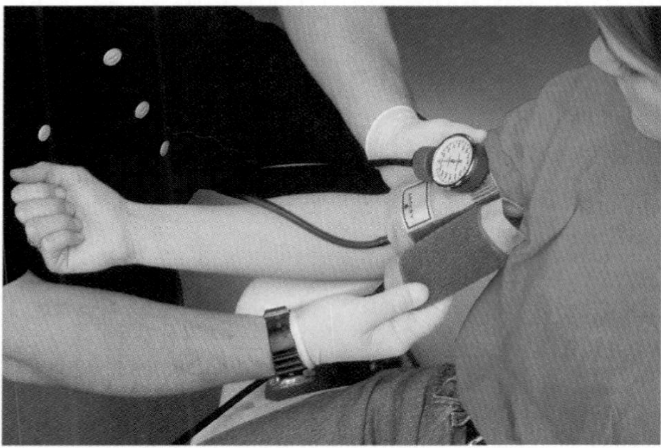

Figure 13-10a
Proper placement of the blood pressure cuff.

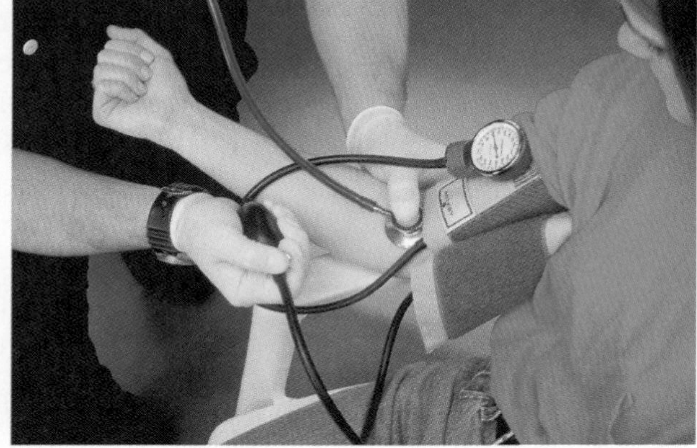

Figure 13-10b
Taking blood pressure by auscultation.

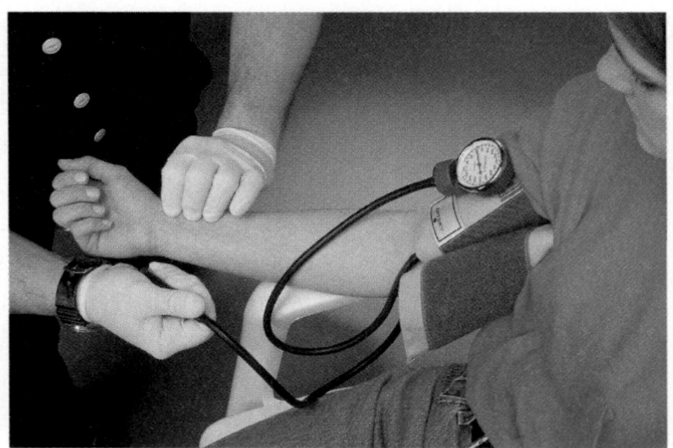

Figure 13-11
Taking blood pressure by palpation.

1. Choose a blood pressure cuff that is the correct size for your patient. It should circle the patient's arm without overlapping and cover about two-thirds of the upper arm. Center it above the brachial artery and about one inch above the inside of the elbow. The cuff should be snug, but one finger should be able to fit easily under its bottom edge.
2. Inflate the cuff to 30 mmHg above the point where you no longer feel a radial pulse.
3. Apply the stethoscope to the brachial pulse, and deflate the cuff at about 2 mmHg per second. Watch the pressure indicator drop.
4. When you hear the first few beats, record the pressure reading. This is the systolic pressure. Continue deflating the cuff.
5. When you hear the last beats, record the pressure reading. This is the diastolic pressure.

Assessing Blood Pressure by Palpation

For a palpated blood pressure use a blood pressure cuff while you palpate the radial artery. This method isn't as accurate as an auscultated measurement, because it provides only a systolic reading. However, it can be very useful if scene noise prevents you from using the stethoscope properly.

To take blood pressure by palpation, take all proper BSI precautions and follow these steps (Figure 13-11):

1. Inflate the cuff to about 30 mmHg above the level where the radial pulse can no longer be felt.
2. Slowly deflate the cuff, making a note of the point at which the radial pulse returns. Because you don't have a diastolic reading, you can record this measurement as 120/P for example.

CONCLUSION

This chapter has introduced you to the physical exam and treatment, which includes a SAMPLE history, the head-to-toe exam, and vital signs. This step of your call is performed after your scene size-up and initial assessment and treatment. It's designed to give you more in-depth patient information from which to make good patient care decisions. As important as this step is, never forget that assessment and treatment of the patient's ABCs always take priority.

THE PHYSICAL EXAM

- Gather a SAMPLE history.

  S—Signs and symptoms

  A—Allergies

  M—Medications

  P—Pertinent past history

  L—Last oral intake

  E—Events leading to the injury or illness

- Perform a head-to-toe exam.
  - Head
  - Neck
  - Chest
  - Abdomen
  - Pelvis
  - Extremities
- Take vital signs.
  - Level of responsiveness
  - Airway
  - Breathing
  - Pulse
  - Skin
  - Blood pressure (optional)

KEY TERMS

You may wish to use this list to review your understanding of key terms introduced in the chapter.

auscultated blood pressure a method of taking blood pressure using a blood pressure cuff and stethoscope.

capillary refill a measurement of perfusion usually used with infants and children under six years old; the time it takes for skin or nail beds that have been compressed to return to their normal color.

diastolic blood pressure the pressure being exerted by the blood in the arteries during relaxation or when the heart is at rest (diastole).

DOTS an acronym meant to help the rescuer remember what to look for when conducting a physical exam; the letters stand for deformities, open injuries, tenderness, and swelling.

palpate to examine by touch; to feel.

palpated blood pressure a method of taking blood pressure using a blood pressure cuff while palpating the radial artery.

PQRST a mnemonic used to help the rescuer get an accurate description of a patient's pain; the letters stand for provocation, quality, region and radiation, severity, and time.

SAMPLE history a patient history taken by using the acronym SAMPLE to help the rescuer remember the categories of questioning; the letters stand for signs and symptoms, allergies, medications, pertinent past history, last oral intake, and events leading to the injury or illness.

sign refers to any medical or trauma condition that the rescuer can observe in the patient, such as sounds of respiratory distress or bleeding.

symptom refers to conditions that only the patient can observe, such as headache, pain, itching, and so on.

systolic blood pressure the pressure being exerted by the blood in the arteries during a contraction of the heart (systole).

vital signs the traditional signs of life, or key indicators of the patient's airway, breathing, and circulation status.

APPLICATION QUESTIONS

You may wish to use these questions to review your understanding of the chapter. For answers with page references, see Appendix 2.

1. A First Responder once said that "everybody gets a SAMPLE history taken, a head-to-toe exam, and assessment of vital signs. If you fail to do this, you have not provided adequate care." Is this statement true or false? Explain your answer.
2. You are in the middle of a head-to-toe exam of a 35-year-old female, who is complaining of a painful leg. Suddenly your patient slumps over and becomes unresponsive. What should your next step be?
3. You're managing an agitated patient who has pale, cool, moist skin. His radial pulses are weak at best, and his level of responsiveness keeps changing. Should determining the patient's blood pressure readings be a priority?

CHAPTER 14 ONGOING ASSESSMENT

FIRST RESPONSE

It takes Malik only a few seconds to realize that something is wrong at one end of the pool. Some sort of rough game has been going on. From his lifeguard tower he now sees swimmers suddenly gather around one of their mates in the water. Several parents vault out of their sun chairs and crowd the side of the pool.

Malik grabs his jump kit and investigates. "It's Janell," someone shouts. "She's having another asthma attack." Indeed she was. With the help of a few parents, Malik hauls Janell out of the water and onto a pool chair. Janell looks around anxiously, bolt upright and wide eyed. Her chest and shoulders are heaving as she tries to pull air into her lungs. "Her mom's not here. She forgot her inhaler," he hears from the crowd.

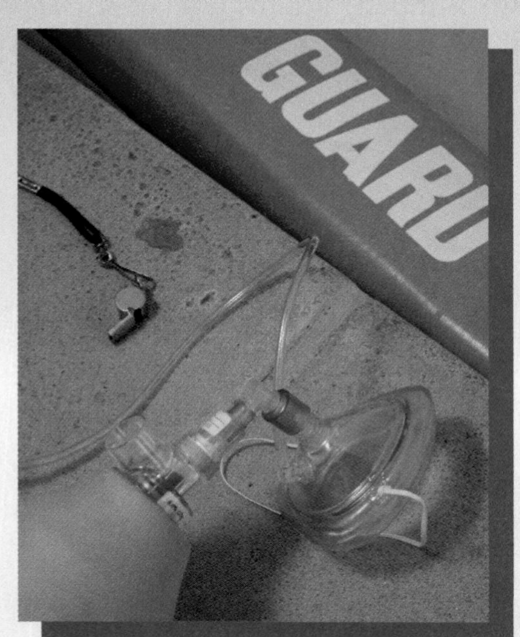

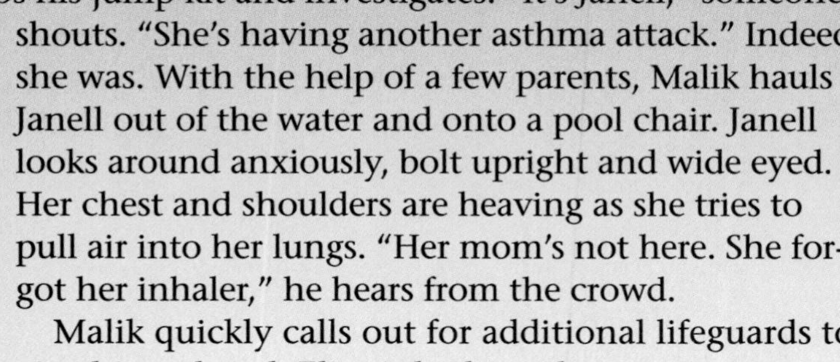

Malik quickly calls out for additional lifeguards to give him a hand. Elise is by his side in an instant. "This girl's really having a tough time breathing," Malik says to her. "Bring me the oxygen and call 9-1-1." He proceeds through the initial assessment and treatment. In seconds, he's able to apply high-flow oxygen using a nonrebreather. Elise assures him that an ambulance is on the way.

Malik quickly completes a SAMPLE history. He's about ready to finish a head-to-toe exam when he notices that Janell looks as if she's getting too tired to breathe. He mumbles under his breath. "Reassess, reassess," he coaches himself. "Janell, are you with me here?" Janell looks at him with glassy eyes, exhausted, gasping weakly, desperate. Malik quickly repeats the initial assessment and realizes that Janell is in serious trouble. "Elise, I need help." Janell stops breathing. Malik positions her head, inserts a nasopharyngeal airway, and with Elise's help begins artificial ventilation with a bag-valve-mask.

EMT-Paramedics arrive a few minutes later. They pass a breathing tube directly into Janell's trachea and administer drugs to combat the asthma. "I think we got to her in time," a Paramedic says. Malik and Elise help load Janell into the ambulance, and then go to locate her parents.

SCENE SIZE UP

INITIAL ASSESSMENT and TREATMENT

PHYSICAL EXAM and TREATMENT

ONGOING ASSESSMENT and TREATMENT

PATIENT HAND-OFF

LEARNING OBJECTIVES

You've done your scene size-up. You've completed your initial assessment and treatment, and you've run through the physical exam and treatment. Other EMS workers are still 10 minutes away. Now what? Perform ongoing assessment and treatment. You can catch changes in your patient's condition before they become life-threatening. What should you reassess? How often should you reassess? This chapter will answer those questions.

By the end of the chapter, you should be able to:†

- 3-1.20 Discuss the components of the ongoing assessment (pp. 187-190)
- * Identify how often reassessment of the patient should be performed. (pp. 187-188, 189, 191)
- * Describe ongoing patient management. (p. 190)

AN OVERVIEW OF THE ONGOING ASSESSMENT

Ideally the ongoing assessment is done after the physical exam and treatment. However, just as in the scenario on the previous page, the patient's condition can stop you from moving onto the ongoing assessment. In general while you wait for the EMTs to arrive, continue to assess the patient. Focus on the reassessment of your patient's ABCs. Then and only then address the patient's chief complaint and your interventions. Remember that the following holds true no matter what your patient's problem:

- *Assess* your patient.
- *Intervene* with treatments as necessary.
- *Reassess* your patient to check the effectiveness of your interventions and to monitor changes in your patient's condition.

REPEATING THE INITIAL ASSESSMENT

The most important part of the ongoing assessment is to repeat the initial assessment (Figure 14-1). Repeat it for a *low priority, stable patient* every 15 minutes. A low priority, stable patient is

†Numbered objectives are from the 1995 U.S. DOT "First Responder: National Standard Curriculum." Asterisks indicate supplemental material.

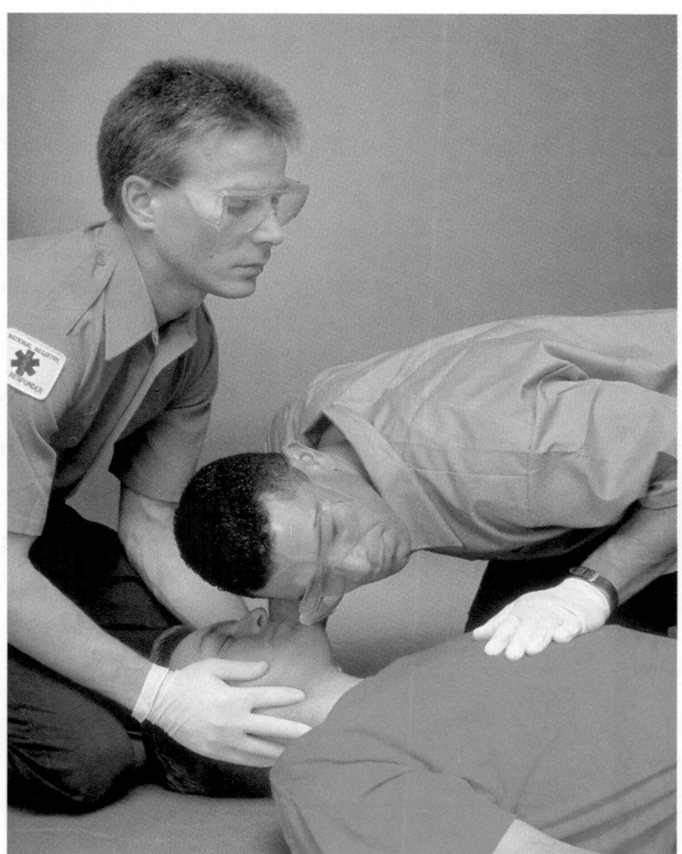

Figure 14-1
The most important part of the ongoing assessment is to repeat the initial assessment.

one who is alert with normal ABCs, is only mildly ill or injured, and doesn't appear to be getting worse.

Repeat the initial assessment for a *high priority, unstable patient* every five minutes. A high priority, unstable patient is one who has problems with or changes in mental status or the status of the ABCs. That includes the patient who becomes confused or unresponsive; who has an increase in airway, breathing, and circulation problems; or who has an increase in the severity of his or her chief complaint.

When you repeat the initial assessment, include the following:

- Recheck your general impression of the patient.
  - What is my patient's posture? Is it slouched, slumped, sprawled? Does it suggest the patient is doing well?
  - What is my patient's overall level of distress?
- Reassess the patient's mental status.
  - What is the level of responsiveness (AVPU)?
  - Is the patient confused, combative, or otherwise behaving abnormally?

- Reassess the ABCs.
  - Is the airway clear?
  - Is there breathing? Is it adequate? Is there any breathing difficulty?
  - Is there a pulse? Is it too weak, rapid, or slow?
  - Is there major external bleeding?
  - What is the patient's skin condition?
- Reprioritize the patient as necessary.

It's also critical that you reassess interventions. For example, is significant bleeding under control? Is bag-valve-mask ventilation achieving adequate chest rise? Has the patient's skin color improved with oxygen administration?

The key to successful ongoing assessment is to pay attention to changes in your patient. Always be flexible. If you find that the patient has a serious problem with his or her ABCs, scrap your previous patient care plan and adopt a new one. Remember, ongoing assessment also includes treatment as required.

Remember *Repeat the initial assessment every 15 minutes on low priority, stable patients and every five minutes on high priority, unstable patients. Also repeat it after any critical intervention and after any major status change.*

REPEATING THE PHYSICAL EXAM

After repeating the initial assessment, perform another physical exam every 10 to 15 minutes. Be sure to check any interventions you made during this exam.

Focus first on your patient's chief complaint. Let's say you're managing a patient with chest pain. Now that the patient is calm and on high-flow oxygen, ask him or her to tell you how it feels. Has it gotten better or worse? Has the pain changed? While it isn't necessary for you to repeat your entire SAMPLE history, reconfirm important information. For the chest-pain patient, this would include repeating the PQRST to get an update on a description of the pain.

It's unnecessary to repeat your entire head-to-toe exam. Focus instead on any important findings from your original exam. For example, if you've bandaged open wounds, check to see if the bleeding still appears to be under control.

Vital signs should be repeated at this time. Focus on your patient's mental status, airway patency, breathing rate and quality, pulse rate and quality, and skin condition. Remember that blood pressure is the least helpful vital sign of all. Be sure to consider the patient's chief complaint. For example, if it's shortness of breath, reassess breathing rate and quality in particular. If it's altered mental status, watch the level of responsiveness closely.

Finally, reassess your interventions. Make sure they're effective. Check to see, for example, if manual stabilization of the spine is being held correctly or if an ice pack is still in position. Reassess all treatments, no matter how minor they may be.

ONGOING PATIENT MANAGEMENT

While you're waiting for other rescuers to arrive, try to give the patient your full attention. Continue to reassure your patient and make him or her as comfortable possible. Person-to-person contact and emotional support help the patient gain confidence in your care. This is as important as reassessing vital signs. Here is how one patient described her experience:

> I wasn't hurt badly, just a neck strain and some bumps and bruises from a car crash. But I remember sitting in the car with steam rising from the crumpled hood and honking, blaring traffic all around me. I felt so scared. The First Responders were really wonderful. They took care of my injuries, and they stayed with me and let me know that I wasn't alone. In fact one of them held my hand. They talked me through everything and really held me together emotionally. I'm not sure what I would've done if they hadn't been there.

Effective ongoing assessment skills help you to become organized on calls that aren't going well. If you find that you're the proverbial chicken running around with your head cut off, "go back to home base." An organized reassessment will help you to answer these questions: What is the patient's status? Airway? Breathing? Circulation? Have interventions been successful? An organized reassessment also will help you to get back on track, prioritizing those tasks that need to be completed first, next, and last.

CONCLUSION

Ongoing assessment of your patients—especially high priority patients—is essential for determining the effectiveness of your interventions and for monitoring any status changes. It also will help you to stay organized.

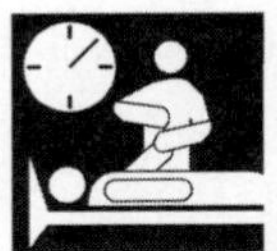

ONGOING ASSESSMENT AND TREATMENT

- Repeat the initial assessment every five minutes for a high priority, unstable patient and every 15 minutes for a low priority, stable patient.
  - Recheck your general impression of the patient.
  - Reassess mental status.
  - Reassess the ABCs.
  - Reprioritize as necessary.
- Repeat the physical exam every 10 to 15 minutes.
- Continue to provide reassurance and emotional support.

Remember that the following holds true no matter what your patient's problem: *Assess* your patient. *Intervene* with treatments as necessary. *Reassess* your patient to check the effectiveness of your treatment and to monitor changes in your patient's condition.

APPLICATION QUESTIONS

You may wish to use these questions to review your understanding of the chapter. For answers with page references, see Appendix 2.

1. You're managing a 16-year-old who fell off his skateboard. The patient has a large bruise on his head and he was "knocked out" for several minutes. You've completed the initial assessment and physical exam and treatments. Now you're waiting for the arrival of a Paramedic ambulance. The patient is awake but very confused and agitated. Which of the following vital signs—level of responsiveness, respiratory rate, skin condition, or blood pressure—would you consider the top priority for monitoring this patient? Why?
2. You're managing a patient who fell from a tree and sustained multiple injuries. You've completed your initial assessment and you're about to complete your physical exam, when your patient becomes silent. Up until this moment, she's been talking to you appropriately and in complete sentences. What should your next step be? Why?

CHAPTER 15 PATIENT HAND-OFF

FIRST RESPONSE

Jimmy Lee just started working as a volunteer firefighter. So it's the first time ever he's completed a patient hand-off to another EMS worker. Today he's responded to a 47-year-old patient who is complaining of chest pain. Patient assessment and treatment goes well, but as soon as he tries to turn over his patient to the transporting EMTs, he starts stepping on his tongue.

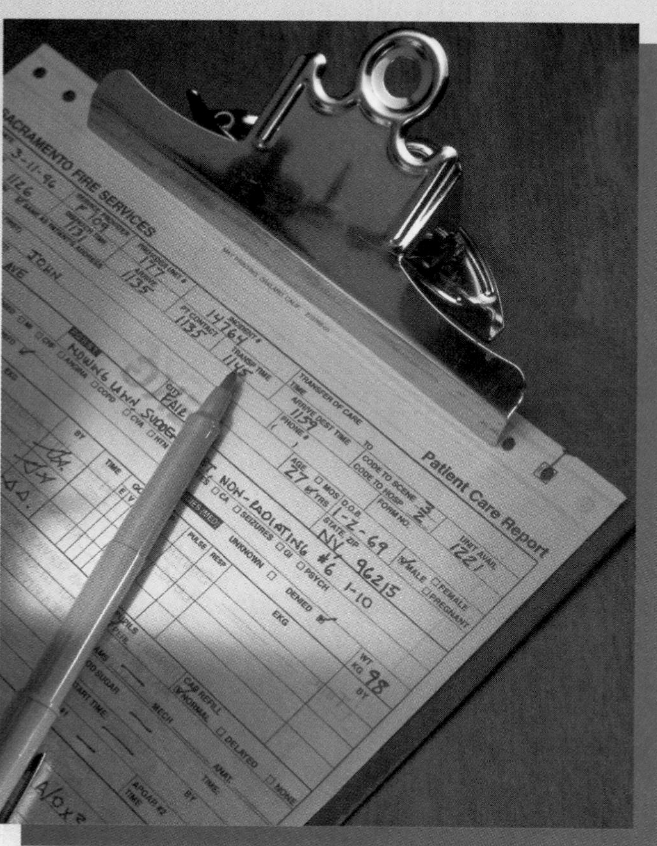

Jimmy Lee forgets to introduce the patient to the EMTs. All in all, his report is a mess, disorganized and rambling. To top that he nearly drops the patient when he helps to extricate her from her house. On the way to the station after the call, his partner says to him, "Despite your best efforts, Jimmy Lee, everything turned out fine!"

When Jimmy Lee reports to his supervisor, they go over the call. After a thorough review, Jimmy Lee sees the areas where he needs improvement. "I spent too much time getting information on operations the patient had 10 and 20 years ago. I also spent too much time on whether or not the patient was allergic to particular types of medications. When I was giving my report, the EMT I was speaking to must have just had enough. He brushed right past me and went directly to the patient. My feelings were hurt, but I understand where this guy is coming from. He needed concise information presented to him in an organized way. I'll work on it."

Before his next volunteer shift, Jimmy Lee develops a patient hand-off worksheet for himself. He feels that at least for a while he could use it to help him stay focused and organized.

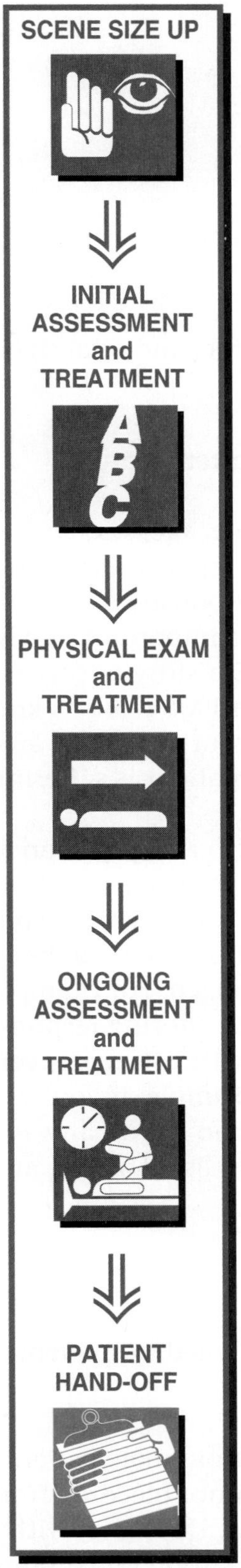

SCENE SIZE UP

INITIAL ASSESSMENT and TREATMENT

PHYSICAL EXAM and TREATMENT

ONGOING ASSESSMENT and TREATMENT

PATIENT HAND-OFF

LEARNING OBJECTIVES

Jimmy Lee's experience is not unusual. New First Responders often put so much effort into assessing and treating patients that patient hand-off often gets ignored. In fact this fifth and final step of the patient care plan is a crucial link in the patient's chain of survival.

By the end of the chapter, you should be able to:[†]

- 3-1.21 Describe the information included in the First Responder "hand-off" report. (pp. 193-194)
- * Identify the key components of a successful patient hand-off. (pp. 194-197)
- * Describe the role of the First Responder in patient extrication to the transporting ambulance. (p. 197)

OVERVIEW OF PATIENT HAND-OFF

Patient hand-off occurs when EMS workers with more training than you arrive at the scene to take over patient care. It's critical that you give them accurate and complete information. It's also critical that the transfer of care occurs in a way that avoids delays in patient treatment and transport. A successful patient hand-off allows the EMTs to build on your work rather than start over at square one. Patient hand-off includes:

- A patient report.
- Transfer of care from you to the transporting EMTs.
- Your assistance with extrication and transport.

PATIENT REPORT

The patient report sums up all the information you've gathered from the patient, the care you started, and the patient's response to that care. Good patient reports are organized, short, and to the point. They "paint a picture" of the emergency so that others can understand the patient's chief complaint, status, and condition. Your patient reports will vary. However, they should all include the following:

[†]Numbered objectives are from the 1995 U.S. DOT "First Responder: National Standard Curriculum." Asterisks indicate supplemental material.

- Patient's name, age, and sex.
- Chief complaint.
- Priority.
- Level of responsiveness.
- Airway and breathing status.
- Circulation status.
- Physical exam (SAMPLE history, head-to-toe, and vital signs).
- Interventions provided.
- Patient's response to interventions and current status.

Note that after reporting the patient's name, age, sex, and chief complaint, this format requires you to report on the patient's priority level (high or low), level of responsiveness, and airway, breathing, and circulation status. It is important to cover these indicators before the patient's SAMPLE history or physical findings so that other EMS workers know how sick or injured your patient is, and whether or not your patient is suffering from any life-threats.

End your report with an update on the patient's response to your treatments as well as the patient's current status. This last piece of information is critical because your patient's condition may have changed. For example, you may have arrived to find the patient with snoring respirations, which were then cleared up with a jaw-thrust maneuver.

Tailor your report to the emergency. For example, if you're fighting to establish an airway in a patient who has an airway full of blood, you may not get to all the items listed above, at least not at first.

STREET NOTES

When reporting your patient's SAMPLE history, give the "E" (events leading to the illness or injury) first. It'll make your report more logical. After the "E," go through the rest of the history.

THE ORAL REPORT

The following are illustrations of trauma and medical patient reports you would give orally:

> **Trauma report**: This is Anthony, a 35-year-old male patient complaining of neck and back pain and minor bleeding from the scalp. Anthony is a low priority patient. He is alert with a patent airway, unlabored breathing, and a strong radial pulse. His skin is pink, warm, and dry, and he has no major bleeding. The story here is that Anthony was pruning a tree when he

slipped and fell about 10 feet onto grass, landing on his back. He had no loss of consciousness. He states that he has left-sided neck pain and pain throughout his entire back. He has no medication allergies, takes no medications, and has no previous medical history. His last meal was about four hours ago. Our physical exam reveals only the neck and back pain. His vital signs are: alert mental status, a patent airway with unlabored breathing at 16 per minute, a strong pulse of 88, and normal skin signs. We didn't take a blood pressure. We're maintaining manual stabilization of the spine. Anthony appears to be resting comfortably, and there are no changes in his status.

Medical report: This is Gladys Maynard, a 74-year-old female patient with altered mental status. Gladys is a high priority patient who is unresponsive to any stimuli. We found her with snoring respirations at 6 per minute. After opening her airway, the snoring stopped and breathing became adequate. Gladys has a rapid, weak radial pulse. Her skin is pale, cool, and moist. The family states that Gladys was last seen about two hours ago when she left to take a nap. They found her in bed in her current state about 10 minutes ago. Gladys has no medication allergies. She takes medication for high blood pressure and diabetes. She last ate this morning. We found no signs of trauma in the physical exam. We have just started mouth-to-mask ventilation because her breathing rate began to fail. We have an oropharyngeal airway in place. She remains unresponsive.

Whenever you can, shorten your reports. Look at the medical report above. Notice that the details on the physical exam are very brief, pointing out only that no trauma was found. If you're short-handed and very busy managing a patient's airway and breathing, your report might sound like the following:

Shortened medical report: This is Gladys Maynard. She's a 74-year-old female with an altered mental status. Gladys is a high priority patient. She's unresponsive to any stimuli. We found her with snoring respirations at 6 per minute. She has a rapid, weak radial pulse. Her skin condition is pale, cool, and moist. Family states they found her in bed in her current state about 10 minutes ago. We've just started ventilating her because her respiratory rate began to fail. We have an oropharyngeal airway in place. She remains unresponsive.

Note that the short version focuses on the patient's chief complaint, ABCs, and the current treatment. Full reports are helpful. However, your primary responsibility is to support your patient's

ABCs. Incoming rescuers will always look for this information above all else.

THE WRITTEN REPORT

Many EMS systems require the First Responder to fill in a standard patient report. Even if your system doesn't require such a report, be sure to keep accurate and complete notes. Follow local protocols.

Your written report can provide what is called a "baseline" for measurements of your patient's condition. It's important for the EMTs and other medical personnel to know how the patient has changed since the onset of the emergency. Has the patient improved? Has the patient gotten worse? Has the patient responded to care? This information can help them determine the best possible patient care plan.

The patient report or your notes also could become a legal document. For example, if your patient was injured as a result of a crime or is involved in a lawsuit related to the emergency, you may be called to testify as a witness. Your accurate and complete documentation would be very valuable.

TRANSFER OF CARE

When you transfer responsibility for the care of your patient to personnel with more training, keep two issues in mind. One is a legal one. The other involves using strategies that help the patient feel supported and safe. Here's an example:

> You happened upon a traffic collision. Michael, your patient, is a 49-year-old who spun his car out on the wet roadway and slammed into an embankment. He's complaining of pain to his face, neck, and shoulder. He's also quite scared. As you hold manual stabilization of the spine, you talk to him softly to calm him. An ambulance and fire truck soon arrive at the scene. One of the EMTs asks, "What have you got?" You give her a patient report.
>
> After you read the EMT's name tag, you end your report by turning to the patient. "This is Patricia," you tell him. "She's an EMT with the ambulance service. She's going to check you out further." Michael looks at Patricia. He has confidence in you, but now he's being asked to trust another EMS provider. He's obviously not too sure about this.
>
> Hi, Michael," Patricia says. She smiles at the patient and moves in to complete an assessment. Michael relaxes. Patricia

turns to you. "Do you mind continuing to hold manual stabilization of the spine while I examine Michael?"

As mentioned above, there are legal obligations involved in patient hand-off. In order to avoid abandonment, it's important for you to be clear when you turn over patient care to another EMS worker. In the brief scenario above, this was done when the rescuers acknowledged each other, when the patient report was made, and when the EMT moved into the call and began to run it.

The second issue involves ways to help your patient feel supported and safe. Notice above that the incoming EMT is introduced and allowed to establish herself as the new caregiver. It's extremely important that your patients feel that the standard of care is being maintained. By introducing both rescuer and patient by name, you help the patient feel less alone. You also send a clear message that the patient's feelings matter and that you care enough to make the transfer go smoothly.

PATIENT EXTRICATION

It may be necessary to extricate a patient from a collapsed structure or other hazardous environment before emergency care can be provided. (See Chapter 8 "Scene Size-up.") However, extrication usually occurs after a patient has been assessed, treated, and *packaged* (fitted in scoop stretcher, on a backboard, or on a wheeled stretcher; see Figure 15-1). The role of the First Responder is to assist other rescuers as needed. Remember that clear communication is the key to success. You may want to refer to Chapter 6 "Lifting and Moving" for specific techniques.

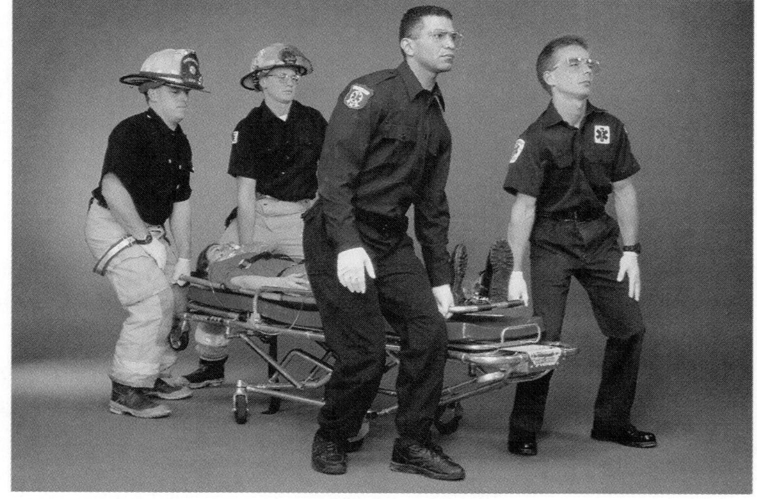

Figure 15-1
Extrication usually occurs after a patient has been assessed, treated, and packaged.

CONCLUSION

Patient hand-off is the last crucial step to managing patients in the field. It's critical for accurate information to be transmitted to other rescuers. It's also important that a smooth transfer of care occurs so that there are no delays in treatment or transport. The key to successful patient hand-off is to allow the incoming EMS rescuers to build on your work. By accomplishing this, you will have a direct positive impact on the outcome of the patients in your EMS system. In summary:

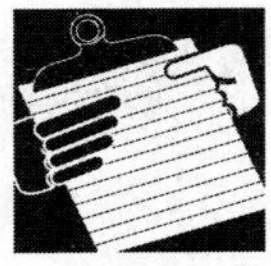

PATIENT HAND-OFF

- Give a patient report. Include:
  - Patient's name, age, and sex.
  - Chief complaint.
  - Priority.
  - Level of responsiveness.
  - Airway and breathing status.
  - Circulation status.
  - Physical exam (SAMPLE history, head-to-toe, and vital signs).
  - Interventions provided.
  - Patient's response to interventions and current status.
- Conduct the transfer of care.
- Provide assistance in extrication and transport.

APPLICATION QUESTIONS

You may wish to use these questions to review your understanding of the chapter. For answers with page references, see Appendix 2.

1. Reorganize the following patient report so that it will provide relevant information in an orderly way and get to the point quickly.

   Henry was stepping up onto the curb when he fell forward, striking his head and chest on the sidewalk. He has a patent airway and normal, unlabored breathing. He had no loss of consciousness. He had a large bruise to his forehead and abrasions to his chest and hands. He appears to be awake and alert. He has no allergies to medications. His chief complaint is pain to his head, chest, and hands. He is a low priority patient, 87 years old, who takes medication for high blood pressure, arthritis, and Parkinson's disease. He has had a stroke and a heart attack in the past year. Henry last ate this morning. We are holding manual stabilization of his spine and have bandaged his abrasions.

2. You are managing a trauma patient who has an airway full of blood due to massive injuries to her mouth. You are busily suctioning the airway when other rescuers arrive. You give them a quick patient report, describing mechanism of injury and the patient's mental status and the status of airway, breathing, and circulation. One of the rescuers asks you why you can't give him a rundown on the patient's injuries, of which there are many. What is your response to him?

SECTION 3 FIRST RESPONDER EMERGENCY CARE PLANS

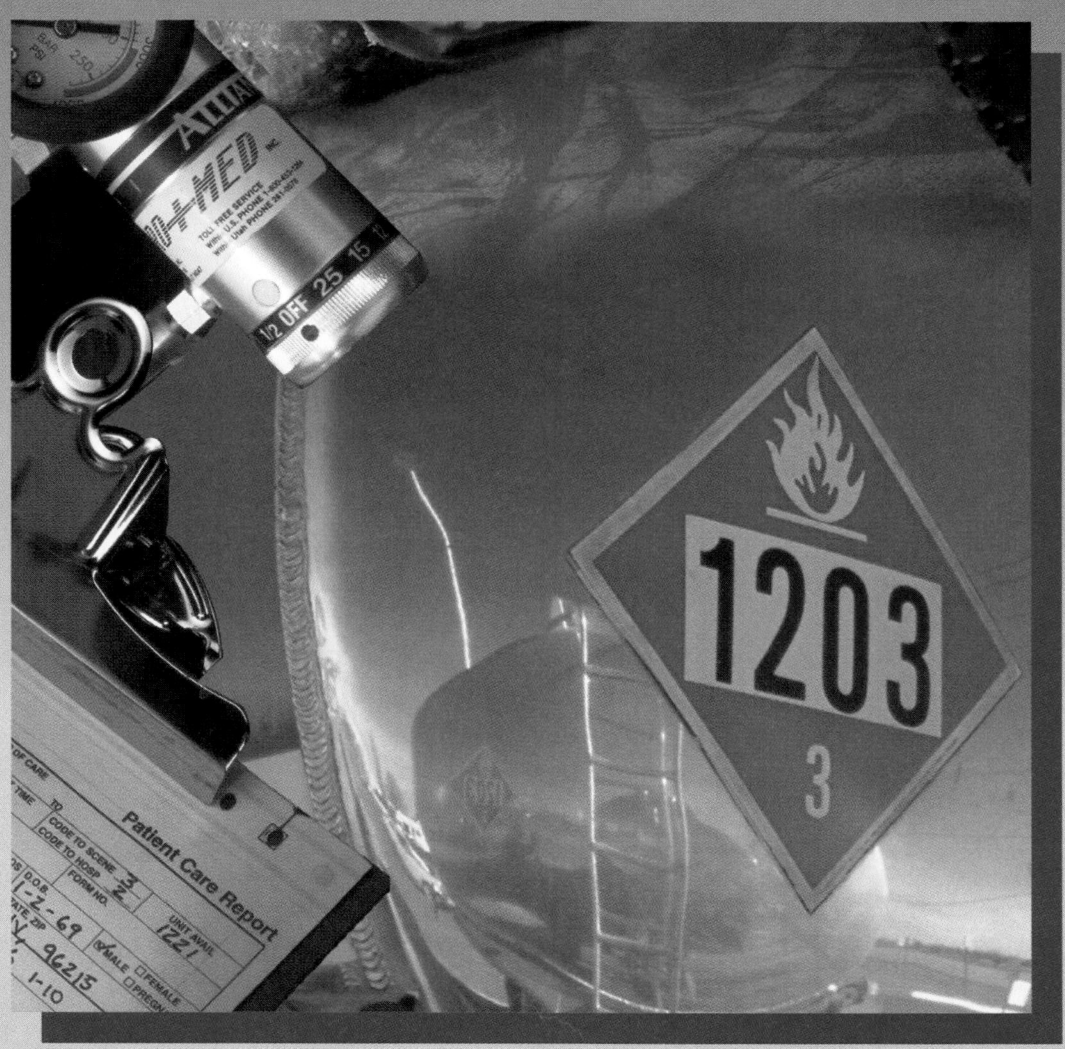

Should I figure out why a patient has a headache or stomach pain? How should I treat a patient who fell off a roof? Will I know what to do, when to do it, or if I'm doing it right? Each chapter in Section 3 provides you with an overview of a specific patient complaint. Each overview is then followed by an "Emergency Care Plan" which shows how to apply your skills to manage the patient in an organized way. Note that both the medical and trauma parts of this section begin with an introductory chapter that highlights the important aspects of managing either type of patient.

CHAPTER 16 OVERVIEW TO MANAGING MEDICAL PATIENTS

FIRST RESPONSE

Patty has been a First Responder at a large amusement park for three years. She's been training Eric for the past 10 days. During their first set of shifts, Patty allowed Erik to observe medical calls. Today it's time for Eric to take a turn managing a patient by himself. So when dispatch calls after lunch, Patty and Eric respond. They take the electric cart to the Ferris wheel where an elderly patient is complaining of weakness and dizziness. EMS has been notified and is on the way.

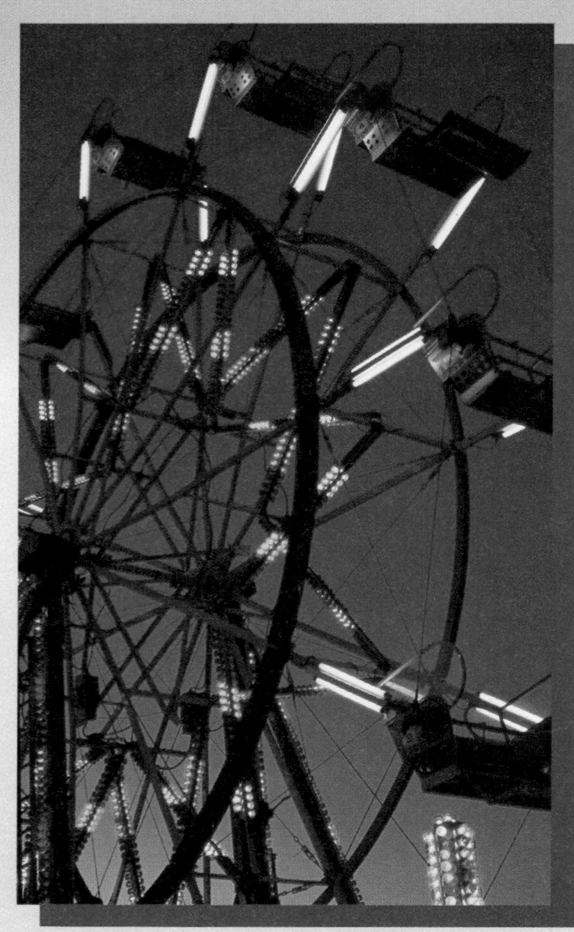

After making sure the scene is safe, Eric puts on a pair of latex gloves. Then he approaches the patient. He forms a general impression and begins the initial assessment and treatment. As he evaluates his patient's mental status, he starts to plan for the head-to-toe exam. Distracted by this leap-frog thinking, he doesn't hear his patient say that she feels as if she's going to pass out.

Flustered and confused, Eric begins to panic. "She said she's dizzy? Weak? What's going on with her?" Suddenly he realizes, "I have no idea!" He starts to ask the patient every question that pops into his head, hoping that one will give him the clue he needs to get back on track. Just as he feels the whole call slip away ("What do I do now?"), Patty puts her hand on his shoulder.

"Let's have her lie down, Eric. She says she's going to pass out and she looks pale to me."

Together Patty and Eric help the patient to the ground. Without missing a beat, Patty moves in. She introduces herself to the patient and performs an initial assessment. She directs Eric to apply high-flow oxygen. Then she begins the physical exam, recording a SAMPLE history, examining the patient from head to toe, and taking vital signs.

By now the patient is feeling better. When the EMT-Paramedics arrive, Patty quickly performs a patient hand-off.

LEARNING OBJECTIVES

Eric's story is not unusual. Emergency care of patients in the field can be overwhelming at first. Medical patients especially can appear to have a host of complaints, old and new. Whatever the problem, stick to the five-step plan you studied in Section 2 of this book.

In this chapter, you'll be introduced to a general emergency care plan for medical patients. In Chapters 17 to 25, you'll learn how to manage specific medical emergencies.

By the end of the chapter, you should be able to:†

- 5-1.1 Identify the patient who presents with a general medical complaint. (pp. 203-205)
- 5-1.2 Explain the steps in providing emergency medical care to a patient with a general medical complaint. (pp. 204-210)

* Discuss the medical complaints that most commonly occur in the out-of-hospital setting. (pp. 203-204)

WHAT IS A MEDICAL COMPLAINT?

Simply, a **medical complaint** is any complaint that isn't caused by trauma. Will you have more medical patients than trauma patients? That depends on the region in which you work. You'll probably run more medical calls in areas with large retirement communities. You'll probably run more trauma calls in rural, industrial, or high-density urban areas.

The types of medical calls you'll run also will vary. For example, in areas with many elderly people you'll see more chest-pain and shortness-of-breath calls. Both of these problems are symptoms of heart and lung diseases, which commonly afflict the elderly.

In general, some of the most common medical complaints include:

- Chest pain.
- Shortness of breath.
- Altered mental status.
- Abdominal pain.
- Poisoning and overdose.

---

†Numbered objectives are from the 1995 U.S. DOT "First Responder: National Standard Curriculum." Asterisks indicate supplemental material.

- Allergic reactions.
- Dizziness and fainting.
- Heat and cold emergencies.

Notice that this list does not include names of diseases. Your training isn't designed to teach you how to tell the difference between heart attack and heartburn, for example. A physician must do that. Your job is to recognize your patient's chest pain and then plan for the worst case scenario. By planning for the worst,

EMERGENCY CARE PLAN | PATIENTS WITH MEDICAL COMPLAINTS

PRIORITIES

Your top priorities as a First Responder are to assure the safety of all those on scene and to assess and treat your patient for any life-threats. Note that a high priority medical patient may not appear to be a high priority at first. For example, an elderly patient with a chief complaint of "I don't feel well" may already be suffering from shock. Be alert. Don't take medical patients for granted. Always assess your patient fully for life-threats, no matter what the complaint.

Top priorities for managing all medical patients include:

- Early recognition of airway, breathing, and circulation problems.
- Early activation of the EMS system.
- Aggressive treatment for airway, breathing, and circulation problems.
- Continuous reassessment.
- Accurate patient histories and physical exams.

PATIENT CARE APPROACH

Medical patients may feel varying degrees of panic, denial, pain, and mistrust. However, the patient with a chronic illness may be just as upset as the patient with an acute problem. To

you'll be prepared if the patient actually does have a heart attack. If it turns out to be only heartburn, no harm done.

The patient in the scenario at the beginning of the chapter was both weak and dizzy. These two symptoms can be caused by any number of chronic conditions. They also can be caused by an **acute** (sudden onset) **problem** such as stroke or heart attack. However, the First Responder in the scenario didn't try to figure out which is which. She did her job by treating the symptoms until more highly trained EMS personnel could take over care.

help you determine the best patient care approach, ask these questions:

- What does my patient think and feel?
- What does my patient need?
- What do I need to get done as a First Responder?

While it's critical to care for the patient's physical problems, don't forget to manage the patient's emotional state as well. A gentle, empathetic approach will go a long way toward comforting your patient. It'll also encourage the patient to comply with your emergency care plan.

DANGER SIGNS

Always "go back to home base" when in doubt. Constantly reassess your patient's level of responsiveness, airway, breathing, and circulation. They'll help you find out if the patient is critical and a high priority. Remember, the following holds true no matter what your patient's problem:

- *Assess* your patient.
- *Intervene* with treatments as necessary.
- *Reassess* your patient to check the effectiveness of your interventions and to monitor changes in your patient's condition.

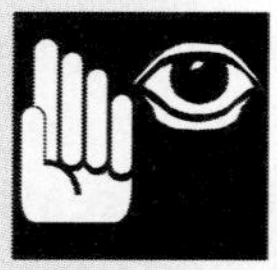

SCENE SIZE-UP

1. **ASSESS SCENE SAFETY.** Unsafe scenes are often associated with trauma calls, such as car crashes. But medical calls also can be hazardous. A patient may be violent, for example. Remember, if the scene isn't safe, either make it safe or stay clear. Be sure to protect yourself.

   Take all BSI precautions now. All body fluids carry a risk of infection. That includes blood, urine, feces, droplets from a sneeze, and so on. It's best to go into a call with your personal protective equipment on (Figure 16-1).

2. **DETERMINE NATURE OF ILLNESS.** What is the nature of your patient's illness? What is the who, what, when, where, why, and how of the problem? Look for clues at the scene such as hospital beds, home oxygen, medications, and bottles of alcohol.

   If it hasn't already been done, activate the EMS system as soon as you know the nature of illness and have some idea about its seriousness.

3. **TRIAGE THE PATIENT.** Even medical calls can have more than one patient. Hazardous materials emergencies and drug overdoses are examples. Always rule out this possibility, or be prepared to triage.

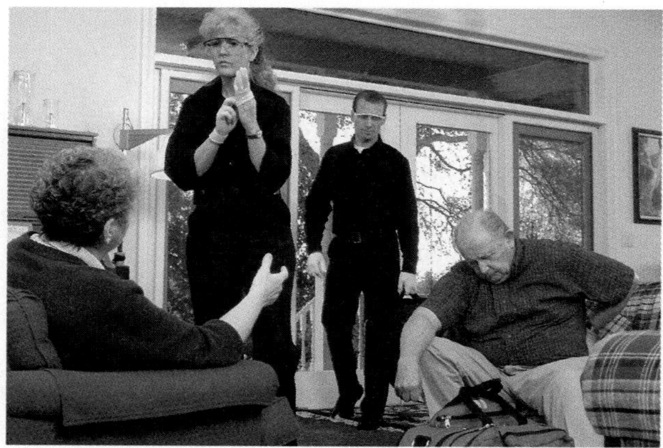

Figure 16-1
During scene size-up, take BSI precautions.

4. **DETERMINE ACCESS AND EXTRICATION NEEDS.** Trying to provide rescue breathing for a patient who has fallen down between a waterbed and a wall can be daunting. Be aware of access and extrication issues even on the most basic of medical calls.

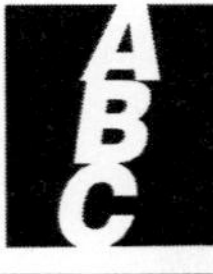

INITIAL ASSESSMENT AND TREATMENT

1. **FORM A GENERAL IMPRESSION.** Determine the patient's sex and approximate his or her age. What is the patient's level of distress? Posture and position will tell you a lot about it. You also may see clues (labored breathing, seizures, etc.) to your patient's chief complaint at this point.

2. **CHECK MENTAL STATUS.** This is one of the most sensitive indicators of your patient's overall status. Use the mnemonic AVPU to help you estimate level of responsiveness. Remember, AVPU stands for alert, verbal, painful, and unresponsive.

3. **ASSESS THE ABCs.**

   - **Airway.** Is the airway open? If it isn't, open it. Keep in mind that medical patients can faint and bang their heads too. Use the jaw-thrust maneuver if there's any indication of trauma.

   - **Breathing.** Is the patient breathing? Is breathing adequate? Is it labored? If your patient needs it, provide rescue breathing or oxygen therapy now.

   - **Circulation.** Does the patient have a pulse? Is it weak, rapid, or slow? At this time, you're interested in the presence or absence of a pulse, and whether or not the patient's pulse indicates shock. If your patient needs it, perform CPR now.

     Control any major external bleeding at this time. Medical patients may have open wounds. They also may have major bleeding from the rectum or mouth caused by a medical condition.

     What is the patient's skin condition (Figure 16-2)? Observe color. Check temperature and moisture. Pale or

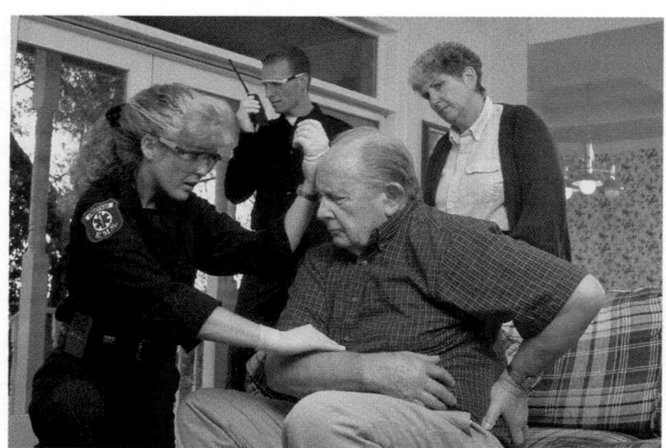

Figure 16-2
Checking skin condition is part of the initial assessment.

ashy skin that is cool and wet may indicate shock. Cyanosis can indicate the patient is not getting enough oxygen.

4. **DETERMINE PRIORITY.** Is the patient a high or low priority? It's critical that you determine priority early in the call. It will influence your assessments, treatment, and patient hand-off report. Make certain that EMS has been activated, if it hasn't been done already.

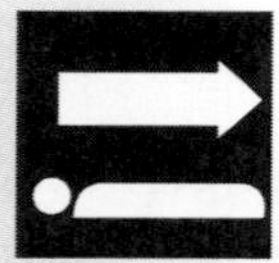

PHYSICAL EXAM AND TREATMENT

1. **GATHER A *SAMPLE* HISTORY.** Record your patient's history at this time. It tends to be more important for a medical patient than for a trauma patient, since it often provides clues specific to the chief complaint.

(S)igns and symptoms? Use the PQRST mnemonic as a way to describe the patient's pain. Remember, PQRST stands for provocation, quality, region and radiation, severity, and time.

(A)llergies? In particular, find out whether or not your patient has any allergies to medications or other substances.

(M)edications? Gather up all medications. They provide valuable insight into the medical patient's problem. Note that it's common for elderly patients to have several "generations" of medications on their shelves. They may have expired medications and ones they're no longer taking. There may be medicines that belong to a deceased spouse.

(P)ertinent past history? Ask if the patient has recently seen a doctor or if he or she has recently been ill or injured. Be sure to gather information that is relevant to the patient's complaint.

(L)ast oral intake? This is especially important if your patient is a diabetic.

(E)vents leading to the illness? Find out what the patient was doing when the problem started.

2. **PERFORM A HEAD-TO-TOE EXAM.** Be organized. Look for signs that will assist you in managing the patient with a medical complaint (Figure 16-3). Also remember to look for a Medic Alert medallion.

3. **TAKE VITAL SIGNS.** Organize vital signs the same way you did in the initial assessment. The difference here is that you need to get more exact measurements. Include level of responsiveness, airway, breathing, pulse, skin, and blood pressure. Recall that blood pressure is the least important of all. Instead depend on level of responsiveness and the ABCs to determine your patient's status.

4. **PROVIDE TREATMENT AS NEEDED** After you've completed the SAMPLE history, the head-to-toe exam, and vital signs, take time to perform any treatments the patient needs. By and large, these are treatments for non-life-threatening problems, such as applying an ice pack to a swollen ankle.

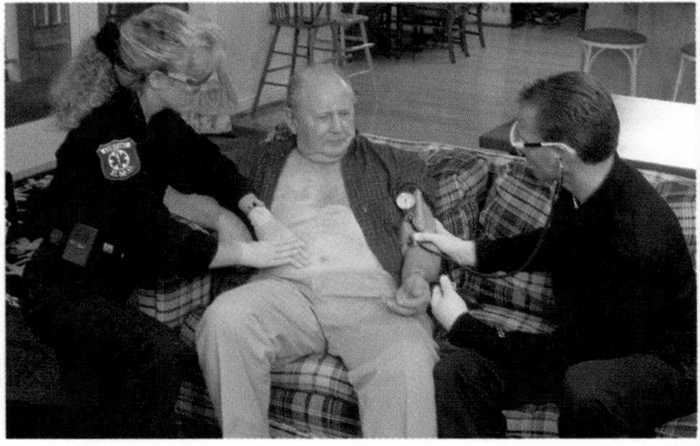

Figure 16-3
During the physical exam, check for signs related to the patient's chief complaint.

ONGOING ASSESSMENT AND TREATMENT

1. **REPEAT THE INITIAL ASSESSMENT.** Repeat it every five minutes for a high priority, unstable patient and every 15 minutes for a low priority, stable patient. Also repeat it if the patient has any significant status change and after any critical intervention, such as rescue breathing. Be sure to constantly assess medical patients who have complaints that can lead to life-threatening problems, such as chest pain, shortness of breath, and altered mental status.

2. **REPEAT THE PHYSICAL EXAM.** Repeat it every 10 to 15 minutes (Figure 16-4). Focus on the patient's chief complaint, and reconfirm important elements of the patient's SAMPLE history. The head-to-toe exam also should focus on any important findings from your original exam. Finally, check your interventions to confirm that they're still effective.

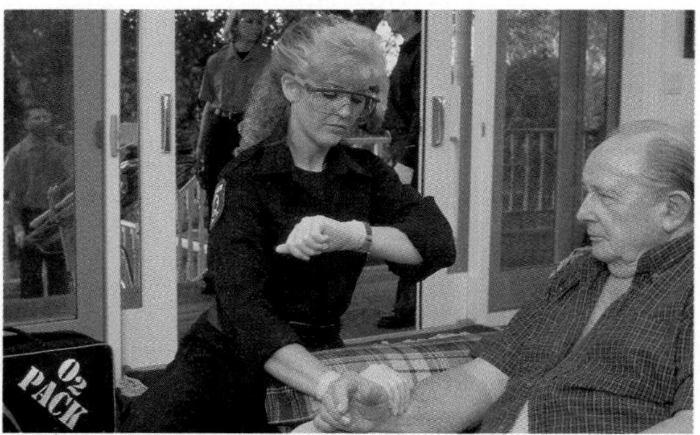

Figure 16-4
Continue to monitor the patient's vital signs during ongoing assessment.

CONCLUSION

It can be overwhelming when you first begin to manage patients in the field. Medical patients in particular can present with a host of complaints. Often you'll need to recognize the patient's chronic problem before you can understand what the current medical problem is.

3. **PROVIDE REASSURANCE.** Don't forget to continually reassure your patient. Providing emotional support is essential to your patient feeling well cared for.

PATIENT HAND-OFF

1. **GIVE A PATIENT REPORT.** Report both orally and in writing (Figure 16-5). Include the patient's name, age, and sex, chief complaint, priority, vital signs, the medical history, interventions provided and the patient's response to those interventions, and the patient's current status.

2. **CONDUCT THE TRANSFER OF CARE.** Be clear about it. Avoid any reduction in the standard of care. Avoid any delays in care and transport.

3. **ASSIST IN EXTRICATION AND TRANSPORT.**

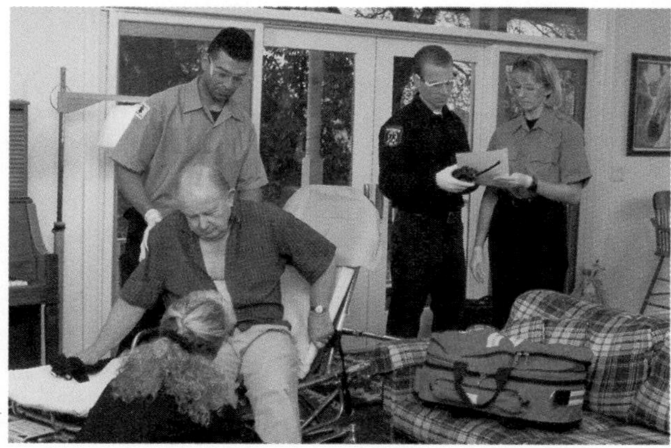

Figure 16-5
Make your patient report both orally and in writing.

Stick to the five-step plan described in Section II of this book and outlined here. Never lose sight of what your job as a First Responder is: to maintain scene safety, assess and treat life-threats, and continue to assess and treat the patient until other EMS workers with more training take over care.

KEY TERMS

You may wish to use this list to review your understanding of key terms introduced in the chapter.

acute problem a medical problem with a sudden onset.

medical complaint a complaint caused by a disease process or any complaint not caused by trauma.

APPLICATION QUESTIONS

You may wish to use these questions to review your understanding of the chapter. For answers with page references, see Appendix 2.

1. You've responded to a 76-year-old female patient who is complaining of acute chest pain. Organize the following tasks in the order in which you should complete them for this patient.

   - Gather a SAMPLE history.
   - Check the scene to see if it's safe.
   - Assess her mental status.
   - Take BSI precautions.
   - Complete a head-to-toe exam.
   - Repeat the initial assessment.
   - Check her airway, breathing, and circulation status, and apply oxygen at this time.
   - Complete a patient hand-off.
   - Form a general impression of the patient.
   - Take vital signs.

2. You responded to a 29-year-old male with shortness of breath. You have completed your patient's initial assessment and treatment, physical exam and treatment, and the patient is resting in a position of comfort. Suddenly you notice that his mental status appears to have changed. What is your very next task?

CHAPTER 17 CHEST PAIN

FIRST RESPONSE

Deanna has just arrived home from work when the phone rings. It's her neighbor, Mrs. Rosen. Aware that Deanna is a volunteer First Responder with the fire department, Mrs. Rosen asks, "Could you come over to see my husband? He's had pain in his chest since lunch, and he won't let me call the doctor. He's being a stubborn, old fool."

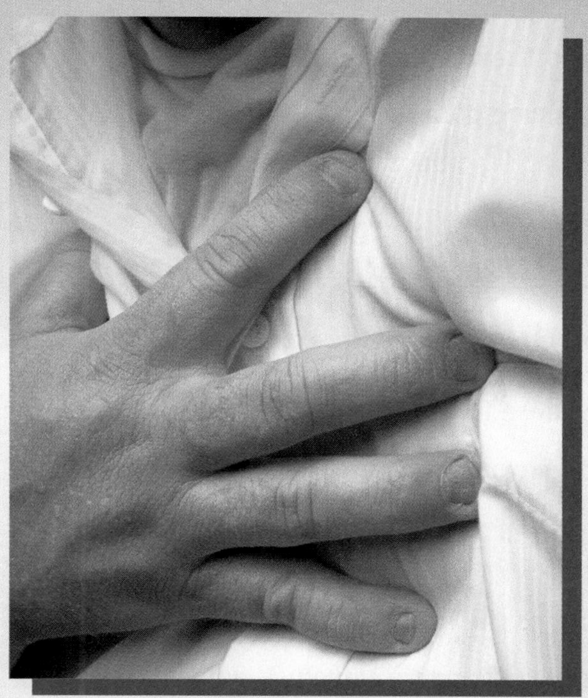

As soon as Deanna sees Mr. Rosen, she realizes he's in trouble. Deanna notes his distressed look and pale skin. Mr. Rosen," she says to him, "are you still having chest pain?"

"Just a little indigestion, I think," he replies. He seems annoyed by all the attention he's getting. "Look, I'm really fine. If I don't feel better in a bit, I'll go see my doctor."

Moments later Mr. Rosen breaks out into a cold sweat. Deanna immediately calls 9-1-1 and then returns to Mr. Rosen's side. As she begins the initial assessment, Mr. Rosen becomes unresponsive, breathless, and pulseless.

Deanna begins CPR as the anguished Mrs. Rosen looks on. Within minutes First Responders from Deanna's fire house arrive. They apply an automatic defibrillator and shock Mr. Rosen three times. The third shock does the trick. "I've got a carotid pulse," calls out one of the First Responders.

By the time the Paramedics arrive, Mr. Rosen has regained consciousness. Though still not speaking, he's awake. Soon he's rushed to the hospital, where tests will show he's had a major heart attack.

Mr. Rosen will spend several days in the hospital. The heart attack left permanent damage to his heart. Despite this, Mr. Rosen is glad to be alive, and he credits both his wife and Deanna both for saving him. He's especially grateful to Deanna for sticking with him even when he tried to send her packing.

LEARNING OBJECTIVES

Patients with chest pain typically wait several hours before accessing the EMS system. This delay often proves fatal. Heart disease is the number-one cause of death in the U.S. The American Heart Association reports that hundreds of thousands of heart disease patients die from heart attacks every year and most of them die before they ever reach a hospital. The key to helping patients survive a heart attack is early recognition and aggressive treatment.

Now is a good time to review the circulatory system as described in Chapter 4.

***By the end of the chapter, you should be able to:*†**

* List the different causes of chest pain. (pp. 214-215)
* Define heart attack. (p. 215)
* List the warning signs of heart attack. (pp. 216-217)
* Describe an emergency care plan for assessing and treating the patient with chest pain. (pp. 218-221)

CAUSES OF CHEST PAIN

It's natural to think of all chest pain as the pain of a heart attack. In fact there are many reasons why a patient experiences chest pain. Chest pain can be caused by:

- Injuries to the ribs and **intercostal muscles** (muscles between the ribs).
- Lung infections (*pneumonia*).
- Infections of the lining of the lungs (*pleurisy*).
- Blood clots in the lungs (*pulmonary embolus*).
- Infections of the sac surrounding the heart (*pericarditis*).
- A partial or total collapse of the lung (*pneumothorax*).
- Heartburn.
- Problems associated with abdominal organs such as the gall bladder.
- Heart attack.

---

†Asterisks indicate material supplemental to the 1995 U.S. DOT "First Responder: National Standard Curriculum."

Many of the conditions listed above can mimic the signs and symptoms of heart attack. Even so, your job as a First Responder is to identify the chest pain and treat the patient, not to diagnose the exact cause. Leave it to the physician to make the specific diagnosis.

HEART ATTACK

Just like the rest of the body, the heart needs a constant supply of oxygen-rich blood in order to survive and function properly. The **coronary arteries** supply the heart with blood. These arteries can become narrowed or blocked by a buildup of fatty substances called *plaque*. When this occurs, oxygenated blood can't get to the heart and the patient experiences chest pain.

Chest pain caused by lack of oxygen to the heart is called **angina pectoris**. Stopping physical exertion or stress often relieves this pain. **Heart attack** occurs when the heart muscle is so deprived of oxygen that it actually dies. It isn't necessary for you to distinguish between angina and heart attack in the field. There's no way for you to do so.

Sudden death from heart attack most often is caused by disturbances in the electrical conduction system of the heart.

Caution *Unless your patient is suffering from an obvious external injury to the chest, always consider any patient with chest pain to be a possible heart-attack victim until proven otherwise.*

The muscle of the heart is called the **myocardium**. A simple rule to remember when managing the possible heart-attack patient is this:

Time = myocardium

The longer a clot blocks the blood supply to the myocardium, the greater the chance of permanent damage to the heart. Recall from above that many heart-attack victims will wait several hours after signs and symptoms occur before seeking medical care. This places the heart-attack victim squarely behind the eight ball. In those few precious hours, the patient's heart muscle is dying and the risk of sudden death is great.

Signs and symptoms of heart attack include (Figure 17-1):

- Chest pain or pressure. This is often described as a constant, dull pain or pressure located in the center of the chest, moderate to severe in intensity, often radiating to the jaw, shoulder, or arm (most commonly to the left arm).

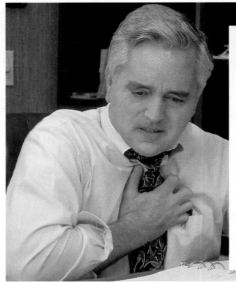

• Squeezing, dull pressure in chest, commonly radiating down arms or up to jaw.

• Abnormal pulse.
• Stomachache.

Figure 17-1
A medical patient may complain of chest pain or pressure.

EMERGENCY CARE PLAN | PATIENTS WITH CHEST PAIN

PRIORITIES

Your top priorities in caring for a patient with chest pain are:

- Early recognition of the signs and symptoms of chest pain.
- Early activation of the EMS system.
- Assurance of a patent airway and adequacy of breathing and circulation. If possible, administer oxygen.
- Continuous reassessment.

PATIENT CARE APPROACH

As you saw in the scenario at the beginning of the chapter, patients with chest pain often deny it. Approach these patients in a calm, supportive, and reassuring manner. To help reduce the

- Jaw, neck, shoulder pain.
- Shortness of breath.
- Dizziness or fainting episodes.
- Heart *palpitations* (abnormally rapid throbbing or fluttering).
- Nausea and vomiting.
- Sudden onset of sweatiness.
- Shock.
- Epigastric (between the navel and sternum) pain.
- Anxiety, irritability, feelings of impending doom.

strain on the heart, attempt to reduce the patient's anxiety as much as possible. Don't allow unnecessary movement. Place the patient in a position of comfort, which will likely be a sitting or semi-reclined position.

■ *DANGER SIGNS*

Chest-pain patients who are experiencing a heart attack or other cardiac emergency can worsen rapidly. Be on the lookout for any sudden changes in mental status and level of distress. Be especially alert to any changes in airway, breathing, or circulation status. Poor skin condition is often a sign of chest pain in a patient who is denying it. If your patient begins to describe any change in symptoms or says something like "I think I'm going to die," take it seriously.

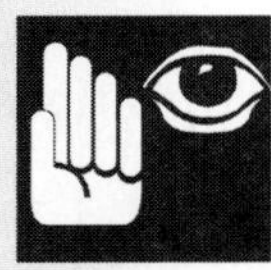

SCENE SIZE-UP

1. **ASSESS SCENE SAFETY.** Is the scene safe to enter? Protect yourself, and take all BSI precautions now.

2. **DETERMINE THE NATURE OF ILLNESS.** Once you've determined that your patient is complaining of chest pain, activate the EMS system if someone hasn't already done so.

3. **TRIAGE THE PATIENT.** How ill does the patient appear to be? Are the proper resources responding to the call?

4. **DETERMINE ACCESS OR EXTRICATION NEEDS.** Are there problems preventing you from getting to the patient? Will there be problems getting the patient to an ambulance?

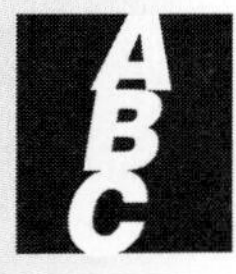

INITIAL ASSESSMENT AND TREATMENT

1. **FORM A GENERAL IMPRESSION.** What is the patient's age and sex? Are there any clues to help you understand the patient's chief complaint? What is the patient's body position? Is the patient clutching his or her chest? Does the patient appear anxious? What is the patient's overall level of distress?

2. **CHECK MENTAL STATUS.** Is the patient awake and answering all questions appropriately? Does the patient answer and respond to your questions and verbal commands? If the patient is showing signs of an altered mental status, it may be due to **hypoxia** (too little oxygen in the patient's blood). If you're allowed to do so, administer high flow oxygen.

3. **ASSESS THE ABCs.**

   - Airway. Is the airway open and clear? If necessary, open the airway.

- **Breathing.** Is your patient breathing? Is your patient's rate and quality of breathing adequate? Is the breathing labored? Provide your patient with ventilations if necessary. All chest-pain and shortness-of-breath patients should receive high-flow oxygen by nonrebreather mask.

- **Circulation.** Does your patient have a pulse? If not, start CPR. Be sure advanced life support (ALS) personnel are being dispatched to the scene. If you're equipped and trained to use an *automated external defibrillator (AED)*, attach it to the patient to determine if he or she qualifies for defibrillation. Follow all local protocols on the use of this equipment!

  If the patient has a pulse, is it too fast, slow, or weak? What is the condition of your patient's skin? Is it cool, pale, or sweaty? Treat for shock as necessary.

4. **DETERMINE PRIORITY.** All chest-pain patients should be considered high priority.

PHYSICAL EXAM AND TREATMENT

1. **GATHER A *SAMPLE* HISTORY.**

(S)igns and symptoms? Does the patient have chest pain? Use the PQRST mnemonic as a way to describe it. Are there any other signs or symptoms such as shortness of breath, dizziness, nausea/vomiting, heart palpitations?

(A)llergies? What medications is the patient allergic to?

(M)edications? What prescription medications does your patient take? Patients with heart problems also may take medications to control high blood pressure. Some patients have been directed by their physician to take nitroglycerin in case of chest pain. It's possible that the patient may want to take this medication during your care. Encourage him or her to take it as prescribed, but you are not allowed to administer it.

(P)ertinent past history? Has the patient been diagnosed with a heart problem? Does the patient have a history of heart attack? Has the patient ever had this kind of episode before? When was the last time? What was done to treat it?

(L)ast oral intake? How long ago did the patient eat? Was it anything unusual? Could this food have caused an upset stomach and heartburn?

(E)vents leading to the chest pain? What was your patient doing when the chest pain began?

2. **PERFORM A HEAD-TO-TOE EXAM.** Focus on the neck, chest, and abdomen. Look for accessory muscle use in the neck. Palpate and examine the chest. Does the patient's chest hurt when you touch it? Are there any surgical scars that indicate previous heart surgery? Is there any accessory muscle use in the chest? Palpate and examine the abdomen.

3. **TAKE VITAL SIGNS.** Check your patient's level of responsiveness. Is the airway open? What is the respiratory rate and quality, pulse rate and quality, skin condition, and blood pressure (if you're equipped)? A patient having a heart attack may be in shock if the heart is damaged. So look for signs of shock.

4. **PROVIDE TREATMENT AS NEEDED.** Does your patient need to be repositioned? Have you determined that your patient is in shock and requires treatment?

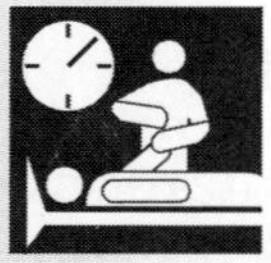

ONGOING ASSESSMENT AND TREATMENT

1. **REPEAT THE INITIAL ASSESSMENT.** Remember that the status of chest-pain patients can change rapidly. Repeat this assessment every five minutes, if there are changes in your patient's status and after critical interventions.

2. **REPEAT THE PHYSICAL EXAM.** Is your patient's chest pain changing? Focus on the pain complaint. Reconfirm other pertinent elements of the patient's medical history.

3. **PROVIDE REASSURANCE.** Chest-pain patients can be quite anxious. Calm and reassure them. This actually can reduce the stress on their hearts.

PATIENT HAND-OFF

1. **GIVE A PATIENT REPORT.** Deanna, the First Responder in the scenario at the beginning of the chapter, may have given the following priority report to the First Responders who took over care of her patient.

   Mr. Rosen is 65 years old and has been pulseless for the past three to four minutes. He became unresponsive and pulseless in my presence. I immediately began CPR. I've been ventilating him with good success with a pocket face mask. Prior to this he was complaining of chest pain for several hours. I arrived to find him quite pale and distressed. Mr. Rosen has had previous heart attacks.

2. **CONDUCT THE TRANSFER OF CARE.**

3. **ASSIST IN EXTRICATION AND TRANSPORT.** Chest-pain patients should not walk or move around unnecessarily. Be as gentle and reassuring as possible during extrication and transport. It's often harmful to transport these patients with lights and sirens, since it increases their anxiety.

CONCLUSION

Chest pain is a frequently encountered medical complaint in the out-of-hospital setting. As a First Responder, you can truly make a difference between life and death through early recognition and prompt medical care of these patients.

KEY TERMS

You may wish to use this list to review your understanding of key terms introduced in the chapter.

angina pectoris chest pain caused by a deficiency of oxygen to the heart.

coronary arteries arteries that supply blood to the myocardium of the heart; reduced blood flow through these arteries can cause angina pectoris.

heart attack heart muscle death caused by blockage of one or more of the coronary arteries.

hypoxia condition caused by a deficiency of oxygen.

intercostal muscles muscles between the ribs.

myocardium heart muscle.

APPLICATION QUESTIONS

You may wish to use these questions to review your understanding of the chapter. For answers with page references, see Appendix 2.

1. You've been called to care for an elderly man who has collapsed on a golf course. The patient is awake and has a pulse that is extremely fast. He's sweaty and states that he has chest pain. How will you treat this patient?
2. You're doing an assessment on a 56-year-old female coworker with chest pain and shortness of breath. She has nitroglycerin prescribed to her by her physician. She asks you to tell her if she should take it or not. What is your reply?

CHAPTER 18 SHORTNESS OF BREATH

FIRST RESPONSE

It's Ed's first month on the job and he and his partner, Krista, have been called to a "female feeling ill." They enter the apartment and find the patient in a bedroom surrounded by concerned family and friends. Krista speaks to relatives as Ed approaches the patient.

"What's going on today?" Ed asks. Ed finds Lucille, a 72-year-old patient, lying in bed. He immediately sees the telltale coil of oxygen tubing, which probably means Lucille has chronic lung disease. Lucille appears tired. Her eyes are closed, and she's able to muster only a weak one- or two-word reply to Ed's questions. She has a pale, dusky appearance. Her breathing rate is only about 20 times per minute, but it appears quite labored. "Don't worry, Lucille," Ed says, "we're going to help you."

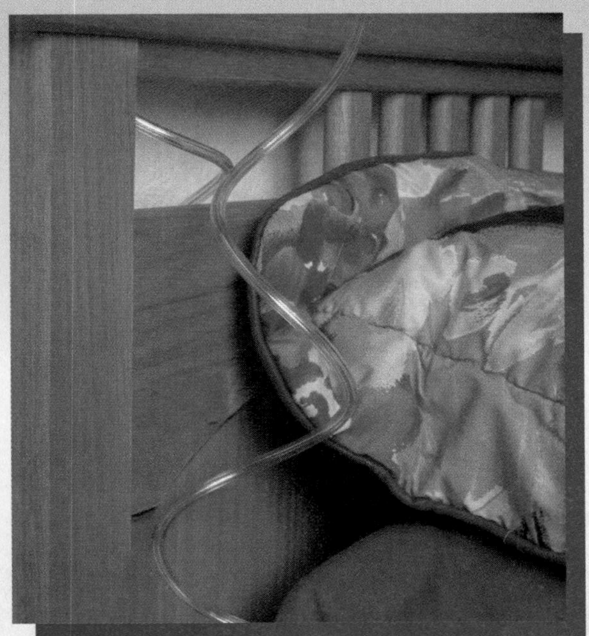

"Please, can't you do something?" pleads one of Lucille's relatives, "Grandma's never looked like this before." After a moment of indecision, Ed decides to complete a physical exam.

As Ed completes his exam, Krista joins him at the bedside. "What have you got?" she asks as she looks at Lucille. Before Ed can respond, she continues. "Ed, this patient looks pretty short of breath. Do you see how she's using accessory muscles to breathe? And how tired she appears? She needs high-flow oxygen. How much oxygen do you have on her?"

"I was waiting to put her on oxygen until I completed the physical exam."

"The physical exam can wait," answers Krista. "This patient needs help now. Help me sit her up, and then break out a nonrebreather mask. Let's put her on high flow oxygen. Also get the BVM out. She may get too tired to breathe for herself before the Paramedics get here." Struggling to keep up with Krista, Ed feels his face getting hot. Is Lucille really that bad? After all, her respiratory *rate* is normal. Ed isn't quite sure what to think.

LEARNING OBJECTIVES

As Ed found out, shortness of breath calls can be very stressful. Patients who are short of breath are often anxious and panicky. They can worsen quickly as they tire from the effort of breathing. In fact, they have a high risk of sudden death.

Short-of-breath calls represent a high percent of the calls in any EMS system. It's a common complaint among all age groups. In fact, respiratory distress is a leading cause of medical emergencies in infants and children. In addition, elderly patients often suffer from chronic lung disease.

By the end of the chapter, you should be able to:[†]

- * Recognize signs and symptoms of shortness of breath. (pp. 224-226)
- * Recognize danger signals that indicate a patient may stop breathing. (pp. 225-226)
- * Discuss common causes of shortness of breath. (pp. 226-227)
- * Describe an emergency care plan for assessing and treating the short-of-breath patient. (pp. 228-233)

RECOGNIZING SHORTNESS OF BREATH

Recall from Chapters 9 and 10 that normal breathing at rest is effortless. A patient who is breathing normally appears to be relaxed. The patient's chest expands adequately, and breath sounds are full and clear with no whistling (wheezy) or bubbling sounds.

Short-of-breath patients may present with a variety of signs and symptoms. Remember Lucille, the patient in the scenario on the previous page? Imagine you're witnessing the onset of her problem. First she'll feel slightly air hungry. She'll respond by breathing more rapidly. As her shortness of breath worsens, she'll become anxious and agitated. This occurs because the oxygen supply to her brain is decreasing. As Lucille's breathing deteriorates even more, she may sit bolt upright and use accessory muscles to help her breathe. Lucille will become more and more anxious as her brain becomes further deprived of oxygen. Then she'll become increasingly pale and able to speak only in short sentences.

[†]Asterisks indicate material supplemental to the 1995 U.S. DOT "First Responder: National Standard Curriculum."

By the time Ed and Krista reach her, Lucille has begun to tire from the exertion of breathing. She's no longer able to hold herself in an upright position. She's too tired to talk more than a word or two at a time, and her respiratory rate is decreasing as she becomes more and more fatigued.

If the First Responders hadn't intervened, Lucille's respirations would have decreased along with her level of responsiveness. Her skin would have become cyanotic. At some point, a lack of oxygen to her brain may have caused her to lose consciousness. Her breathing would have become more irregular and gasping, and she finally would have gone into respiratory arrest. Cardiac arrest would have followed within minutes.

Patients with shortness of breath can present with any of the following signs and symptoms:

- Air hunger.
- Labored breathing.
- Noisy breathing.
- Unusually rapid, slow, or irregular breathing.
- Increased pulse rate.
- Pale or cyanotic skin.
- Use of the muscles of the neck, ribs, or abdomen to breathe. (This is called using the **accessory muscles of breathing** or breathing with retractions.)
- Sitting in a tripod position (Figure 18-1).
- Restlessness, confusion, unresponsiveness.
- Fatigue.

If your patient has any of the following signs or symptoms, assume they may stop breathing and plan to breathe for them:

- Gasping respirations.
- Unusually slow breathing (less than 10 breaths per minute).
- Extreme fatigue.
- Inability to speak.
- Cyanosis.
- Inability to maintain an upright position.

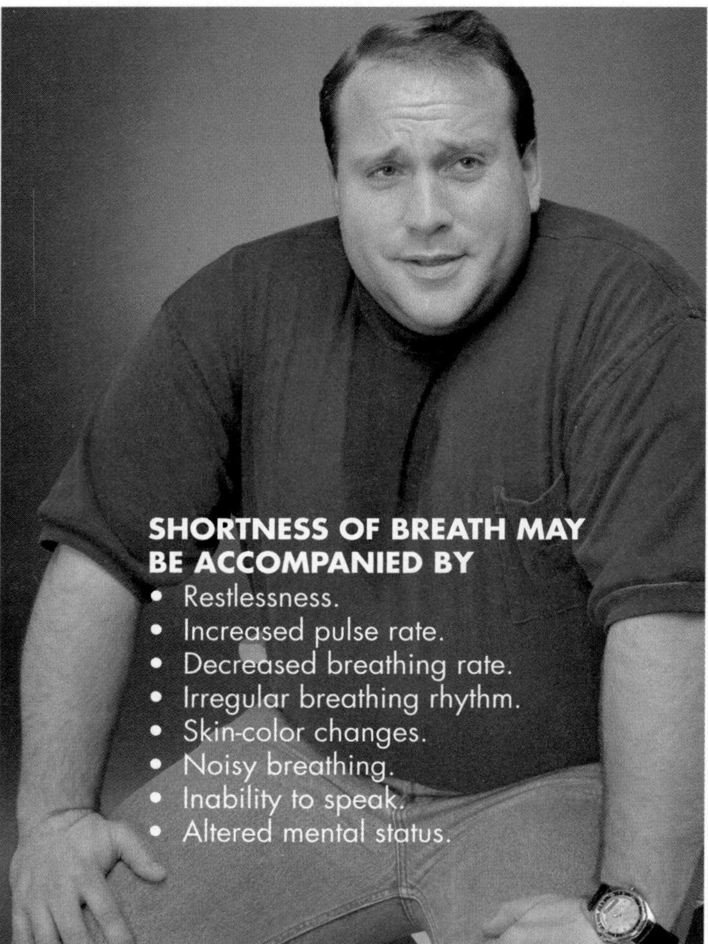

SHORTNESS OF BREATH MAY
BE ACCOMPANIED BY
• Restlessness.
• Increased pulse rate.
• Decreased breathing rate.
• Irregular breathing rhythm.
• Skin-color changes.
• Noisy breathing.
• Inability to speak.
• Altered mental status.

Figure 18-1
A patient with shortness of breath may sit in a tripod position.

Signs of breathing problems may be difficult to detect in infants and children. Look for seesaw breathing, where the chest and abdomen appear to move in opposite directions with each breath. Also check for nasal flaring and grunting sounds with breathing. Infants and children also have much more pronounced use of accessory muscles than adult patients.

CAUSES OF SHORTNESS OF BREATH

Ultimately, it isn't important for you to determine specifically why a patient is short of breath. For the First Responder, it's more important to recognize shortness of breath and to provide timely, appropriate care to the patient. However, the following information will help you to identify patients who are commonly short of breath. It'll also help you to develop a better SAMPLE history.

PULMONARY (LUNG) CAUSES

Shortness of breath can be caused by any blockage in the flow of air in the respiratory system. This blockage can be caused by a foreign body obstruction, trauma, or disease. Diseases of the respiratory system can lead to **inflammation**, **constriction**, or the buildup of mucus or fluid in the *bronchiole tubes* or *alveoli* (air sacs in the lungs). Common lung diseases include *asthma, emphysema, chronic bronchitis*, and *pneumonia*. Childhood respiratory diseases include *bronchiolitis, croup*, and *epiglottitis*.

Shortness of breath also can be caused by *hyperventilation*. Hyperventilation can occur when a patient becomes upset and begins to breathe faster than necessary. This rapid breathing causes the patient to exhale too much carbon dioxide, leading to shortness of breath, dizziness, and tingling of the fingers and mouth. Not all rapid breathing is hyperventilation. Patients may breathe rapidly when suffering from a severe cardiovascular or pulmonary problem.

> ***Caution*** *Hyperventilation should be treated the same as any other breathing problem. Don't ever deny oxygen to a patient by directing him or her to breathe into a paper bag. Many patients with severe medical emergencies may appear to be hyperventilating. Short-of-breath patients who are breathing rapidly should be treated with high-flow oxygen, even if you believe they're hyperventilating.*

CIRCULATORY CAUSES

Shortness of breath can be caused when a patient's circulatory system fails to deliver enough oxygen-rich blood to the body. Heart attacks, which interrupt the supply of oxygen to the heart, can cause a patient to feel short of breath. Patients with diseased hearts may become short of breath when their lungs fill with fluid. Shock patients often are short of breath too. This is true whatever the cause of the patient's shock—blood loss, infection, a severe allergic reaction, or heart failure.

EMERGENCY CARE PLAN | PATIENTS WITH SHORTNESS OF BREATH

■ PRIORITIES

The keys to successfully managing the short-of-breath patient include:

- Early recognition.
- Early activation of the EMS system.
- Aggressive airway, ventilation, and oxygen therapy.
- Continuous reassessment.

■ PATIENT CARE APPROACH

The short-of-breath patient often is panicky, anxious, and may be irrational if his or her brain is getting too little oxygen. Focus on a rapid assessment along with a reassuring approach. Stay with your patient. Constantly reassess your patient's breathing status and use a calm, even approach.

■ DANGER SIGNS

Remember that a short-of-breath patient who is too tired to speak, appears exhausted, is cyanotic, or unable to maintain his or her own upright position may be close to respiratory arrest. Be prepared to breathe for this type of patient.

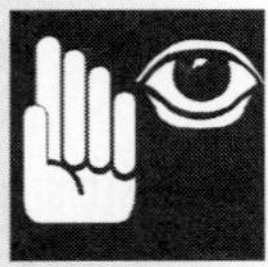

SCENE SIZE-UP

1. **ASSESS SCENE SAFETY.** Patients who are severely short of breath can be panicky, even combative. Assess your patient to make sure that he or she can be approached safely. Take all BSI precautions now. Mask up to protect yourself against droplet infection from a sneeze or cough. Keep an approved HEPA respirator on hand in case you suspect an infectious respiratory condition such as TB.

2. **DETERMINE THE NATURE OF ILLNESS.** Do scene clues indicate that this patient is having an acute episode of a chronic breathing problem? Do you see a hospital bed, home oxygen, or inhalers ("puffers"), which indicate your patient has a chronic condition?

3. **TRIAGE THE PATIENT.** How ill does the patient appear to be? Are the proper resources responding to the call?

4. **DETERMINE ACCESS AND EXTRICATION NEEDS.**

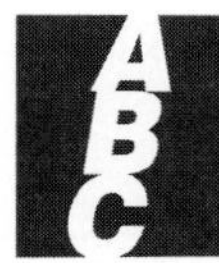

INITIAL ASSESSMENT AND TREATMENT

1. **FORM A GENERAL IMPRESSION.** Note your patient's sex and approximate age. What is your patient's overall level of distress? What position do you find your patient in? In the tripod position? Unable to sit upright due to fatigue? Is your patient able or unable to speak in full sentences?

2. **CHECK MENTAL STATUS.** Watch for the short-of-breath patient who appears confused, agitated, or slow to respond. Remember that your patient's mental status is a very sensitive indicator of how much oxygen is reaching the brain.

3. **ASSESS THE ABCs.**

   - **Airway.** Is the airway open? If not, open it using the head-tilt/chin-lift or jaw-thrust maneuver. Remember that a noisy airway is an obstructed airway.

   - **Breathing.** Is your patient breathing? If so, is it adequate? Is it labored? If necessary, ventilate your patient now. Otherwise, apply high-flow oxygen if you're allowed to do so. If your patient is alert, he or she will benefit by sitting in an upright position.

   - **Circulation.** Does your patient have a pulse? Is it weak, rapid, or slow? What is your patient's skin condition? Remember cyanosis indicates that your patient is not getting enough oxygen to support life. Treat your patient for shock if necessary.

The leading cause of abnormally slow heart rates in children is hypoxia (too little oxygen). So be alert for extremely slow heart rates. If your patient is an infant or child, check capillary refill.

4. DETERMINE PRIORITY.

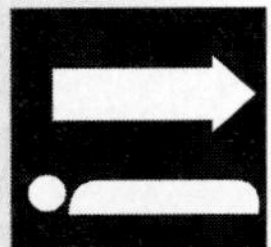

PHYSICAL EXAM AND TREATMENT

1. GATHER A *SAMPLE* HISTORY.

(S)igns and symptoms? How short of breath is the patient? Sometimes it helps to have the patient rate his or her own shortness of breath on a scale of 1 to 10. The number 1 would indicate no shortness of breath. The number 10 would indicate extreme shortness of breath. Also, find out if there is any chest pain or other complaints such as cough or fever.

(A)llergies to medications?

(M)edications? Look for aerosolized inhaler ("puffer") medications, which indicate a history of respiratory disease. Common respiratory medications include: Proventil®, Albuterol®, Alupent®, Bronkosol®, Prednisone®, Theophylline®, Atrovent®.

(P)ertinent past history? Does the patient have a history of respiratory or cardiac problems? Is there a history of smoking?

(L)ast oral intake?

(E)vents leading to the illness? When did your patient's shortness of breath first occur? What was the patient doing at the time? Has the shortness of breath stayed the same or gotten better or worse? Does anything make your patient's shortness of breath better?

2. **PERFORM A HEAD-TO-TOE EXAM.** Focus on the following:

   - **Head.** Are there any signs of cyanosis? Is the airway still open?

   - **Neck.** Are there any signs of accessory muscle use at the base of the neck?

   - **Chest.** Are there any signs of accessory muscle use between or around the ribs? Any surgical scars? Is there any pain with palpation?

   - **Abdomen.** Are there any signs of accessory muscle use with breathing? In particular, watch for seesaw breathing.

   - **Pelvis.** Are there any signs of *incontinence* (the inability to hold the urine or feces). Extremely short-of-breath patients may become incontinent as they lose consciousness.

   - **Extremities.** Can the patient move all extremities? Is there a Medic Alert bracelet?

3. **TAKE VITAL SIGNS.** Include level of responsiveness, airway, breathing rate and quality, pulse rate and quality, skin condition, and blood pressure (if you're equipped and trained to do so). Remember that blood pressure is the least important of all vital signs.

4. **PROVIDE TREATMENT AS NEEDED.** If you haven't applied oxygen and are allowed to do so, apply high-flow oxygen now. Deal with any other complaints as needed.

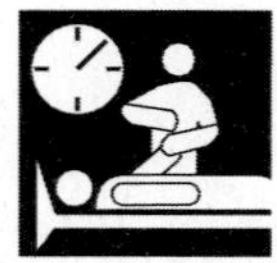

ONGOING ASSESSMENT AND TREATMENT

1. **REPEAT THE INITIAL ASSESSMENT.** Do so every five minutes. Also repeat the initial assessment if your patient has a sudden status change or after providing critical interventions such as ventilations or oxygen.

Is your patient's breathing getting better or worse? Are danger signs developing? Do you need to consider ventilating your patient? If your patient has self-administered medications, have they helped? Pay particular attention to your patient's level of responsiveness, skin condition, and respiratory rate and effort.

2. **REPEAT THE PHYSICAL EXAM.** Repeat it every 10 to 15 minutes. Is your patient's shortness of breath better or worse? Confirm key SAMPLE history elements, including signs and symptoms and the events leading to the shortness of breath. Focus the head-to-toe exam on the neck and chest. Look for accessory muscle use and monitor the work of breathing. Reassess vital signs.

3. **PROVIDE REASSURANCE.**

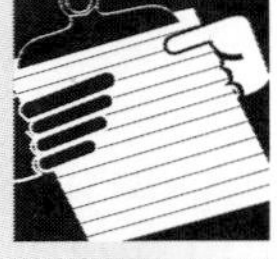

PATIENT HAND-OFF

1. **GIVE A PATIENT REPORT.** The following is a sample of a patient report based on the scenario from the beginning of the chapter:

CONCLUSION

Recall the scenario at the beginning of the chapter. While Ed did a good job of reassuring Lucille, he clearly misprioritized his assessment and treatment. Although he was being careful about his history taking and physical exam, he prioritized them above an accurate initial assessment of Lucille's level of distress and breathing status. He also delayed critical interventions, such as oxygen administration and correct positioning. It was only when his partner intervened that Lucille began to receive the prioritized care that severely short-of-breath patients need.

Never forget that your job is primarily to support your patient's airway, breathing, and circulation until other EMS rescuers with more equipment and training arrive to manage the patient. The keys to successfully managing the short-of-breath patient include:

This is Lucille. She's 72 years old. Lucille's complaining of severe shortness of breath. She says that she also feels some chest tightness. Lucille is a high priority patient. She's awake, but tired and is speaking in one- or two-word sentences. Her airway is open. Lucille has labored, rapid breathing at 32 breaths per minute and marked accessory muscle use. Her pulse is rapid and strong at 120 beats per minute. Her skin is warm and pale. Lucille has been short of breath since this morning. It came on at rest. Lucille has no mediation allergies. She takes the following medications: Proventil®, Ventolin®, Prednisone®, Premarin®, HCTZ®, and Lasix®. Lucille has a chronic history of shortness of breath and states that she has emphysema. Lucille had breakfast this morning. Her physical exam reveals accessory muscles use in her neck and chest. We have Lucille sitting up and we're administering high flow oxygen by mask. There has been no change in her status for the past 10 minutes or so.

2. **CONDUCT THE TRANSFER OF CARE.**

3. **ASSIST IN EXTRICATION AND TRANSPORT.** Don't let a short-of-breath patient walk if at all possible. Walking often makes the patient's distress worse, particularly if the shortness of breath is caused by a heart problem.

- *Assess* your patient. Rapid recognition of the patient's shortness of breath and level of distress is essential.
- *Intervene* with aggressive airway and breathing intervention.
- *Reassess* the patient to gauge the effectiveness of your interventions.

KEY TERMS

You may wish to use this list to review your understanding of key terms introduced in the chapter.

accessory muscles of breathing muscles of the neck, ribs, and abdomen used to help breathing; this is a sign of a breathing problem.

constriction a binding or squeezing of a part.
inflammation swelling and irritation.

APPLICATION QUESTIONS

You may wish to use these questions to review your understanding of the chapter. For answers with page references, see Appendix 2.

1. Review the scenario at the beginning of the chapter. How would you have run this call correctly?
2. Recall all the information about Lucille from this chapter. What would a shortened, prioritized patient report cover?

CHAPTER 19 ALTERED MENTAL STATUS

FIRST RESPONSE

Steve is dispatched to investigate a "possible drunk" sleeping on a bus stop bench. Steve's spent much of his first two years on the police force patrolling this beat and knows many of the "regulars." As he arrives on scene, Steve immediately sees a middle-aged man lying on his side with his legs drawn up.

From his unit Steve scans the area. It looks safe. As Steve approaches the man, he notices that he's well groomed and dressed in a good suit and coat. Steve also sees a small pool of saliva on the bench next to the man's head.

"Hey partner," Steve says, "Are you okay?" The man doesn't respond. Steve taps the man's foot. Still no response. Steve puts on gloves and bends down. He doesn't smell alcohol, but he hears snoring respirations. He quickly repositions the man's head to open the airway. This clears up the snoring sounds.

Steve rubs the man's chest with his fist. The man groans a little and lifts up his left arm as if to bat something away. "This patient has got to be checked out by the Paramedics," Steve thinks to himself. He asks the police dispatcher to have an ambulance dispatched to the scene.

As he waits for the ambulance to arrive, Steve does a rapid head-to-toe exam to look for anything that might give a clue about this person's condition. Nothing turns up, so Steve focuses on reassessing the patient's mental status, and airway, breathing, and circulation status.

When the EMT-Paramedics arrive, Steve gives a patient report and helps them package and load the patient into the ambulance. As they drive away, Steve disposes of his gloves, gets into his unit, and continues his patrol.

LEARNING OBJECTIVES

Caring for patients with an altered mental status can be challenging. These patients can be combative. They may give a poor history, and they may be uncooperative during the physical exam. You also have the challenge of determining if the mental status you observe is normal for the patient or not. Whatever the cause of the altered mental status, the most important thing you can do is assure this patient's airway, breathing, and circulation.

By the end of the chapter, you should be able to:[†]

- 5-1.3 Identify the patient who presents with a specific medical complaint of altered mental status. (pp. 236-237)
- 5-1.4 Explain the steps in providing emergency medical care to a patient with an altered mental status. (pp. 241-245)
- 5-1.5 Identify the patient who presents with a specific medical complaint of seizures. (pp. 238-239)
- 5-1.6 Explain the steps in providing emergency medical care to a patient with seizures. (pp. 241-245)

* Define altered mental status. (pp. 236-237)
* List the common causes of altered mental status. (pp. 237-238)

WHAT IS ALTERED MENTAL STATUS?

The term **altered mental status** means a change in behavior or demeanor that is different from the patient's norm. The patient with altered mental status may show changes in mood, judgment, and the ability to make sense. These changes may be gradual or sudden, brief or prolonged. They may indicate an underlying problem that's not immediately obvious.

One of the most important components of the initial assessment is to check the patient's ability to respond and understand what's going on around him or her. You can do this by asking questions such as:

- What is your name?
- What day is it?

[†]Numbered objectives are from the 1995 U.S. DOT "First Responder: National Standard Curriculum." Asterisks indicate supplemental material.

- Where are you?
- What happened to you?

Sometimes unusual responses or unusual behaviors are normal for a patient. For example, a patient who lives in a convalescent home may not know his or her own name. Is that normal for this patient? You may have to ask someone who knows, such as a family member or the patient's caregiver. If the patient doesn't appear to be responding normally, you'll need to get a sense of how far from normal he or she is. In other words, does the patient just seem a little sleepy and slow or is the patient completely disoriented or even unresponsive?

Always be cautious around any patient who has an altered mental status. These patients may not be in complete control of their behavior. They may do things or take actions that you don't expect. If you need help, don't hesitate to call for it.

CAUSES OF ALTERED MENTAL STATUS

There are many causes of altered mental status. They include decreased levels of oxygen in the brain (hypoxia), fever, poisoning, head injury, and many more. One way to remember the possible causes is by using the mnemonic **AEIOU-TIPS**. Each letter stands for the following:

A — Alcohol

E — Epilepsy (a **seizure** disorder)

I — **Insulin** (diabetes)

O — Overdose (alcohol or prescription and illegal drugs)

U — Underdose (prescribed amounts of medications aren't being taken)

T — Trauma

I — Infections (a common cause in the elderly patient)

P — Psychiatric problems

S — Shock or stroke

As part of the history, you may learn the patient has a medical condition that could be the reason for the current altered mental status. For example, patients with diabetes can develop low or high levels of sugar in their blood. This can cause them to be confused or even unresponsive.

Ultimately, it isn't important for you as a First Responder to discover why a patient has an altered mental status. It's more important for you to recognize it and to provide appropriate care to the patient. Understand, however, that at least two causes of altered mental status—hypoxia and shock—are life-threatening conditions. When you observe signs of either one, treat the patient aggressively.

SEIZURES

One of the more common causes of altered mental status is seizures (Figure 19-1). Seizures are caused by sudden chaotic electrical activity in the brain resulting from:

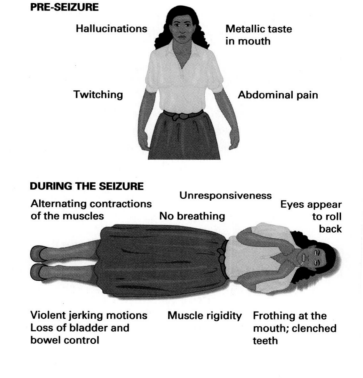

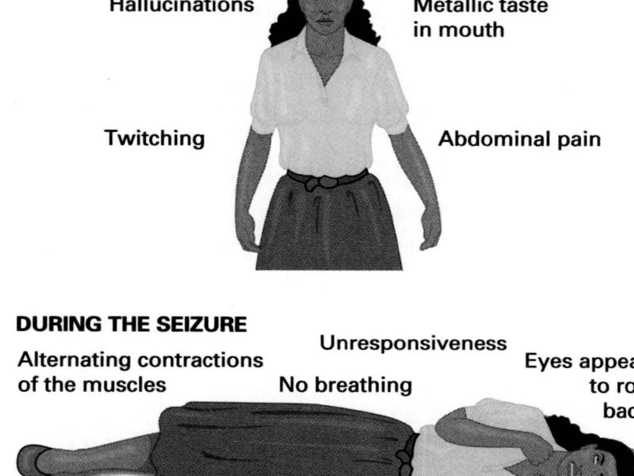

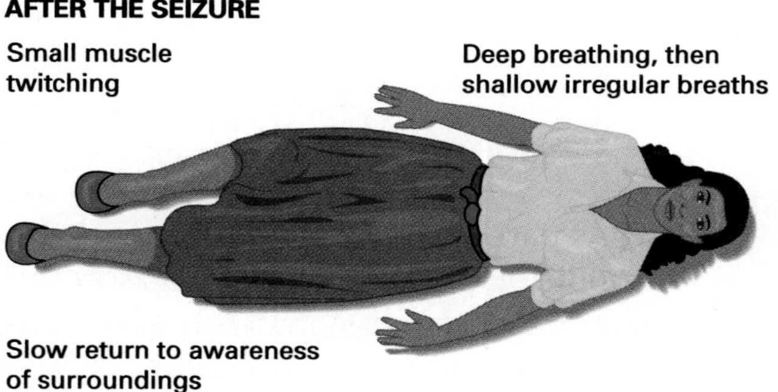

Figure 19-1
Signs and symptoms of seizures.

- Chronic medical conditions.
- Fever.
- Infections.
- Poisoning, including drugs and alcohol poisoning.
- Low blood sugar.
- Head injury.
- Decreased level of oxygen (hypoxia).
- Brain tumors.
- Complications of pregnancy.
- Unknown causes. (Many patients have seizure disorders with no obvious cause.)

Though most aren't life-threatening, a prolonged seizure called *status epilepticus* can be.

Most seizures last only a few minutes and stop on their own. Generally, they look more frightening than they are dangerous. After a seizure, patients typically are confused, tired, and will fall asleep. Protect them from onlookers and assure them that you are there to help. As one First Responder describes it:

> The patient told me that he was going to have a seizure He said he was having an "aura" that he described as a funny taste in his mouth. Then he suddenly went unconscious. His body went rigid. His teeth clenched, and his eyes rolled back in his head. He began shaking violently from head to toe. This lasted for a minute or two, and then he went limp. He slowly regained consciousness, and after about 10 minutes he was able to talk to me. The first words out of his mouth were "What happened?" People who have this type of seizure never remember it. They don't even know they had one.

During a seizure your priority is to protect the patient from injury. Never restrain the seizure patient. Move furniture and other objects away from the seizing patient. Keep everything out of the seizure patient's mouth. If during the seizure the patient shows signs of inadequate breathing, ventilate if possible. Once the seizure has stopped, maintain an open airway, ventilate if necessary, and provide high flow oxygen if you are equipped to do so.

EMERGENCY CARE PLAN | PATIENTS WITH ALTERED MENTAL STATUS

PRIORITIES

Your top priorities in caring for the altered-mental-status patient are:

- Early activation of the EMS system.
- Aggressive treatment for airway, breathing, and circulation problems.
- Continuous reassessment.
- An accurate patient history and physical exam.

PATIENT CARE APPROACH

Patients with altered mental status range from slightly confused to unresponsive. As a rule, they require clear, simple communication. However, you may need to repeat your questions more than once. Do so patiently. Work slowly. Realize that their perceptions are altered, and you may get only irrational responses. If you see a potential for violence, stay clear and call the police for help immediately.

DANGER SIGNS

Danger signs in patients with altered mental status include

- Sudden change in level of responsiveness.
- Seizure activity lasting more than five minutes.
- Signs of airway, breathing, and circulation problems.

Never leave the completely unresponsive patient unattended. Remember, unresponsive patients cannot manage their own airways! Consider the use of airway adjuncts for the patient with altered mental status. If there are no signs of spinal injury and your patient doesn't need an airway maneuver or airway adjuncts, place the unresponsive patient in the recovery position and keep suction readily available (Figure 19-2).

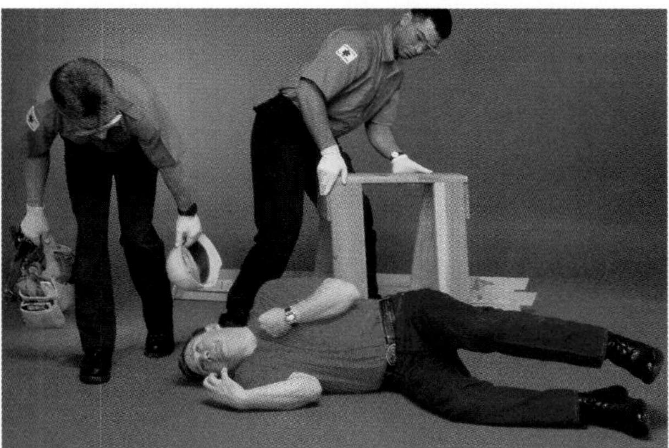

Figure 19-2a
Move objects away from the seizing patient.

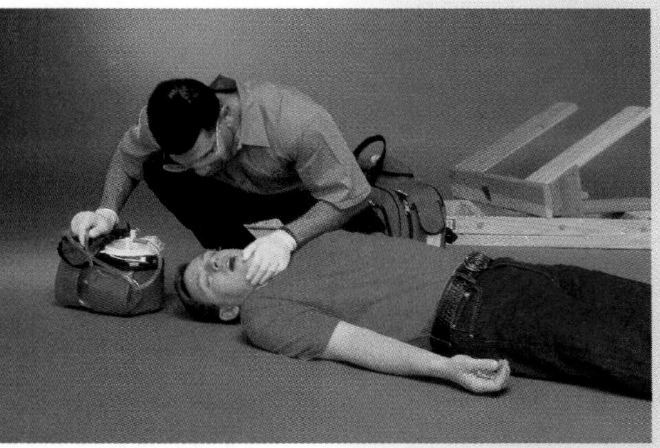

Figure 19-2b
Keep suction equipment close by.

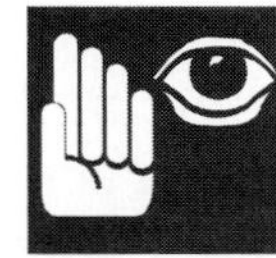

SCENE SIZE-UP

1. **ASSESS SCENE SAFETY.** Do you see any dangers? Is the patient behaving in a threatening way? Size up the patient before you move into his or her personal space. Can you get away from the patient if he or she strikes out at you? Have you identified and moved away all objects that the seizing patient could bump into? Take all BSI precautions now.

2. **DETERMINE NATURE OF ILLNESS.** Look for clues at the scene such as seizure medication, illegal drug paraphernalia, bottles of alcohol, use of hazardous materials. If it hasn't already been done, activate the EMS system as soon as you know the nature of illness and have some idea about its seriousness.

3. **TRIAGE THE PATIENT.** Is there more than one patient on the scene? If so, the emergency may be caused by hazardous materials exposure. Protect yourself and other rescuers first. Don't enter the scene until you are adequately protected.

4. **DETERMINE ACCESS AND EXTRICATION NEEDS.** One of the most common mistakes is to begin to assess and treat the unresponsive patient in poor lighting or in an extremely confined space. Remember that it's important to have plenty of light and clear access before assessing and treating the patient.

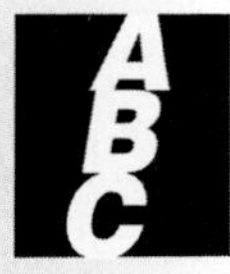

INITIAL ASSESSMENT AND TREATMENT

1. **FORM A GENERAL IMPRESSION.** What is the patient's sex and approximate age? Is the patient curled up in a tight ball with eyes squeezed shut? Is the patient lying limp? Posture and position can give you a lot of information about a patient's overall level of distress.

2. **CHECK MENTAL STATUS.** Use the AVPU scale (alert, verbal, painful, unresponsive) to help you identify the patient's level of responsiveness (Figure 19-3). For completely unresponsive patients, make sure EMS has been activated prior to any assessment. Apply high flow oxygen if you're equipped.

3. **ASSESS THE ABCs.**

   - **Airway.** Keep in mind that seizure patients may have fallen. Use the jaw-thrust maneuver to open the airway and maintain manual stabilization of the patient's head and neck, if they're indicated. Patients with an altered mental status need you to help them maintain a clear, open airway, especially if there is vomit or other secretions. So if there is no possibility of spinal injury, place the patient in the recovery position. Remember that if the patient requires aggressive suctioning, airway maneuvers, and ventilation, you must keep him or her supine. Suction should always be kept nearby. Never place anything into the patient's mouth unless an airway adjunct is indicated and you're trained to insert it. Never insert an airway while the patient is seizing.

   - **Breathing.** If breathing is fast or slow, continually reassess respirations. Open the airway of patients who have loud or snoring respirations. Administer high flow oxygen or intervene with artificial ventilation if necessary.

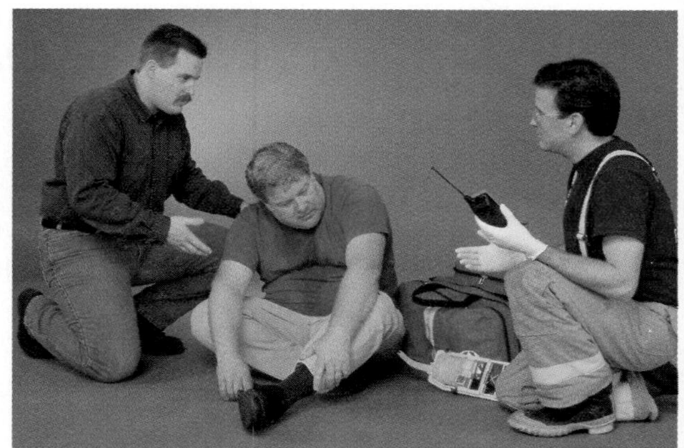

Figure 19-3
Use the AVPU scale to help you determine mental status.

- **Circulation.** Does the patient have a pulse? Is it weak, rapid, or slow? What is the patient's skin condition? Observe color. Check temperature and moisture. Pale or ashy skin that is cool and wet may indicate shock. Cyanosis can indicate the patient is not getting enough oxygen. Treat for shock as indicated.

4. **DETERMINE PRIORITY.** All patients with altered mental status are a high priority.

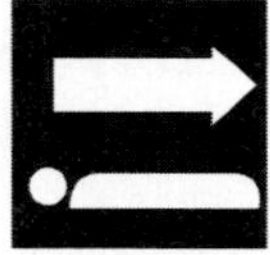

PHYSICAL EXAM AND TREATMENT

1. **GATHER A *SAMPLE* HISTORY.**

(S)igns and symptoms? How altered is the patient? Is there any shaking or seizure activity? Is there any sign or symptom of overdose on drugs or alcohol? Are there any signs of trauma?

(A)llergies to medications or other substances?

(M)edications? Does the patient appear to be taking any medications that are related to the altered mental status? Is the patient taking insulin for a diabetic condition or an anti-seizure medication? Look in the refrigerator for insulin. Common anti-convulsant medications include Dilantin®, Tegretol®, Klonopin®, *valproic acid*, or Depakote®.

(P)ertinent past history? Has the patient ever had this kind of episode before? When was the last time?

(L)ast oral intake? This information is particularly important if your patient is a diabetic. The most common diabetic emergency is low blood sugar, which can be caused by not eating.

(E)vents leading to the injury or illness? When did the patient become altered? Did it occur gradually or suddenly? Did the patient fall or strike his or her head? Was there any seizure activity?

2. PERFORM A HEAD-TO-TOE EXAM.

- **Head.** Are there any secretions from the mouth? Vomiting in the airway? Is there a smell of alcohol or any odd odors indicating poisoning? Is there any trauma?
- **Neck.** Are there any signs of trauma? Are there any signs of retractions at the base of the neck? Is there a Medic Alert necklace?
- **Chest.** Are there any signs of accessory muscle use with breathing? Is there any pain with palpation? Is there any evidence of trauma?
- **Abdomen.** Are there any signs of accessory muscle use with breathing? Is there any pain with palpation? Is there any evidence of trauma?
- **Pelvis.** Are there any signs of *incontinence* (the inability to hold urine or feces)? If so, this may indicate that the patient had a period of unconsciousness.
- **Extremities.** Can the patient move all extremities? Does the patient move one side of the body more than the other? If so, the patient may have had a stroke. Are there any signs of trauma? Puncture wounds that could indicate IV drug use?

3. TAKE VITAL SIGNS. Measure all vital signs, paying particular attention to level of responsiveness.

4. PROVIDE TREATMENT AS NEEDED. Continue airway, breathing, and circulation support as necessary. If the patient is a suspected diabetic, offer orange juice, candy, or another sugary food *only* if the patient can administer it himself. Follow all local protocols!

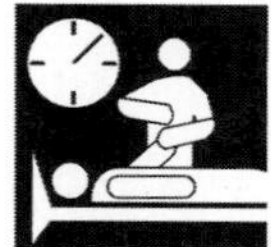

ONGOING ASSESSMENT AND TREATMENT

1. **REPEAT THE INITIAL ASSESSMENT.** Reassess the patient every five minutes. Watch for abrupt changes in mental status.

2. **REPEAT THE PHYSICAL EXAM.** Repeat the physical exam every 10 to 15 minutes. Focus on the patient's airway, and reconfirm important elements of the patient's SAMPLE history if possible. The head-to-toe exam also should focus on any important findings from your original exam. Finally, check your interventions to confirm that they're effective.

3. **PROVIDE REASSURANCE.**

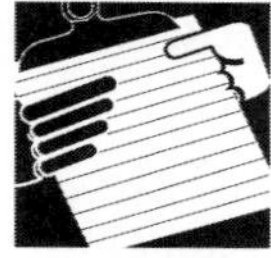

PATIENT HAND-OFF

1. **GIVE A PATIENT REPORT.** The following is an example of the report Steve might give for the patient in the scenario at the beginning of the chapter:

   The patient is male, probably in his 40s. I found him in this position on the bench. The patient has been unresponsive to my voice but groans with painful stimulation. Initially he had snoring respirations, which cleared up when I repositioned his airway. His breathing and circulation seem adequate. I was unable to obtain a SAMPLE history. There has been no witnessed seizure activity and there appears to be no smell of alcohol or any indication that the patient may have ingested anything else. I found nothing in the head-to-toe exam. His vital signs are respirations 16 and pulse 88. The patient's level of responsiveness has not improved since my arrival.

2. **CONDUCT THE TRANSFER OF CARE.**

3. **ASSIST IN EXTRICATION AND TRANSPORT.** The patient with altered mental status may be combative and uncooperative. You may be asked to assist the EMTs with restraining the patient prior to transport.

CONCLUSION

You can provide the most benefit to patients with altered mental status by focusing on their ABCs and protecting them from injury. Keep in mind that your priorities are:

- Early activation of the EMS system.
- Aggressive treatment for airway, breathing, and circulation problems.
- Continuous reassessment.
- An accurate patient history and physical exam.

KEY TERMS

You may wish to use this list to review your understanding of key terms introduced in the chapter.

AEIOU-TIPS a mnemonic used to remember common causes of altered mental status; the letters stand for alcohol, epilepsy, insulin, overdose, underdose, trauma, infections, psychiatric problems, shock or stroke.

altered mental status a sudden or gradual decrease in a patient's normal level of responsiveness.

insulin a hormone secreted by the pancreas essential for the proper metabolism of blood sugar.

APPLICATION QUESTIONS

You may wish to use these questions to review your understanding of the chapter. For answers with page references, see Appendix 2.

1. You're caring for a 19-year-old male who was found in the backyard of a neighborhood residence where a large party was being held. The patient cannot sit up and only groans when you pinch his shoulder. He has a strong smell of alcohol on his breath. As you finish your assessment, you're told by one of his friends that he is a diabetic and takes insulin. He would like to give the patient some orange juice, since this usually "wakes him right up." Will you allow this? What are your priorities for this patient?

2. While you're caring for a 71-year-old female with a high fever, the patient suddenly stops speaking, gazes upward, and begins to have a full-body convulsion. How will you treat the patient until the seizure stops?

CHAPTER 20 ABDOMINAL PAIN

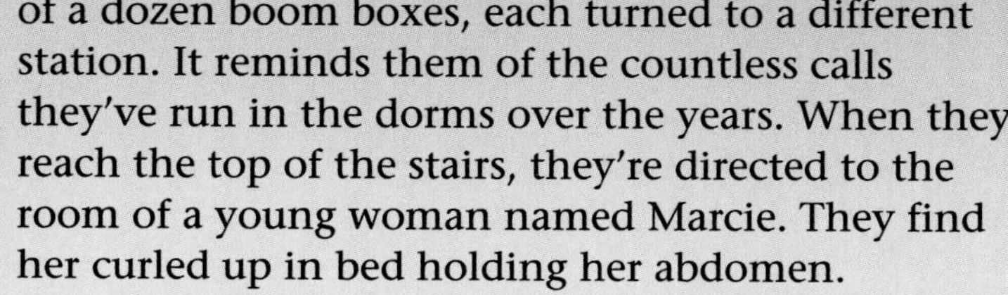

FIRST RESPONSE

John and his partner Rosie are just about to sit down to eat when they're called to a medical emergency at the university. As their fire engine roars up the hill toward the dormitory complex, dispatch reports that the patient is a 19-year-old female with abdominal pain. They're told an ambulance is on the way.

As John and Rosie walk up the dorm stairs, they hear the blare of a dozen boom boxes, each turned to a different station. It reminds them of the countless calls they've run in the dorms over the years. When they reach the top of the stairs, they're directed to the room of a young woman named Marcie. They find her curled up in bed holding her abdomen.

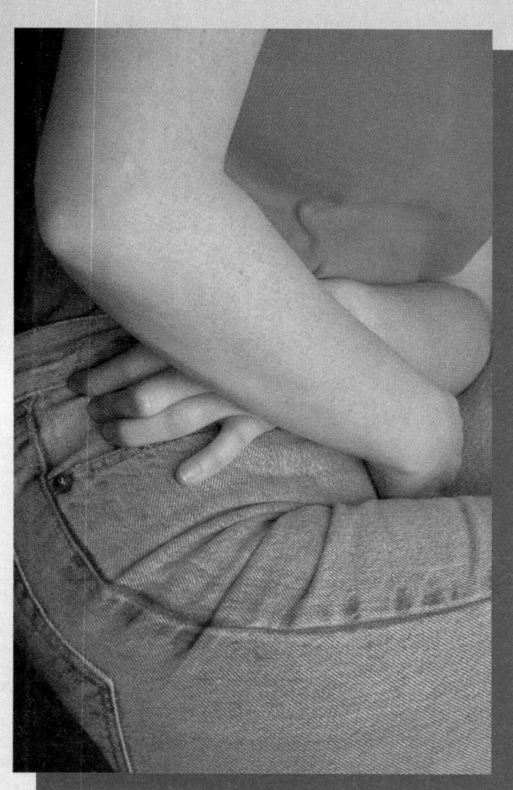

As John begins to assess Marcie, Rosie clears the room of onlookers. The patient appears to be very pale and seems to have been crying. His initial assessment shows no airway, breathing, or circulation problems.

John then asks Marcie questions about her pain. She whispers it's getting worse and curls up more tightly. After a few seconds, she manages to tell John that the pain is a constant intense feeling on her right side, radiating around to her back. She says when the pain gets really bad, she feels a wave of nausea. She says she hasn't vomited.

Marcie is guarding her abdomen and won't let John touch or examine it. However, he is able to determine that the pain came on suddenly. It was not accompanied by any unusual bowel changes, and she had a normal period about two weeks ago. He continues to ask questions, but it's difficult to get any more information from her.

John notices that Marcie's forehead is now moist. He touches it with the back of his hand and realizes her skin also is cool. So he places her on oxygen and, without success, attempts to help her into the shock position. At this point, he knows that the best he can do for her until the ambulance arrives is monitor her vital signs and try to keep her as comfortable as possible.

LEARNING OBJECTIVES

A patient who complains of having abdominal pain can have any number of underlying problems. As a First Responder your top priorities for this patient are to assure the ABCs and gather accurate information from the physical exam.

By the end of the chapter, you should be able to:[†]

* List common causes of abdominal pain. (pp. 248-249)
* Describe an emergency care plan for assessing and treating the patient with abdominal pain. (pp. 250-253)

CAUSES OF ABDOMINAL PAIN

There are dozens of causes of abdominal pain. So, understanding the exact cause of the pain is not your role. Your job is to assess and support the patient's ABCs, gather an accurate history, and

[†]Asterisks indicate material supplemental to the 1995 U.S. DOT "First Responder: National Standard Curriculum."

EMERGENCY CARE PLAN | PATIENTS WITH ABDOMINAL PAIN

PRIORITIES

Your top priorities for managing patients with abdominal pain include:

- Early recognition of the patient's chief complaint and level of distress.
- Early activation of the EMS system.
- Aggressive treatment for airway, breathing, and circulation problems.

help your patient remain as comfortable as possible until EMS workers with more training take over.

However, the following information may help you gather better histories and identify patients who have a serious underlying problem.

- *Gastroenteritis* — An inflammation of the stomach and intestinal tract, this condition usually causes patients to have pain, nausea, and vomiting. They may have eaten something that is now making them sick, or they may be suffering from a viral infection such as the "flu bug."
- *Gastrointestinal bleeding* — This may occur in the esophagus, stomach, intestines, rectum, or anus. Causes may include alcohol abuse, ulcers, cancer, and hemorrhoids.
- *Pregnancy problems* — Patients who are pregnant can develop a number of conditions that cause abdominal pain. One of the most serious occurs when the ovum (egg) attaches itself to the wrong place in the abdominal cavity. When the ovum grows large enough, it can cause the surrounding tissues to rupture and bleed.
- *Other abdominal problems* — There are many causes of abdominal pain that involve organs such as the liver, pancreas, and spleen. Most of them tend to be chronic and may be described to you as part of the patient's history.

- Continuous reassessment with a focus on watching for the signs and symptoms of shock.

PATIENT CARE APPROACH

Patients with abdominal pain may wish to remain quiet and motionless. Handle them with care. A calm, supportive, reassuring approach will help these patients cooperate with your questions, assessments, and treatment.

DANGER SIGNS

Most abdominal pain—even severe pain—is not life-threatening. However, the top life threat associated with abdominal pain is shock. Continually reassess the patient's airway, breathing, and circulation. Be prepared to treat the patient for shock.

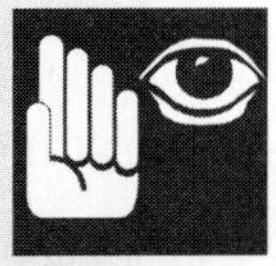

SCENE SIZE-UP

1. **ASSESS SCENE SAFETY.** Some patients with abdominal pain may bleed from the mouth or the rectum. Take all BSI precautions before approaching the patient.

2. **DETERMINE THE NATURE OF ILLNESS.** Look for clues to the possible causes of the patient's abdominal pain. Activate the EMS if you haven't done so already.

3. **TRIAGE THE PATIENT.** How ill does the patient appear to be? Do you have the proper resources arriving?

4. **DETERMINE ACCESS AND EXTRICATION NEEDS.**

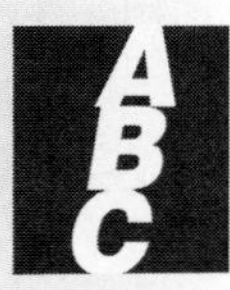

INITIAL ASSESSMENT AND TREATMENT

1. **FORM A GENERAL IMPRESSION.** Determine the patient's sex and approximate age. What is the patient's level of distress? Posture and position will tell you a lot. If the patient has abdominal pain, he or she will likely be in a **guarding position** (Figure 20-1).

2. **CHECK MENTAL STATUS.** Does the patient respond to your questions and verbal commands? Use the mnemonic AVPU to help you estimate level of responsiveness.

ABDOMINAL PAIN MAY BE ACCOMPANIED BY

- Anxiety, fear.
- Rapid breathing and pulse rates.
- Nausea, vomiting, diarrhea.
- Signs of internal bleeding and shock.

Figure 20-1
Patient in a guarding position.

3. ASSESS THE ABCs.

- **Airway.** Patients with abdominal pain may vomit. Reassess the airway often and be sure suction is readily available.
- **Breathing.** Is breathing adequate? Labored? Patients with severe pain may breathe rapidly.
- **Circulation.** Assess the patient for signs of shock and treat appropriately.

4. DETERMINE PRIORITY. If the abdominal-pain patient is extremely distressed or has signs of shock, he or she is a high priority.

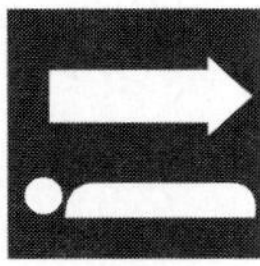

PHYSICAL EXAM AND TREATMENT

1. GATHER A *SAMPLE* HISTORY.

(S)igns and symptoms? Has the patient been vomiting? Did the vomit have blood in it or look like coffee grounds? Has there been diarrhea or rectal bleeding? How does the pain feel? Use the PQRST mnemonic as a way to describe the patient's pain. If the patient is thirsty and asks for something to drink, do *not* provide it. The patient should *not* be given anything by mouth until after being assessed by a physician.

(A)llergies to medications? Is there a Medic Alert medallion present?

(M)edications? Does the patient appear to be taking any medications that are related to the abdominal pain? Look for over-the-counter and prescription medications for ulcers or stomach acid problems. Common medications include Maalox®, Riopan®, Tagamet®, and Zantac®.

(P)ertinent past history? Has the patient ever had this kind of episode before? When was the last time?

(L)ast oral intake? How long ago did the patient last eat? Was it anything unusual? Did the patient share a meal with someone who also has abdominal pain?

(E)vents leading to the illness? What was the patient doing when the pain started? Did the patient lift anything heavy? How long has the pain been going on? Has there been recent abdominal trauma? If the patient is a female, is it possible that she's pregnant?

2. **PERFORM A HEAD-TO-TOE EXAM.** Focus on the patient's chest and abdomen. Is there any pain with palpation? Is there any distention? Rigidity? Masses?

3. **TAKE VITAL SIGNS.** Reassess vital signs as appropriate. Be on the lookout for signs and symptoms of shock.

4. **PROVIDE TREATMENT AS NEEDED.** Don't give the patient anything by mouth. If he or she is shocky, place the patient in the shock position and treat as appropriate. If the patient is not shocky and isn't vomiting, place him or her in a position of comfort.

ONGOING ASSESSMENT AND TREATMENT

1. **REPEAT THE INITIAL ASSESSMENT.**

2. **REPEAT THE PHYSICAL EXAM.**

3. **PROVIDE REASSURANCE.** Remember patients in a lot of pain require a lot of reassurance.

PATIENT HAND-OFF

1. **GIVE A PATIENT REPORT.** The following is an example of a patient report based on the scenario at the beginning of the chapter:

   This is Marcie Goldstein. She's 19 years old with abdominal pain that started about 30 minutes ago. She's alert but is finding it very difficult to communicate through the pain. Her vital signs are respiration 24, pulse 108, and blood pressure 100/70. Her skin is pale, cool, and moist. She was studying at her desk when she had a sudden onset of dull cramping abdominal pain about 30 minutes ago. It's located in the lower right of the abdomen, and it's gotten worse since we've been with her. The patient states that the pain is constant and radiates to her back. She says she feel nauseous but has not vomited. She describes the pain as a "10" on a scale of 1 to 10. The patient ate dinner about an hour ago but had nothing out of the ordinary. We attempted to put her in a shock position, but the patient won't tolerate it. She appears most comfortable in the position she's in, on her side and guarding her abdomen. We started her on oxygen via nasal cannula. She refused the nonrebreather mask. She asked for a glass of water to drink, but we told her she'd have to wait until a doctor could see her.

2. **CONDUCT THE TRANSFER OF CARE.**

3. **ASSIST IN EXTRICATION AND TRANSPORT.** Patients with abdominal pain should not walk or move around unnecessarily. They may have dizziness or weakness associated with their condition. So to avoid a fall, the patient should be assisted at all times. If the patient has a weak pulse or low blood pressure, transport the patient in the shock position. If the patient is nauseated or vomiting, transport the patient on his or her side to allow drainage.

CONCLUSION

Caring for a patient in severe pain can be overwhelming. So never lose sight of what your job as a First Responder is: to maintain scene safety, assess and treat life-threats, and continue to assess and treat the patient until other EMS workers with more training take over care.

KEY TERMS

You may wish to use this list to review your understanding of key terms introduced in the chapter.

guarding position patient is on his or her side with knees drawn up and arms folded over abdomen.

APPLICATION QUESTIONS

You may wish to use these questions to review your understanding of the chapter. For answers with page references, see Appendix 2.

1. You're caring for a 56-year-old male who has had a dull pain in his abdomen for about four hours. The patient states that he has vomited bright red blood several times in the last hour. What kind of BSI precautions should you consider?
2. You're caring for a 68-year-old female with abdominal pain. The patient is extremely pale, sweaty, and has a very weak radial pulse. Your partner informs you that the patient's blood pressure is low. What are your treatment priorities for this patient?

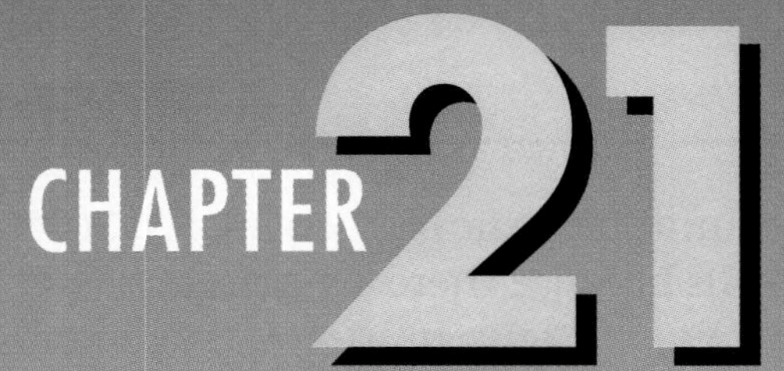

CHAPTER 21 POISONING AND OVERDOSE

FIRST RESPONSE

Nathan and Greg are lifeguards at the local state beach. They're just ending their shift when a dispatcher informs them of a possible overdose in the women's bathroom. Arriving in a jeep a few minutes later, they first make sure the scene is safe.

When Nathan and Greg approach the patient, they find Lydia, a 41-year-old, sitting on the bathroom floor. Their general impression is that she's in a moderate level of emotional distress. The initial assessment reveals that she's alert with an open airway, unlabored breathing, and normal circulation. However, she admits that she's swallowed the contents of a bottle of antidepressants.

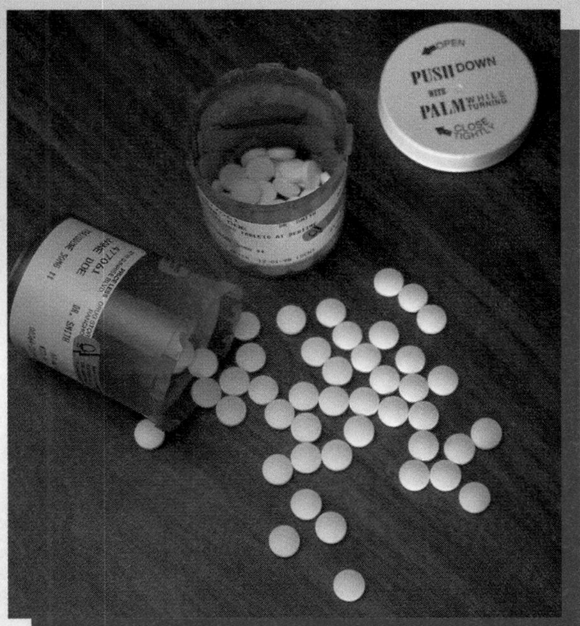

"How many pills have you taken, and when did you take them?" Greg asks Lydia.

"Most of a bottle, I think," Lydia tells him. "Probably 30 or 40 pills. Guess I took them about half an hour ago. I thought if one is supposed to even out my moods, maybe a whole bottle will get me feeling right. Pretty stupid, huh?"

As Greg completes a physical exam, he's startled to see that Lydia has suddenly become pale and sweaty. "I don't feel so good," she says, "It's like I'm going to pass out."

Greg and Nathan help her down to a supine position. Nathan administers high flow oxygen. Greg performs another initial assessment only to find that her pulse is weak and rapid. Within minutes, Lydia is unresponsive and Greg is ventilating her.

A blur of activity occurs when the ambulance arrives. An advanced airway is inserted into Lydia's trachea. She's packaged and whisked into the unit, as the Paramedics busily reassess her status, establish IVs, and administer medications.

Later, Greg and Nathan would learn that Lydia went into cardiac arrest en route. All resuscitation efforts were unsuccessful.

LEARNING OBJECTIVES

Poisoning and overdose are common medical emergencies. Such calls really can stretch your skills because there are so many issues to be addressed. For example, not only must you try to identify the poison, you also have to make sure there are no threats to other rescuers.

Your top duties as usual are scene safety and support of the patient's airway, breathing, and circulation. However, it's also critical that you gather an accurate history of the patient's exposure to the poison. This information often guides the patient's treatment all the way up to and including treatment in the hospital emergency department.

By the end of the chapter, you should be able to:[†]

* Define poisoning and overdose. (pp. 256-257)

* List different types of poisonings and describe their routes of absorption. (pp. 256-259)

* Describe an emergency care plan for assessing and treating the poisoning or overdose patient. (pp. 260-265)

WHAT IS A POISONING EMERGENCY?

A **poison** is any substance that causes harm to a patient's health. An overdose refers to any drug, but usually a drug of abuse, that is taken in quantities large enough to cause an acute reaction or even death. Poisons can range from medications and illegal drugs to cleaning products and insecticides. They can be liquid, solid, or gas.

As a First Responder you will see three types of poisoning or overdose situations:

- *Intentional poisoning*—Patients may try to commit suicide by ingesting large amounts of medications. They'll often wash the pills down with alcohol (Figure 21-1). Some patients may even ingest household cleaners or chemicals in an attempt to hurt themselves.
- *Accidental poisoning*—Accidental poisoning can be caused by farm products, cleaning agents (Figure 21-2), insecticides,

[†]Asterisks indicate material supplemental to the 1995 U.S. DOT "First Responder: National Standard Curriculum."

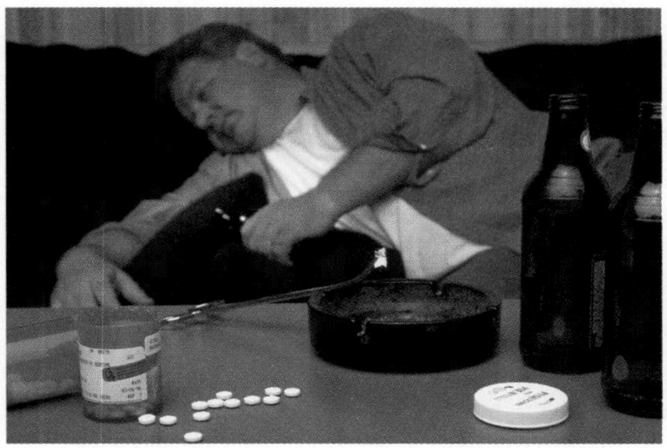

Figure 21-1
Patients may mix prescription drugs and alcohol.

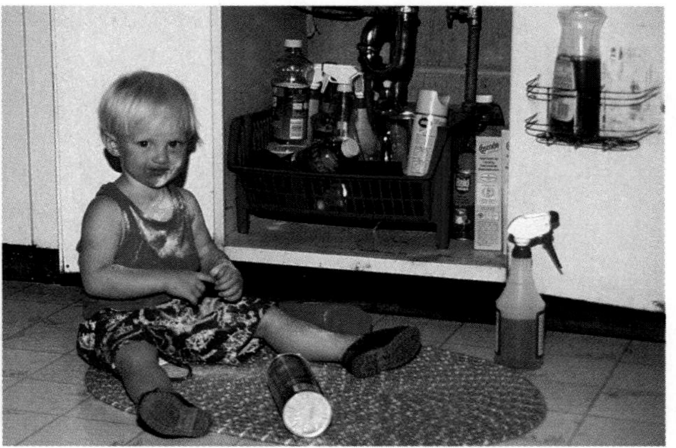

Figure 21-2
Accidental poisoning is common among children, especially toddlers.

even poisonous plants and animals. It also can occur when patients are prescribed several medications, which together cause a toxic reaction.

- *Illegal drug use*—Patients may expose themselves to illegal drugs such as cocaine or heroin that either are mixed with a toxic substance or are simply too strong for the patient.

ASSESSMENT CONSIDERATIONS

How severe a poisoning is depends on three factors: route of exposure (in what way was the patient poisoned), properties of the poison, and the amount of poison involved.

- *Route of exposure*—Exposure to poisons can occur through **ingestion** by mouth, **injection** into a vein or muscle, **inhalation** into the lungs, or **absorption** through the skin. In general, symptoms occur most rapidly when a poison is injected into a vein or inhaled into the lungs.
- *Properties of the poison*—For example, ingesting a bottle of ibuprofen such as Advil® or Motrin® may cause bleeding in the stomach. Ingesting a bottle of acetaminophen such as Tylenol® or Panadol® can lead to liver failure and death in a matter of days.
- *Amount of poison involved*—For example, recall the scenario at the beginning of the chapter. Lydia had few symptoms at first. But once the large quantity of antidepressants was absorbed into her bloodstream, it affected her very quickly and with deadly results.

In any poisoning emergency, *assume the worst.* If you have no information about a poison, assume it can cause life threats until someone with more medical training tells you otherwise. If a suicidal patient claims to have swallowed three or four pills, assume he or she has swallowed the entire bottle. If a patient isn't sure how much of a chemical splashed onto his or her skin, assume it was enough to make the patient very ill.

It's also important for you to take **over-the-counter (OTC) medications** seriously. One of the most dangerous types of overdose is acetaminophen (mentioned above). As few as 15 extra-strength (500 mg) tablets can cause toxic symptoms in an adult. Common OTC sleeping pills such as Nytol® and Sominex® can cause fatal seizures if taken in large enough doses. Tile and oven cleaners can cause severe mouth, throat, and stomach burns if ingested.

EMERGENCY CARE PLAN | POISONING OR OVERDOSE PATIENTS

PRIORITIES

Don't become a casualty of someone else's poisoning emergency. Remember: scene safety, scene safety, scene safety! Patient priorities include:

- Early activation of the EMS system.
- Maintenance of the patient's airway, breathing, and circulation.
- Frequent reassessment of the patient's status.
- An accurate history of the route of exposure, the name or type of poison, and the quantity involved.

PATIENT CARE APPROACH

Poisoned patients may respond in a variety of ways. Anticipate your patient's needs by putting yourself in his or her shoes. The poisoned patient who has tried to commit suicide may be in complete emotional crisis and may even be violent. The poisoned patient who has been taking illegal drugs may be afraid of getting arrested. Depending on the drug, this patient also may be violent.

Caution *Many EMS rescuers have become victims of poisoning by accidental exposure to the same poison that sickened their patients. So protect yourself! Careful scene size-up is essential, especially if the poison is in a form that can be inhaled into the lungs or absorbed through the skin.*

Regional **poison control centers** provide information about poisons to both lay people and EMS professionals. Staffed by highly trained personnel, the centers have access to information about thousands of poisons and chemicals. They can tell you whether or not a substance is dangerous, the signs and symptoms to watch for, and what treatment should be provided. Learn the phone number of the regional poison control center nearest you.

Scenes where an infant or child has been accidentally poisoned may include several people in need of a calm hand. In general, poisoned patients will respond best to a calm, reassuring approach. Communicate with body language, your tone of voice, and your words. Make sure patients know that you aren't a threat and that you're there to meet their medical needs, not to judge or to scold them.

DANGER SIGNS

Danger signs include the following:

- Any problems with level of responsiveness, airway, breathing, or circulation.
- Rapid changes in level of responsiveness, airway, breathing, or circulation status.
- Evidence that more than one drug has been ingested. Commonly this includes alcohol and sedatives. Illicit drug users also may inject heroin and cocaine together. If the patient has taken more than one drug, his or her physical and emotional reactions will be unpredictable.

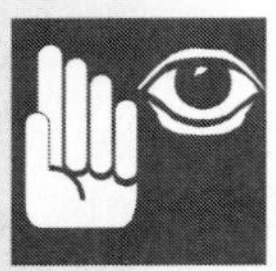

SCENE SIZE-UP

1. **ASSESS SCENE SAFETY.** Is the scene safe to enter? Remember that scenes with illicit drug use or intentional poisoning can be extremely dangerous. If a hazardous material is suspected, don't enter the scene until trained hazmat personnel say it's safe. When in doubt, pull back from the scene and wait for law enforcement to establish a safe scene. Take all BSI precautions now.

   Warning *If you suspect your patient has been injecting drugs, be on the lookout for IV needles. Many an unsuspecting rescuer has entered such a scene and been stuck by a dirty needle. Watch out!*

2. **DETERMINE NATURE OF ILLNESS.** Scan the scene for any clues that would help you identify the poison. Are there empty whiskey or pill bottles? Chemical bottles? Is there evidence of IV drug use? Look at the patient's overall environment. Is there any chance that the poisoning was caused by inhalation? If EMS hasn't been activated, do so now.

3. **TRIAGE THE PATIENT.** Is it possible that more than one patient has been exposed to the poison? How ill do they appear to be? Do you need more resources to manage this emergency? Ask dispatch for help if necessary.

4. **DETERMINE ACCESS AND EXTRICATION NEEDS.** Will there be problems getting to the patient or patients? Will there be problems with extrication?

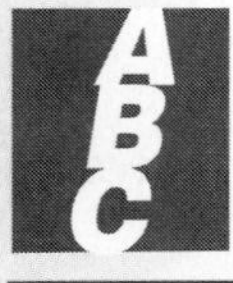

INITIAL ASSESSMENT AND TREATMENT

1. **FORM A GENERAL IMPRESSION.** What is the patient's sex and approximate age? What is the chief complaint? What is the patient's body position? Overall level of distress? Recall

from the scenario at the beginning of the chapter that it isn't necessary for the patient to appear to be very distressed in order to be a high priority.

2. **CHECK MENTAL STATUS.** Using AVPU, perform a quick assessment of the patient's level of responsiveness. If your patient has an altered mental status, apply high flow oxygen. Ingestion patients in particular may vomit, so monitor them closely if you apply a mask. Vomiting into an oxygen mask can cause major airway problems.

3. **ASSESS THE ABCs.**

   - **Airway.** Is the airway open and clear? If necessary, open the airway now.

   - **Breathing.** Is your patient breathing? Is the rate and quality of breathing adequate? Are there any signs of labored breathing? Apply oxygen and ventilate as necessary.

   Remember *Many types of prescription and illicit drugs can cause respiratory difficulties or respiratory arrest if taken in large enough quantities. Some drugs—including codeine, Darvon®, Vicodin®, Percodan®, Valium®, and Klonopin® as well as the illegal drug heroin—can cause respiratory problems, especially if taken with alcohol.*

   - **Circulation.** Does your patient have a pulse? If not, start CPR. If a pulse is present, is it fast, slow, weak? What is the patient's skin condition? Is it showing signs of shock (pale, cool, sweaty)? If so, treat for shock. Alcohol, tranquilizers, and painkillers may cause the patient's pulse to slow. Cocaine and methamphetamines can cause the pulse to be extremely rapid.

4. **DETERMINE PRIORITY.** All poisoning patients should be considered high priority. Determine how stable your patient is by measuring the patient's level of distress, mental status, and status of his or her airway, breathing, and circulation. Stable poisoning patients will show these indicators to be intact and unchanging.

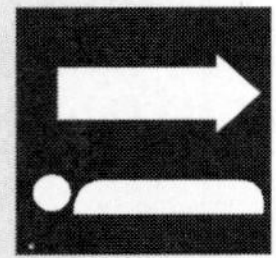

PHYSICAL EXAM AND TREATMENT

1. GATHER A *SAMPLE* HISTORY.

(S)igns and symptoms? What is the patient's chief complaint? Any chest pain, shortness of breath, heart palpitations? Is there any headache, abdominal cramping, nausea or vomiting, dizziness? Is the patient salivating or complaining of a dry mouth?

(A)llergies? Include any allergies to any ingested substance, medications, bee stings, and so on.

(M)edications? Does your patient take any prescription medications? Does he or she take OTC medications? Use this opportunity to rule out an overdose of prescribed medications. To do this, you will need to count the pills remaining in medication vials. All medication containers—both prescription and OTC—will include a pill count on the label. Also look for telltale medication wrappers or any other clue that your patient may have ingested a large quantity of a medication in a short period of time.

(P)ertinent past history? What is the history of ingestion, overdoses, illicit drug use?

(L)ast oral intake?

(E)vents leading to the illness? This requires detective work if the route of exposure isn't clear. Have the patient and witnesses walk through the events leading to the exposure for you.

Remember *The three critical questions that must be answered in a poisoned patient's history are: What were you exposed to? How much were you exposed to? How long ago were you exposed to it?*

2. **PERFORM A HEAD-TO-TOE EXAM.**

   - **Head.** Are there any signs of burns to the mouth or nose? Is there any residue or unusual breath odor from an ingested substance? Is there any vomit or excess oral secretions? Is there any bleeding from the nose (may be from recent cocaine use)? Are there any signs of trauma?

   - **Pupils.** Though checking the pupils isn't a standard part of the First Responder physical exam, in the case of possible poisoning check the patient's pupils. Are they unusually large or small given the available light? Unusually large (*dilated*) pupils may indicate an overdose of alcohol, cocaine, or methamphetamines. Extremely small (*pinpoint*) pupils may indicate the patient has ingested an opiate-derived drug such as heroin.

   - **Neck.** Are there any signs of accessory muscle use at the base of the neck? Are there signs of trauma?

   - **Chest.** Are there any signs of accessory muscle use between the ribs? Are there any signs of trauma?

   - **Abdomen.** Is the patient complaining of abdominal pain? Is there pain with palpation? Is there abdominal rigidity or guarding?

   - **Pelvis.** Are there any signs of incontinence (the inability to hold urine or feces)?

   - **Extremities.** Is there a Medic Alert medallion? Are there any puncture wounds in the arms ("needle tracks") indicating recent IV drug use?

3. **TAKE VITAL SIGNS.** Poisoning can cause a number of problems with a patient's airway, breathing, and circulation. Careful assessment and reassessment of vital signs will help you to catch any problems as they arise.

4. **PROVIDE TREATMENT AS NEEDED.** First Responders are discouraged from administering *ipecac* (a medication that induces vomiting in patients). This treatment is no longer the

preferred way to manage patients who have ingested poisons. Only on the advice of a poison control center, consider administering a glass of water or milk, if your patient has ingested a caustic substance and other rescuers still are some distance away. If trained and local protocols allow, you may assist in the administration of activated charcoal. *Follow all local protocols!*

Any patient who has suffered a possible inhalation poisoning should receive high flow oxygen by nonrebreather mask, even if there's no shortness of breath.

If your patient has suffered poisoning by absorption, verify that all poisons have been washed away. Irrigate the affected areas as needed.

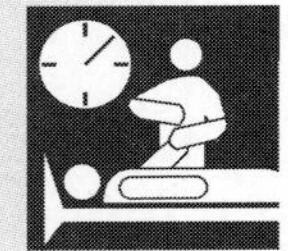

ONGOING ASSESSMENT AND TREATMENT

1. **REPEAT THE INITIAL ASSESSMENT.** Recall from the scenario at the beginning of the chapter that the status of poisoned patients can change rapidly. Repeat the initial assessment at least every five minutes if you are managing an unstable patient.

2. **REPEAT THE PHYSICAL EXAM.** Focus in on your patient's chief complaint as well as any pertinent physical findings. Reassess vital signs.

3. **PROVIDE REASSURANCE.** Patients who have been poisoned intentionally or unintentionally often are quite scared. Provide nonjudgmental reassurance.

PATIENT HAND-OFF

1. **GIVE A PATIENT REPORT.** The following is an example of a patient report based on the scenario at the beginning of the chapter:

   This is Lydia. She's 41 years old. About an hour ago she ingested up to 40 Elavil® tablets because she has been quite depressed. Initially alert and without complaint, she quickly became unresponsive. She's a high priority patient who remains unresponsive. She has a patent airway maintained with positioning and an OPA. Her respiratory effort is minimal and we are ventilating her with 100% oxygen via BVM. Lydia's pulse is rapid and weak. Her skin is pale and sweaty. Before becoming unresponsive, Lydia denied any other drug ingestion. Her allergy status is unknown. She has a history of depression. Her head-to-toe exam shows no significant findings. Her respiratory rate is 6 per minute unassisted. Her pulse is 130 beats per minute. Her skin remains pale and sweaty. We were unable to obtain a blood pressure despite numerous attempts. There has been no change in Lydia's status for the past five minutes.

2. **CONDUCT THE TRANSFER OF CARE.**

3. **ASSIST IN EXTRICATION AND TRANSPORT.** If your patient is combative or threatening, you may be asked to help to restrain him or her. The transporting EMS workers also may want to have an additional rescuer in the ambulance for the ride to the hospital, especially if the patient is undergoing status changes.

CONCLUSION

There are thousands of substances that can cause poisoning. Your job on a poisoning call is to make sure that the scene is safe and that you aggressively support your patient's airway, breathing, and circulation. In addition, it's critical that you find out as much as you can about the poisoning. Specifically, what was the route of exposure, the name or type of poison, and the quantity involved? This information will guide the patient's treatment all the way up to and including the hospital emergency department. Altogether, these steps will help to provide your patient with the best chance of surviving a poisoning emergency.

KEY TERMS

You may wish to use this list to review your understanding of key terms introduced in the chapter.

absorption the passage of a substance through the skin or mucous membranes into the body upon contact.

ingestion swallowing a substance.

inhalation the active process of breathing into the lungs.

injection forced introduction of a substance into the body through the skin and into a vein or muscle by way of a syringe, bite, or sting.

over-the-counter (OTC) medications medications sold to the public without a prescription.

poison any substance that causes a harmful effect on a patient's health.

poison control centers regional centers set up to provide lay people and professionals with information about poisons.

APPLICATION QUESTIONS

You may wish to use these questions to review your understanding of the chapter. For answers with page references, see Appendix 2.

1. You're managing a four-year-old who was found playing with and sampling from a bottle of prescription medication at his grandmother's home. He appears fine. What type of questions would you want to ask the grandmother about this event?

2. You've been asked to check out a patient who is suspected of using IV drugs. The patient is sitting on the ground near a patrol car. As you approach the patient, she suddenly becomes unresponsive. What actions should you take?

CHAPTER 22 ALLERGIC REACTIONS

FIRST RESPONSE

It's hot and sunny and the lines of people streaming into the amusement park seem endless. The park hasn't been open more than 20 minutes when Angel responds to an emergency by the carousel. When she pulls up to the scene, Angel gloves up and spots her patient, a 47-year-old female named Brianne. Brianne has been stung by a bee, and she believes she's having an allergic reaction.

"Please," Brianne screams, "I'm allergic to bee stings!" Angel's general impression is that Brianne appears to be extremely agitated. She's alert with a patent airway. Her breathing is fast, but it appears to be unlabored. Her skin condition is warm and flushed, and Angel can see welts forming on the chest and neck. Angel introduces herself to Brianne and performs an initial assessment.

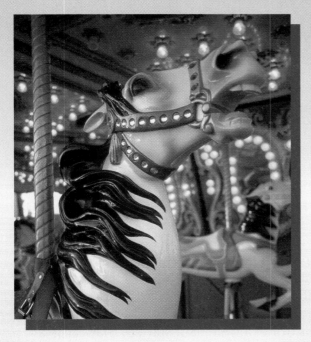

"Ma'am," Angel says, "I know this is upsetting. Try to calm down and tell me what happened." Brianne tells Angel that she was waiting for a carousel ride when a bee landed on her shoulder. It stung her when she tried to brush it away. Angel inspects the site of the sting and finds a large amount of swelling around a raised welt on Brianne's shoulder. The stinger is gone. A quick head-to-toe reveals watery eyes and Brianne reports that she's itching all over.

"Has this ever happened to you before?" Angel asks.

"Once before," Brianne says. "My doctor gave me a bee sting kit, but I lost it some time ago."

"Aside from the itching and swelling where the bee stung you," Angel asks, "are there any other symptoms? Shortness of breath, trouble swallowing, dizziness?"

"No, but that's enough, isn't it?" Brianne manages a weak grin. Angel agrees and repeats the initial assessment. Within a few minutes the Paramedics arrive, establish an IV, and administer an antihistamine. Angel breathes a sigh of relief as she readies herself for her next call.

LEARNING OBJECTIVES

While Brianne's reaction to the bee sting was relatively mild, allergic reactions can be life-threatening medical emergencies that require a rapid, aggressive response.

By the end of the chapter, you should be able to:[†]

* Define allergic reaction. (p. 268)

* List substances that commonly cause allergic reactions. (pp. 269-270)

* Describe the signs and symptoms of an allergic reaction. (pp. 270-271)

* Discuss the difference between a patient having a mild allergic reaction and a patient having a life-threatening allergic reaction. (p. 271)

* Describe an emergency care plan for assessing and treating a patient having an allergic reaction. (pp. 272-277)

WHAT IS AN ALLERGIC REACTION?

The immune system protects the human body from invaders such as viruses and bacteria, which are called **antigens**. The first time an antigen enters the body, the immune system creates antibodies. When the antigen invades the body again, the **antibodies** "remember" it and destroy it. This is called developing an immunity to the antigen.

However, some people have immune systems that respond too aggressively. This overactive response is what produces the signs and symptoms of an allergic reaction. Often an allergic reaction is triggered by substances that are harmless to the body (plant pollens or certain foods, for example). Substances that cause allergic reactions are called **allergens**.

An allergic response occasionally can cause severe, life-threatening airway, breathing, and circulation problems. Known as **anaphylaxis**, this exaggerated allergic reaction can progress rapidly.

[†]Asterisks indicate material supplemental to the 1995 U.S. DOT "First Responder: National Standard Curriculum."

CAUSES OF ALLERGIC REACTION

Nearly any substance in our environment can cause an allergic reaction. Most frequently the substance is a food, drug, or venom from an insect bite or sting. Common examples include:

- Foods
  - Seafood and shellfish
  - Nuts and seeds
  - Fruits such as strawberries and other berries
  - Egg whites
  - Chocolate
  - Milk and other dairy products
- Drugs
  - Antibiotics such as *penicillin*
  - Sulfa drugs
  - Aspirin
  - Dyes used in x-rays
  - Animal serum products such as *gamma globulin*
  - Local anesthetics such as Xylocaine®
- Insect venom
  - Bees
  - Wasps
  - Fire ants
  - Plants
  - Pollen from ragweed and grasses

People who know they're allergic to a substance try to avoid it. However, it isn't always possible to avoid a bee sting, for example. Patients also may accidentally eat a food they're allergic to—when they eat out, for instance, or when food labels don't identify ingredients clearly.

SIGNS AND SYMPTOMS OF ALLERGIC REACTION

An allergic reaction can cause a variety of signs and symptoms (Figure 22-1). They include the following:

- *Skin effects* —The skin is usually the first to show signs and symptoms. Flushing, swelling, itching, and the development of **hives** (large, circular, raised welts) are common. The patient also may complain of a warm tingling feeling in the face, mouth, chest, feet, and hands.
- *Respiratory effects* —Sneezing and coughing may be the first signs of breathing problems. Patients also complain of tightness in the throat or chest and difficulty swallowing and breathing. Voice changes such as hoarseness (losing the voice), shortness of breath, or noisy breathing (wheezing or stridor) are early and serious signs.
- *Circulatory system effects* —Patients may have a rapid heart rate, low blood pressure, and in extreme cases, shock.
- *Gastrointestinal effects* —Your patient may experience nausea, vomiting, abdominal cramps, or diarrhea.
- *Generalized effects* —These include itchy watery eyes, headache and runny nose.

Caution *Most deaths from allergic reaction are due to upper airway obstruction. So monitor the airway carefully and remember, a noisy airway is an obstructed airway! Allergic reactions also may be fatal if the patient slips into shock.*

EMERGENCY CARE PLAN | PATIENTS WITH ALLERGIC REACTIONS

PRIORITIES

Your top priorities in caring for a patient with an allergic reaction are:

- Early recognition of the signs and symptoms of an allergic reaction.

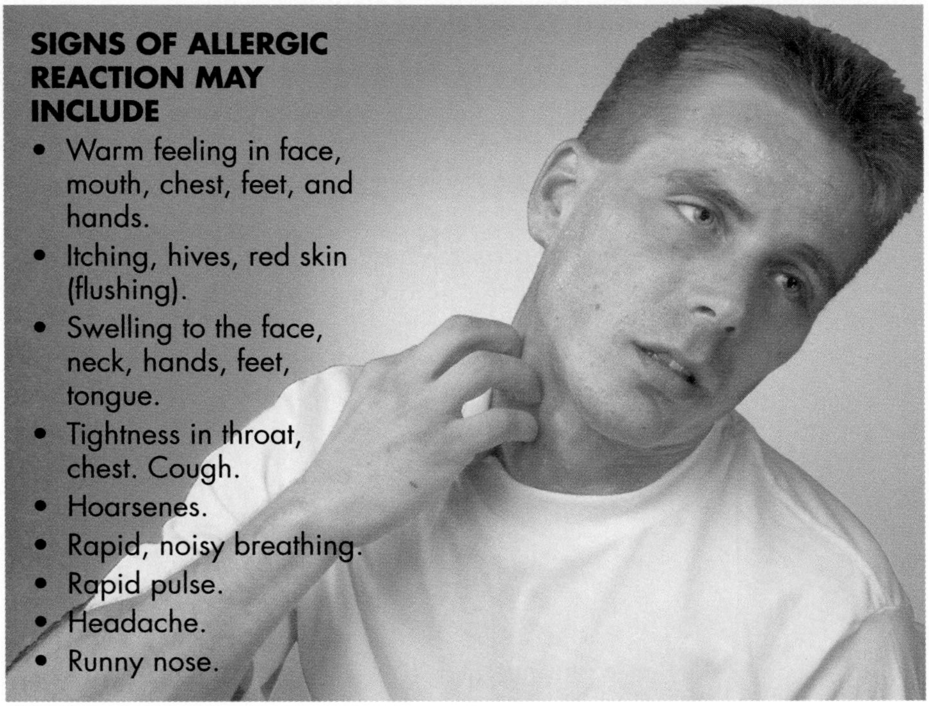

SIGNS OF ALLERGIC REACTION MAY INCLUDE

- Warm feeling in face, mouth, chest, feet, and hands.
- Itching, hives, red skin (flushing).
- Swelling to the face, neck, hands, feet, tongue.
- Tightness in throat, chest. Cough.
- Hoarsenes.
- Rapid, noisy breathing.
- Rapid pulse.
- Headache.
- Runny nose.

Figure 22-1
Signs and symptoms of an allergic reaction.

In general, if a patient has an allergic reaction within minutes after being exposed, expect signs and symptoms to be severe and to progress rapidly. If the allergic reaction develops slowly (over an hour or so), signs and symptoms may be less severe. Mild allergic reactions include swelling at the site of a sting or bite, itching, hives, watery eyes, runny nose, perhaps some abdominal cramping, but no airway, breathing, or circulation problems. Problems with airway, breathing, or circulation characterize a severe allergic reaction.

- Early activation of the EMS system.
- Assurance of an open airway and adequate breathing and circulation.
- Accurate physical exams and continuous reassessment.

PATIENT CARE APPROACH

Approach these patients in a calm, supportive, and reassuring manner. Reducing the patient's anxiety may help to slow the progress of the signs and symptoms. Remember that patients with shortness of breath are often panicky.

DANGER SIGNS

Patients experiencing severe anaphylaxis can deteriorate rapidly. Watch for rapid changes in your patient's status. Monitor your patient for signs of increased airway, breathing, or circulation problems. Noisy breathing, an inability to swallow, fatigue with breathing, and signs of shock are all grave indications.

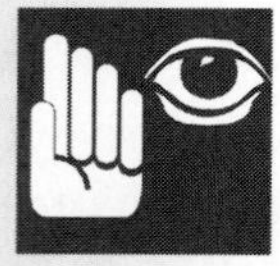

SCENE SIZE-UP

1. **ASSESS SCENE SAFETY.** Is the scene safe to enter? Are there any hazards? Protect yourself, and take all BSI precautions now.

2. **DETERMINE NATURE OF ILLNESS.** Are there any clues that indicate the cause of the allergic reaction? When you've determined that a medical emergency exists, activate the EMS system if someone hasn't already done so.

3. **TRIAGE THE PATIENT.** How ill does the patient appear to be? Are the proper EMS resources responding to the call?

4. **DETERMINE ACCESS AND EXTRICATION NEEDS.**

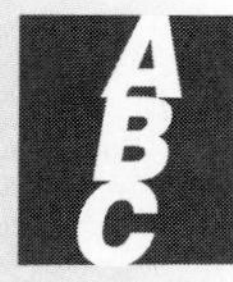

INITIAL ASSESSMENT AND TREATMENT

1. **FORM A GENERAL IMPRESSION.** What is the patient's sex and approximate age? What is the patient's chief complaint? What is the patient's overall level of distress? Patients with significant reactions often will be scratching themselves vigorously.

2. **CHECK MENTAL STATUS.** Is your patient awake and answering your questions appropriately? Use the AVPU scale to measure your patient's level of responsiveness. If the patient shows signs of altered mental status, apply high flow oxygen if you're allowed to do so.

3. **ASSESS THE ABCs.**

   - **Airway.** Is the airway open and clear? Patients experiencing a severe allergic reaction may develop swelling in the throat, which potentially can obstruct the airway. Watch for noisy breathing, particularly stridor. If necessary, open the airway.

   - **Breathing.** Is your patient's breathing adequate? How hard is your patient working to breathe? Is your patient having noisy or obstructed breathing? If so, provide high flow oxygen. Ventilate your patient as necessary.

   - **Circulation.** Does your patient have a pulse? Is it fast, slow, or weak? What is your patient's skin condition? Treat for shock as necessary.

     If your patient is suffering an allergic reaction from an insect sting, make sure the stinger is removed now. Scrape the stinger off the skin using a credit card or similar object (Figure 22-2).

4. **DETERMINE PRIORITY.** All patients with significant levels of distress or with airway, breathing, or circulation problems are high priorities.

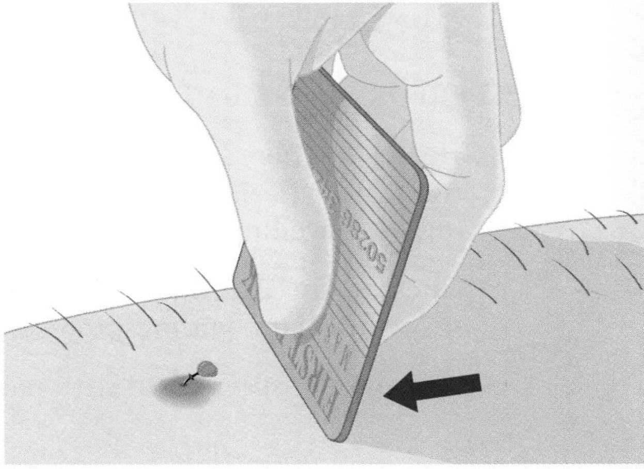

Figure 22-2
Removing the insect's stinger from the wound.

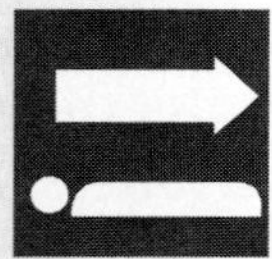

PHYSICAL EXAM AND TREATMENT

1. GATHER A *SAMPLE* HISTORY.

(S)igns and symptoms? Does your patient show flushing, swelling, itching, or hives? Difficulty breathing or noisy respirations? Any dizziness? Any complaints of stomach cramping or nausea? Does your patient have any pain, especially in the chest?

(A)llergies? What is the patient allergic to?

(M)edications? Does your patient take any prescription medications? Has your patient self-administered any medications prior to your arrival? Many patients with severe allergic reactions carry an "allergy kit" or "bee sting kit." This kit contains an injection of **adrenaline**, which can be self-administered, and an **antihistamine** in pill form.

(P)ertinent past history? Has your patient ever had an allergic reaction before? If so, to what? What were the effects? When was the last time? How bad was it? How was the reaction treated?

(L)ast oral intake? How long ago did the patient eat? Any chance that your patient has a food allergy?

(E)vents leading to the illness? What was the patient exposed to and how long ago? By which route was the patient exposed? How much of the substance was the patient exposed to?

2. PERFORM A HEAD-TO-TOE EXAM.

- **Head**. Are there signs of facial swelling? Is there tearing from the eyes? Is the nose runny? Is there difficulty swallowing? Swelling of the tongue? Hives?
- **Chest**. Is the skin flushed? Are there hives? Is there accessory muscle use with respiration?
- **Abdomen**. Is there pain with palpation? Cramping?

- **Pelvis.** Are there any signs of incontinence?

- **Extremities.** Is there a Medic Alert medallion? Are there any hives? Is there swelling or a flushed appearance?

3. **TAKE VITAL SIGNS.** Measure mental status, airway, breathing, and circulation. As always monitor your patient for changes in vital signs. Changes may indicate your patient is getting worse.

4. **PROVIDE TREATMENT AS NEEDED.** Continue supporting your patient's ABCs. You may apply an ice pack to a bite or sting site to help relieve swelling and pain. If the patient has an allergy kit, you may help him or her prepare for self-administration of medication. However, you may not administer medication to any patient. *Follow all local protocols!*

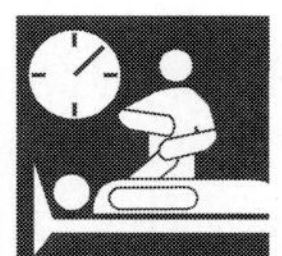

ONGOING ASSESSMENT AND TREAT

1. **REPEAT THE INITIAL ASSESSMENT.** C
airway, breathing, or circulation prob
tient immediately if there are any s

2. **REPEAT THE PHYSICAL EXAM**
and symptoms, such as short
runny nose, and tearing fr
worse? Better?

3. **PROVIDE REASSURA**

PATIENT HA

1. **GIVE A**
patie
beg

ORT. The following is an example of a
rianne, the patient in the scenario at the
e chapter:

Brianne is 47 years old. Fifteen minutes ago she was stung on the shoulder by a bee. Almost immediately she began to experience general itching, eye tearing, and hives. She also has pain and swelling at the site of the sting. She is alert and has a patent airway. Her breathing and circulatory status are normal. She has a history of allergies to bee stings and normally carries a bee sting kit, but not today. This is her only medication. She last ate this morning. Her head-to-toe exam shows some hives on her neck and chest, eye tearing, a runny nose, generalized itching, and swelling at the sting site on her left shoulder. Her vital signs are respiration 16, pulse 110, and blood pressure 120/72. At this time we're

CONCLUSION

Patients having an allergic reaction are suffering from the effects of their own immune system. Signs and symptoms can progress rapidly and can be life-threatening. We know that airway obstruction is the most common cause of death from allergic reaction. However, it's important to assess, intervene, and reassess airway, breathing, and circulation problems, because an allergic reaction can cause all three.

KEY TERMS

You may wish to use this list to review your understanding of key terms introduced in the chapter.

...renaline medication administered to stop an allergic reaction; ...ministered by injection. *Also called* epinephrine.

... substances that cause an allergic reaction.

... a particularly severe allergic reaction that can lead ...tening problems such as airway obstruction, respi... and shock. *Also called* anaphylactic shock.

...es created by the immune system to neutral... ...ng microorganisms or antigens.

antigens ... invade the body and trigger a response from the i...

making her comfortable and have placed an ice pack at the site of the sting. We've seen a decrease in her symptoms in the past few minutes.

2. **CONDUCT THE TRANSFER OF CARE.**

3. **ASSIST IN EXTRICATION AND TRANSPORT.** Severe allergic-reaction patients shouldn't walk or move around unnecessarily. If they are experiencing respiratory distress, have them sit up. If there are signs of shock, put them in the shock position. Otherwise extricate and transport patients in a position of comfort.

---

antihistamine a drug which is used to stop the symptoms of an allergic reaction.

hives large, circular, raised welts or wheals on the sk contact with or ingestion of an allergen.

immunity the state your body reaches when it enough antibodies to fight off an invading virus or bacteria.

APPLICATION QUESTIONS

You may wish to use these question the chapter. For answers with pag

1. You're caring for a 45-ye about 10 minutes ago, face and tongue and and has wheezing ority for this pat

2. You've been is having a al hours a a very l assist posi

...mp to his ... He's hoarse ... top treatment pri-

...or a 61-year-old female who ... to the penicillin she took sever- ... is having trouble breathing and has ... sure. Should you sit the patient up to ... athing or should you place her in a shock

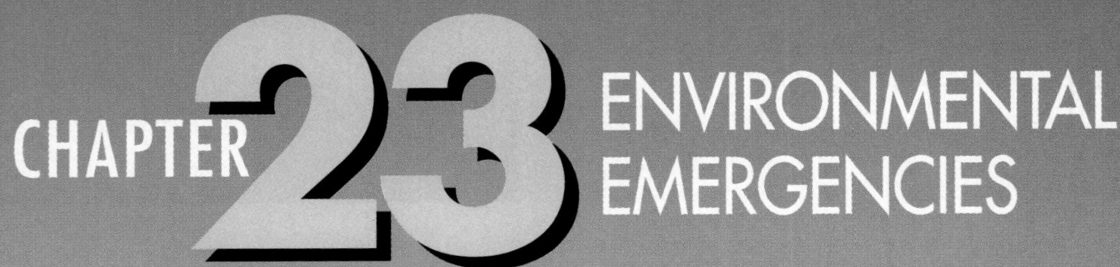

CHAPTER 23 ENVIRONMENTAL EMERGENCIES

FIRST RESPONSE

Volunteer firefighters, Rob and Dave, are dispatched to a "man down" at the back of a nearby grocery store. As they approach the scene, they're met by a police officer. He tells them that the patient is one of the "regular drunks" in town and that he's "out cold." They see a man in his 40s, head tucked deep into the collar of his coat. He's huddled on the wet pavement with dirty blankets wrapped around him. His head and coat also are wet from the morning rain.

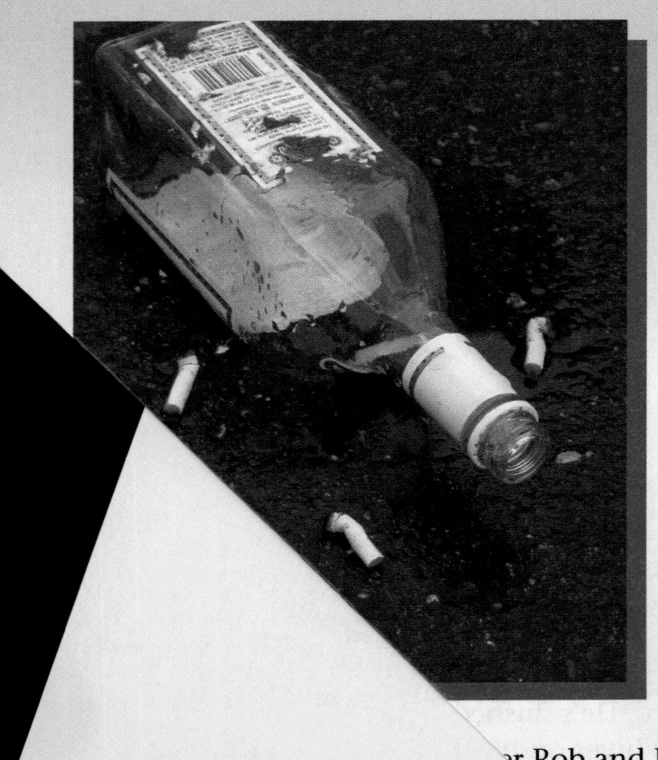

After gloving up, Rob performs an initial assessment. The man only groans when Rob checks his mental status. Rob finds that the man's respiratory and pulse rates are slow and his skin is icy.

After Dave applies high flow oxygen, Rob completes a physical exam. It reveals no major or obvious trauma. The patient's respiration rate is 8-10 breaths per minute. His pulse is 46. Neither Rob nor Dave are able to measure his blood pressure.

Suspecting a cold emergency in addition to intoxication, Rob and Dave strip away the patient's wet clothing and wrap him in heavy blankets from their fire engine. As they begin to ventilate him, the transporting unit arrives. Rob gives the EMTs a patient report. It takes only minutes before the EMTs package the patient and transport him to the hospital.

...r Rob and Dave learn that the patient's body temperature ... After he arrived at the hospital, the emergency depart... ...pent several hours reheating the man with warming ...s, and heated IV fluids.

...erlook heat and cold emergencies," Dave re... ...hen the patient has another problem that's ...ient was drunk. It's easy to focus on that. ...of your patient's signs and symptoms ...rmation about your patient's medical

LEARNING OBJECTIVES

As a First Responder, you'll often treat emergencies related to exposure to the environment. Some of those patients will also have underlying medical conditions. Because environmental emergencies can occur in areas far from hospital emergency departments, it's important for you to learn how to assess and provide adequate emergency care on the scene.

By the end of the chapter, you should be able to:†

- 5-1.7 Identify the patient who presents with a specific medical complaint of exposure to cold. (pp. 280-282)
- 5-1.8 Explain the steps in providing emergency medical care to a patient with an exposure to cold. (pp. 282, 283-284)
- 5-1.9 Identify the patient who presents with a specific medical complaint of exposure to heat. (pp. 284-285)
- 5-1.10 Explain the steps in providing emergency medical care to a patient with an exposure to heat. (p. 285)
- * Describe how the body regulates its temperature. (p. 279)
- * Describe an emergency care plan for assessing and treating environmental emergencies. (pp. 286-290)

BODY TEMPERATURE

The human body tries to keep a constant internal temperature of about 98.6°F. Where does it get that heat? In general all the physical and chemical processes that occur in the body create heat. The body can create extra heat by producing certain hormones and, if necessary, through shivering (muscle movement).

The body loses heat through several processes. Two of them are radiation and evaporation. In radiation, body heat escapes through the skin and into the air. In evaporation, perspiration cools the body's surface as it turns to vapor. Wind, water, and direct contact with cold objects also can take heat away from the body.

The body works to maintain a normal temperature, no matter what the conditions of the environment. However, extreme conditions can overwhelm its ability to do so. If left unchecked, low body temperature (**hypothermia**) or high body temperature (**hyperthermia**) can lead to significant—even deadly—breakdowns of body functions.

†Numbered objectives are from the 1995 U.S. DOT "First Responder: National Standard Curriculum." Asterisks indicate supplemental material.

EXPOSURE TO COLD

GENERALIZED COLD EMERGENCIES

Hypothermia can occur in any setting. It can happen suddenly, such as when someone falls through the ice, or it can occur gradually, such as by wind or wet exposure. Although you might think that cold exposure is always caused by extreme weather, it also occurs to people in poorly heated urban apartments. (See the stages of hypothermia in Figure 23-1.)

Hypothermia occurs when the body loses more heat than it produces. Patients with an internal body temperature between 90°F and 95°F have *mild hypothermia*. Patients with an internal body temperature below 90°F have *severe hypothermia*. Because patients with temperatures as low as 60°F have been resuscitated, EMS personnel abide by this phrase: "A patient is not dead until they're *warm* and dead."

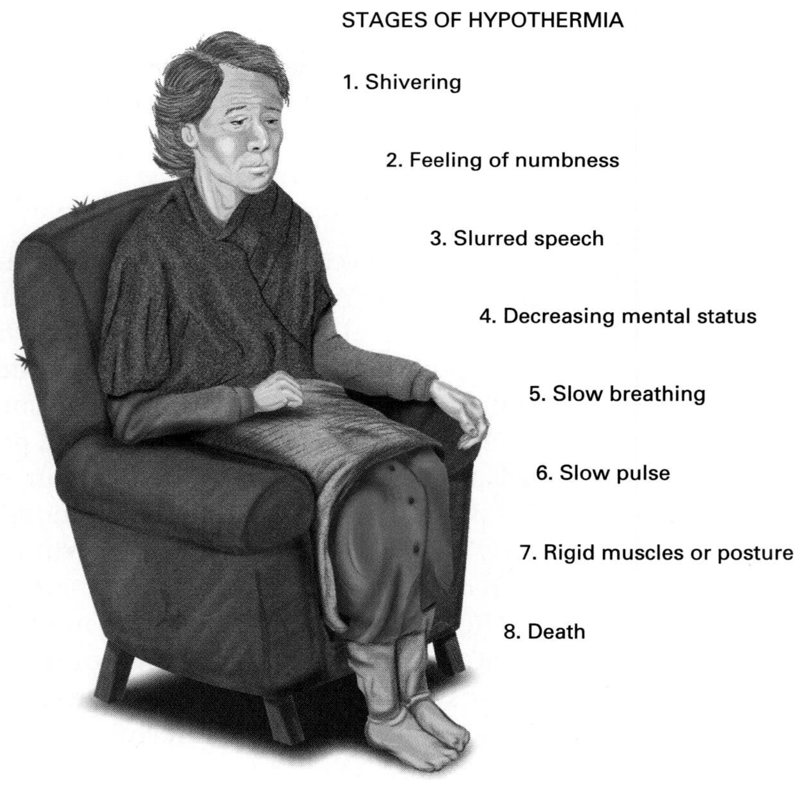

STAGES OF HYPOTHERMIA
1. Shivering
2. Feeling of numbness
3. Slurred speech
4. Decreasing mental status
5. Slow breathing
6. Slow pulse
7. Rigid muscles or posture
8. Death

Figure 23-1
The stages of hypothermia.

Contributing Factors

Some patients are at risk for hypothermia even without exposure to extreme cold. Several factors increase their risk, including the use of substances that alter perception or judgment. The patient that Rob and Dave cared for in the scenario at the beginning of the chapter is a good example.

Elderly patients also are at risk for hypothermia. Their bodies are less able to regulate temperature. They also often have medical conditions that further impair their ability to withstand the cold.

Infants and very young children have an increased risk of hypothermia. Because of their size, they lose heat faster than adults, especially from their heads. They also can't regulate their body temperature as well. Finally, infants and children who have airway, breathing, or circulation problems have much worse outcomes if they get cold and stay cold. So cover them up, especially their heads.

You will most likely encounter hypothermia while managing patients for other complaints. For example, almost all critical trauma patients who lie on the ground in cool or cold conditions become hypothermic. It's common for infants who are delivered in the field to arrive at the hospital mildly hypothermic as well. The key fact here is that all patients do worse if they are cold. Bottom line? Keep all your patients warm.

Signs and Symptoms

Patients with hypothermia may have the following signs and symptoms:

- *Cool or cold skin temperature* — A good way to assess the patient's temperature is to place the back of your hand between the patient's clothing and abdomen.
- *Shivering* — The body attempts to create heat by shivering (this is an early sign).

  Warning *In the field, if the cold-exposure patient is not shivering, he or she is moving from moderate to severe hypothermia.*

- *Decreasing mental status* — Some hypothermia patients become so confused that they begin to remove their clothing because they believe they feel too warm.
- *Rigid muscles or posture* — Your patient also may complain of joint and muscle stiffness.

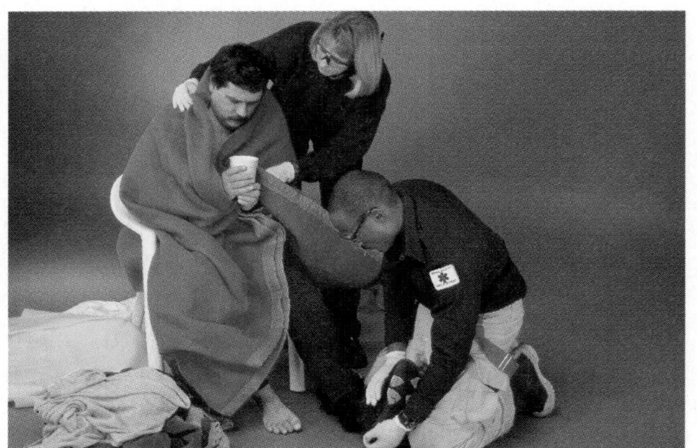

Figure 23-2
After removing the patient from the cold environment, protect him from further heat loss.

- *Vital sign changes* — Hypothermic patients often will develop decreased heart and breathing rates. Because the pulse may be hard to detect, check it for at least 30 to 45 seconds before starting CPR.
- Other related signs and symptoms include:
  - Poor coordination and motor function.
  - Loss of feeling or sensation.
  - Pale or bluish skin color.
  - Mood changes.
  - Dizziness.
  - Difficulty speaking.

PATIENT MANAGEMENT

To manage cold-exposure patients, protect them from any further heat loss. Remove them from the cold environment. Take off their wet clothing. Cover them with warm blankets (Figure 23-2). Handle these patients very gently, and don't massage cold or frozen extremities. Don't allow them to walk or exert themselves in any way. Although it may seem like a good idea to offer a hot drink, don't. It may actually worsen their condition.

LOCALIZED COLD EMERGENCIES

Exposure to cold also can cause **localized** injuries (injuries limited to a specific area). Freezing or near freezing of a body part is called **frostbite**. It most often occurs in the fingers, toes, face, nose, and ears (Figure 23-3).

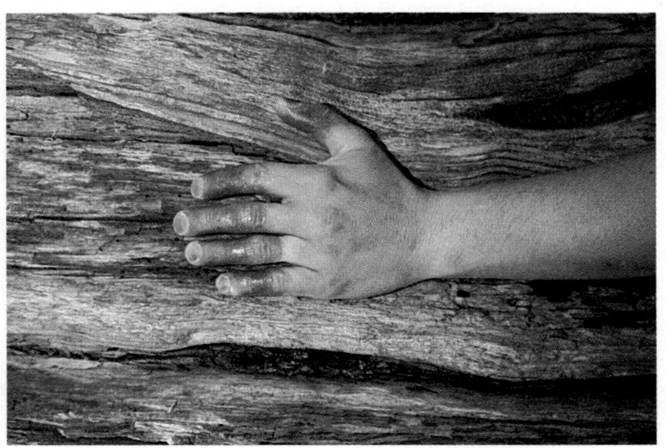

Figure 23-3
Example of a local cold injury.

Signs and Symptoms

Depending on the extent of the exposure, a local cold injury may be **superficial** (confined to the surface) or deep. (In some EMS systems a superficial cold injury is called an "early cold injury" and a deep cold injury is called a "late cold injury.") Signs and symptoms include the following:

- Superficial (early) cold injury
  - Blanching of the skin. That is, when you press on the skin, it doesn't return to its normal color.
  - Loss of feeling and sensation in the injured area.
  - Skin usually remains soft.
  - With rewarming, the patient may experience a tingling sensation in the injured area.
- Deep (late) cold injury
  - White, waxy skin.
  - Firm to frozen feeling when you touch the injured body part.
  - Swelling.
  - Blistering.
  - If thawed or partially thawed, the skin may appear flushed (red) with areas of purple and blanching, or the skin may be mottled and cyanotic.

Patient Management

Once you've determined that the patient has suffered a local cold injury, remove the patient from the cold environment. Remove any wet or restrictive clothing, while protecting the injured body part from further injury. If the injury is an early or superficial cold injury, then manually stabilize and cover the extremity. If the injury is a late or deep cold injury, then cover it with dry dressings.

Avoid exposing the injured part to the cold again. If you see blisters on the injured part, don't break them. Don't rub or massage the affected areas. Don't apply heat or try to rewarm the affected area. Don't allow the patient to walk on a cold-injured extremity.

EXPOSURE TO HEAT

Hyperthermia (high body temperature) occurs when a patient is unable to get rid of excess heat. Heat-related emergencies usually occur when a person is exposed to a hot environment for an extended period of time. This type of emergency is most commonly seen on days when the outside temperature is 100°F or more. Depending on the extent of exposure, the hyperthermic patient's body temperature can rise rapidly to dangerous levels, in some cases as high as 106°F.

CONTRIBUTING FACTORS

The factors that contribute to hyperthermia include:

- *Climate* — A high air temperature can reduce the body's ability to lose heat through radiation. High humidity reduces its ability to lose heat through evaporation.
- *Exercise and activity* — Depending on the level of activity, a person can lose as much as one liter of sweat per hour. This can leave the body dehydrated and less able to regulate temperature.
- *Drugs and alcohol* — Both drugs and alcohol impair the body's ability to regulate its temperature.
- *Age* — Older people are more vulnerable to heat-related emergencies because they don't regulate body temperature as well as they once could. Elderly patients also have preexisting conditions that further impair their ability to withstand a hot environment.

Infants and children are more vulnerable to heat-related emergencies because they don't regulate their temperatures as well as adults. They also may not be able to remove their own clothing.

SIGNS AND SYMPTOMS

A heat emergency may occur on a hot day, especially after strenuous activity. Elderly patients and patients who have preexisting problems are particularly at risk. Signs and symptoms of a heat-related emergency include:

- Altered mental status.
- Muscle cramps.
- Weakness or exhaustion.
- Dizziness or fainting.
- Skin that is either:
  - Moist, pale, normal to cool in temperature.
  - Hot, dry or moist (this is a dire emergency).
- Rapid pulse.

PATIENT MANAGEMENT

As a First Responder, your primary role in a heat emergency is to remove the patient from the hot environment and place him in a cooler one. Administer oxygen, if you're allowed to do so. Help to cool the patient by loosening or removing the patient's clothing and by fanning him. If the patient is responsive and not nauseous, have him drink water. If the patient is unresponsive or is vomiting, place the patient on his side.

If the patient has hot, dry or moist skin, cool him with a wet sheet and fanning (Figure 23-4). Also apply cool packs to the neck, groin, and armpits. As always support the patient's airway, breathing, and circulation. Arrange for immediate transport.

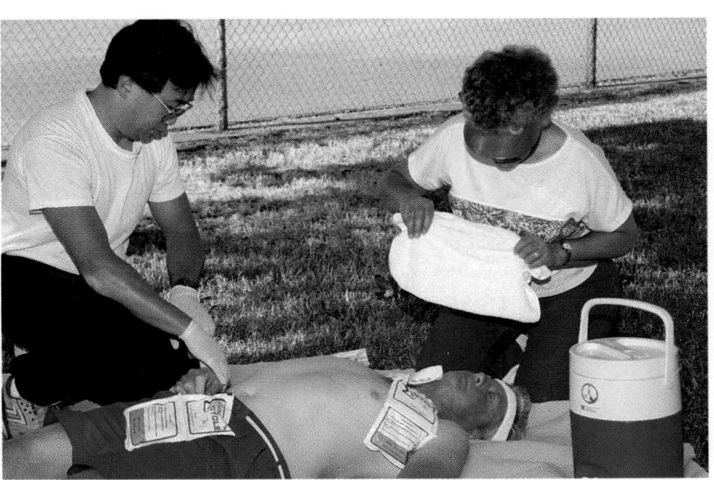

Figure 23-4
Cool the heat-injured patient if he or she is hot to the touch.

EMERGENCY CARE PLAN | PATIENTS WITH ENVIRONMENTAL EMERGENCIES

PRIORITIES

Your top priorities for a patient with a cold or heat emergency are:

- Early recognition of the signs and symptoms.
- Early activation of the EMS system.
- Removing the patient from the harmful environment.
- Assuring an open airway and adequate breathing and circulation.
- Providing simple external cooling or warming measures as appropriate.
- Continuous reassessment.

PATIENT CARE APPROACH

Approach these patients in a calm, supportive, and reassuring manner. Remember that high priority patients will likely have an altered mental status. Treat them accordingly.

DANGER SIGNS

Danger signs include any mental status, airway, breathing, or circulation problems. After removing the patient from the cold or heat, pay attention to changes for the worse. Remember that your patient may have an unrelated medical problem. So watch for any signs and symptoms in addition to those you would expect to see with hypothermia or hyperthermia.

SCENE SIZE-UP

1. **ASSESS SCENE SAFETY.** Is the scene safe to enter? Are there any hazards? Are you protected from the cold or heat? Be sure to perform only the types of rescue you've been trained for. Call for help if needed.

2. **DETERMINE NATURE OF ILLNESS.** Is this a heat or cold emergency? Activate the EMS system if someone hasn't already done so.

3. **TRIAGE THE PATIENT.** How many patients are there? How ill do they appear to be? If you're responding to an outlying area, do you have the resources to effectively manage the patient or patients? Are the proper resources responding to the call?

4. **DETERMINE ACCESS AND EXTRICATION NEEDS.**

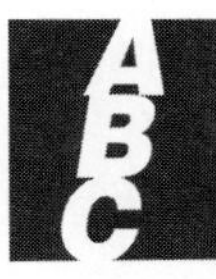

INITIAL ASSESSMENT AND TREATMENT

1. **FORM A GENERAL IMPRESSION.** What is the patient's sex and approximate age? What is the chief complaint? Body position? Overall level of distress?

2. **CHECK MENTAL STATUS.** Is your patient awake and answering all questions appropriately? Is he or she responding to your questions and verbal commands? If your patient has an altered mental status, apply high flow oxygen if you are equipped to do so.

3. **ASSESS THE ABCs.**

   - **Airway.** Is the airway open and clear? If not, open the airway now.

   - **Breathing.** Patients experiencing cold or heat emergencies may have breathing ranging from slow and shallow to deep and rapid. Carefully evaluate the respiratory depth, rate, and effort to determine whether the patient requires oxygen or ventilation.

   - **Circulation.** Assess your patient's pulse and skin condition.

4. **DETERMINE PRIORITY.** Any patient with altered mental status, or with airway, breathing, and circulation problems is a high priority patient. Trust your "gut instincts" on this.

Does your patient appear to be extremely hot or cold? Always err on the side of caution.

5. **PROVIDE TREATMENT.** In all heat and cold emergencies, remove the patient from the harmful environment as soon as possible. Position the patient based on mental status, airway, breathing, and circulation status. If the patient appears to be stable, place him or her in a position of comfort.

   If you are managing a heat-exposed patient who has hot, dry or moist skin, begin cooling procedures immediately. This patient may be suffering from a condition that can be fatal if left untreated.

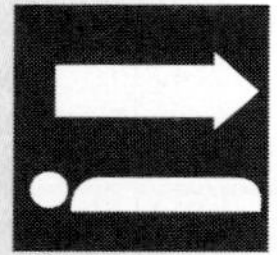

PHYSICAL EXAM AND TREATMENT

1. **GATHER A *SAMPLE* HISTORY.**

   (S)igns and symptoms related to a heat or cold emergency? Are there any related to other emergencies such as intoxication or trauma? Remember that heat and cold emergencies may exist along with other medical problems.

   (A)llergies to medications?

   (M)edications? Is the patient taking any medications that may have contributed to their condition? Did the patient overdose on any drugs or alcohol prior to the exposure?

   (P)ertinent past history? Does the patient have a history of chronic illness? Has that illness made the patient more vulnerable to heat or cold exposure?

   (L)ast oral intake? Has the heat-exposed patient been replacing fluids? Has the cold-exposed patient had any alcohol? When was the patient's last meal?

   (E)vents leading to the illness? To what environment was the patient exposed and for how long?

2. **PERFORM A HEAD-TO-TOE EXAM.** Take time to remove any clothing that is causing the patient to be either hotter or colder now. Continue to protect the patient from the environment.

- **Head.** What is the patient's skin color? Is it pale, flushed, bluish?
- **Neck.** Are there any signs of trauma?
- **Chest.** Are there any signs of trauma? Is there any chest pain?
- **Abdomen.** Is the skin of the abdomen cool or cold?
- **Extremities.** Does the patient have any signs of local cold injury?

3. **TAKE VITAL SIGNS.** Include a more careful check of the patient's mental status, airway, breathing rate and quality, pulse rate and quality, skin condition, and blood pressure.

4. **PROVIDE TREATMENT AS NEEDED.** If the heat-exposed patient has hot, dry or moist skin, continue to cool him or her with a wet sheet and fanning.

   Prevent further heat loss from the cold-exposed patient with additional blankets as needed. If the patient has a superficial cold injury in an extremity, manually stabilize it. If the injury is a deep cold injury, then cover it with dry dressings.

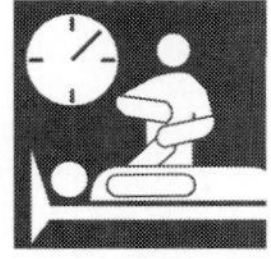

ONGOING ASSESSMENT AND TREATMENT

1. **REPEAT THE INITIAL ASSESSMENT.**
2. **REPEAT THE PHYSICAL EXAM.**
3. **PROVIDE REASSURANCE.**

PATIENT HAND-OFF

1. **GIVE A PATIENT REPORT.** The following is an example of a patient report based on the scenario at the beginning of the chapter:

Our patient is a male in his 40s found lying behind the grocery store. He's been here for an unknown amount of time. He appears to be very cold and smells of alcohol. He responds to verbal stimuli with moaning only. He has a clear airway, but his breathing is 8-10 per minute so we're ventilating him with a BVM and 100% oxygen. His pulse is 46. He's a high priority patient. We smell alcohol on his breath, and he's quite wet from the rain. Otherwise we haven't found any signs of trauma. We don't know his allergy or medication status. We also have no past medical history. We've stripped off his wet clothing and covered him with

CONCLUSION

Environmental emergencies aren't just limited to extreme climates. Become familiar with the signs and symptoms no matter where you work as a First Responder. Your primary role is to remove the patient from the harmful environment, assure the patient's ABCs, and continue supportive treatment until an ambulance arrives.

KEY TERMS

You may wish to use this list to review your understanding of key terms introduced in the chapter.

blanching losing color, usually suddenly.
frostbite local freezing or near freezing of a body part, most often fingers, toes, face, and ears.
hyperthermia having a body temperature above normal.
hypothermia having a body temperature below normal.
localized limited to a specific area.
superficial confined to the surface.

blankets. We've placed him in the recovery position and are continuing to administer high flow oxygen. There have been no changes in the patient's status since our arrival.

2. **CONDUCT THE TRANSFER OF CARE.**

3. **ASSIST IN EXTRICATION AND TRANSPORT.** Cold- or heat-exposed patients shouldn't walk or move around. Don't let a patient with local cold injuries to the feet walk around.

APPLICATION QUESTIONS

You may wish to use these questions to review your understanding of the chapter. For answers with page references, see Appendix 2.

1. You're caring for an elderly man who was found down and confused in his mobile home. His vital signs are as follows: mental status—confused; airway—patent; respiration—8; pulse—50; skin—pale and cold. You and your partner are concerned with his respiratory rate. Your partner believes the top treatment priority is to warm the patient with blankets and a heater. He says this will stimulate your patient to increase his respirations. Do you agree or disagree with this strategy? Why?

2. You're caring for a 45-year-old man who has collapsed while running in a marathon. You find the patient on his back, confused, with very hot, dry skin, and a rapid bounding pulse. As you complete your initial assessment, he vomits and has a seizure. What should you do first?

CHAPTER 24 CHILDBIRTH

FIRST RESPONSE

Larry, a security guard at a hospital, is just beginning his nightly rounds when he hears the insistent blare of a car horn. He finds a young woman in labor parked in front of the hospital's entrance. She has tried to drive herself to the hospital and can make it no farther.

"Are you okay?" Larry asks. "Can I help you to the hospital? My name's Larry, and I'm the hospital security guard. What's your name?"

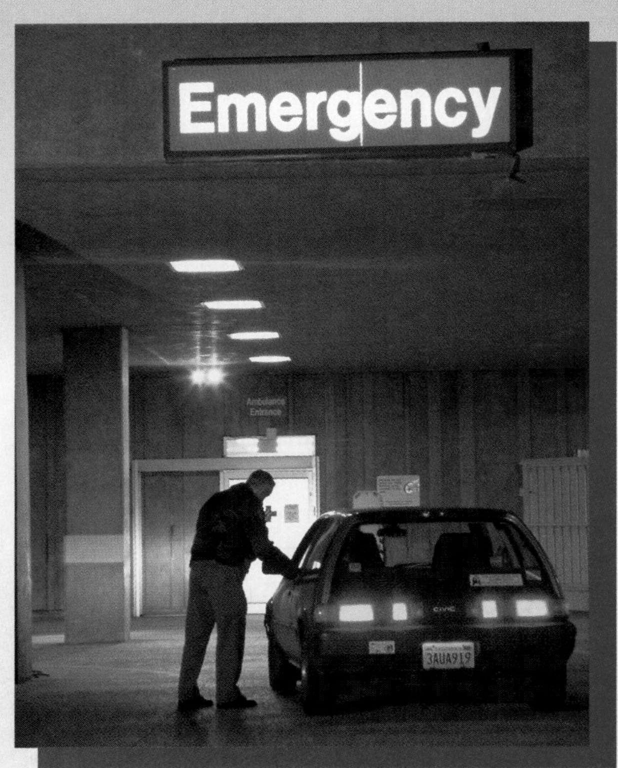

"Maria. I'm having the baby," she cries. "Get help. Now!"

Larry radios the hospital operator to send help. Then he opens the car door. Maria is breathing fast and looks to be in severe distress. "Help will be here in a minute. Are you having a contraction?" he asks.

"Yes!" she gasps. "There's no more time! The baby is coming!"

"I need to see if the baby is crowning," Larry tells her. Maria lies back along the length of the front seat. As she does so, Larry grabs a pair of gloves from the inside pocket of his uniform and puts them on. Sure enough, he can see the top of the baby's head emerging from the birth canal. Larry places the palm of one hand very gently over the baby's head to prevent an "explosive delivery," a birth that occurs so fast that the newborn can actually be injured.

"I have to push," Maria says. She takes a deep breath and begins to push. As the baby's head delivers, Larry removes as much fluid from the baby's face and mouth as he can. In a matter of seconds the baby is born. "It's a girl!" he tells the mother. He dries the slippery infant with a clean beach towel he finds in the back seat. After he performs an initial assessment of the infant, Larry puts the crying newborn on her mother's abdomen.

LEARNING OBJECTIVES

Childbirth in the out-of-hospital setting rarely occurs. When it does occur, complications are rare. So delivering a baby in the field can be a happy and exciting event, as well as a refreshing change from caring for sick and injured patients. However, all this good news doesn't reduce the stress that often surrounds field deliveries. There's lots of emotion and pain, and you'll find yourself caring for two patients instead of one.

As you'll see, assisting with an out-of-hospital birth is much more than calling for hot water and towels. Understanding your role in the birthing process will help you to be less anxious and better able to really help both the delivering patient and the newborn.

By the end of the chapter, you should be able to:[†]

- 6-1.1 Identify the following structures: birth canal, placenta, umbilical cord, amniotic sac. (p. 294)
- 6-1.2 Define the following terms: crowning, bloody show, labor, abortion. (pp. 294-295, 302)
- 6-1.3 State indications of an imminent delivery. (pp. 295-296)
- 6-1.4 State the steps in the pre-delivery preparation of the mother. (p. 296)
- 6-1.5 Establish the relationship between body substance isolation and childbirth. (p. 296)
- 6-1.6 State the steps to assist in the delivery. (pp. 297-299)
- 6-1.7 Describe care of the baby as the head appears. (p. 297)
- 6-1.8 Discuss the steps in delivery of the placenta. (p. 299)
- 6-1.9 List the steps in the emergency medical care of the mother post-delivery. (p. 300)
- 6-1.10 Discuss the steps in caring for a newborn. (pp. 300-301)

* Describe an emergency care plan for assessing and treating patients in childbirth. (pp. 302-307)

[†]Numbered objectives are from the 1995 U.S. DOT "First Responder: National Standard Curriculum." Asterisks indicate supplemental material.

THE PROCESS OF CHILDBIRTH

SPECIALIZED ANATOMY

The specialized anatomy and functions of a woman's reproductive organs include the following:

- **Uterus**—The uterus, or womb, is a pear-shaped smooth muscle within which the fetus grows and develops. After the egg (ovum) is fertilized, it imbeds itself in the lining of the uterus. Development of the fetus begins almost immediately, and the uterus grows and stretches with it. In fact, the uterus will triple in size and weight by the second month of pregnancy.

- **Placenta**—After the egg is implanted, the placenta begins to develop. Very rich in blood vessels, it's responsible for the exchange of oxygen and other gases between the mother and fetus. It's also responsible for the transport of nutrients and wastes.

- **Umbilical cord**—Attached at the baby's navel, this cord is an extension of the placenta. Through it the fetus receives nourishment until it's born.

- **Amniotic sac**—This is the membrane within which the fetus develops. Inside the sac the fetus floats in a clear substance called the **amniotic fluid**. It cushions the fetus against trauma and provides a stable environment in which the baby can grow. Before delivery, the amniotic sac usually breaks and discharges the fluid. When this happens, the mother may report that her "water broke."

- **Cervix**—This is the lowest part of the uterus. It forms an opening that begins to dilate or stretch when labor begins. When this happens, a mucus plug, or the **bloody show**, may be expelled. In order for the baby to be delivered, the cervix must be fully dilated.

- **Birth canal**—The cervix and the vagina form the birth canal. Near the end of a normal pregnancy, the baby usually moves into a head-down position low in the mother's pelvis. When this happens, the baby has "dropped." It's now ready to pass through the cervix and into the vagina. Once in the vagina, it's said that the baby is **crowning**, a sign that the birth is imminent (about to happen).

WHAT IS LABOR?

Labor is the process by which the baby is born. Near the end of pregnancy, the uterus will begin to contract. This signals the first stage of labor. As labor continues, contractions become progressively stronger, more regular, and more frequent. When contractions are about one to two minutes apart and about 45 to 90 seconds each, the baby moves into the birth canal. Very soon after, the baby is delivered. In the final stage of labor, the mother delivers the placenta.

The contractions that signal labor are usually described as cramp-like pain that can radiate around to the mother's back. For some woman, however, labor is an excruciating event. Each woman will have her own unique response to the birthing process and to the level of pain that she experiences.

The length of labor varies from woman to woman. With first pregnancies a woman's labor may last 12 or more hours. Women who already have children tend to proceed more rapidly. A few deliver in only a matter of minutes.

Women also have unique emotional responses to labor and birthing. For example, compare the emotions of a 15-year-old having her first baby after no prenatal care to the 35-year-old who is having her third child. A woman's emotional state will change in the course of her labor too. At times the woman may feel exhausted and unable to continue. Other times, she'll be more confident and relaxed.

BEFORE DELIVERY

WHAT IS AN IMMINENT DELIVERY?

As a First Responder you should make every attempt to get the mother to the hospital safely. However, never try to delay or restrain the delivery in any way.

If any of the following signs or symptoms are present, make preparations to deliver the baby on the scene:

- There are regular contractions one to two minutes apart, lasting 45-90 seconds each. (An interval is measured by timing the beginning of one contraction to the beginning of the next.)
- The mother reports the urge to bear down or to have a bowel movement.
- You see a large bloody show.
- The mother tells you that the baby is coming.

Take BSI precautions and examine the patient to see if the baby's head is emerging from the birth canal (crowning). Be sure not to touch the vaginal area except during delivery and only if your partner is present. If crowning is present, prepare for delivery.

PREPARING FOR DELIVERY

If there's time, attempt to find a private, clean area in which to assist in the delivery of the baby. Position the mother on her back with her knees bent, legs spread apart, and her buttocks slightly elevated with a pillow (Figure 24-1). Place absorbent, clean materials such as sheets or towels directly under the mother's buttocks. Drape the area and the mother with sterile or clean towels. If you have an "OB kit" available (Figure 24-2), open it and assemble the equipment within easy reach. If more than one baby is expected, request the necessary additional resources from EMS dispatch.

> ***Caution*** *It's essential that you wear personal protective equipment when assisting in the delivery of a baby. There's always a great deal of body fluid and blood involved. Protect yourself against exposure to infectious disease by wearing gloves, goggles, face mask, and gown. By draping the mother, you'll also help to protect her and the baby from contaminants.*

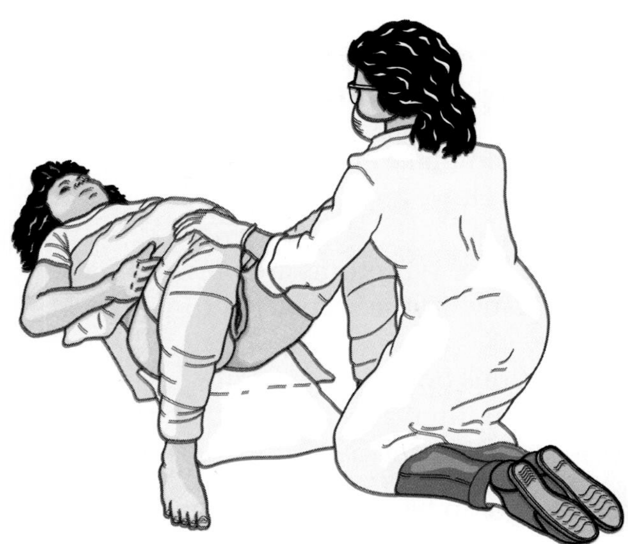

Figure 24-1
Position the mother with her buttocks slightly elevated on a pillow

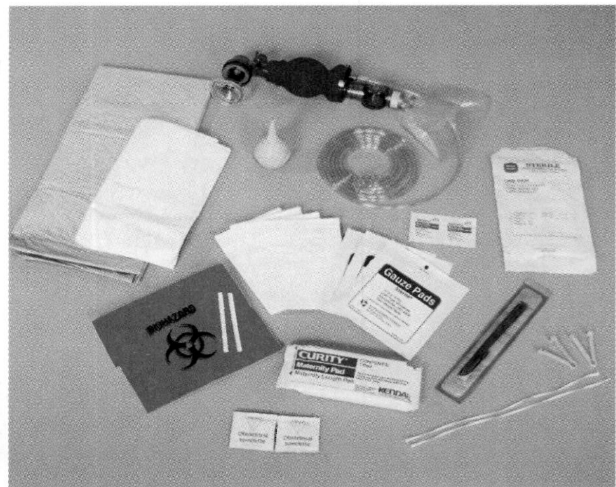

Figure 24-2
An obstetrics (OB) kit includes a bulb syringe, towels, blankets, dressings, surgical scissors, and cord clamps.

THE DELIVERY

ASSISTING WITH DELIVERY

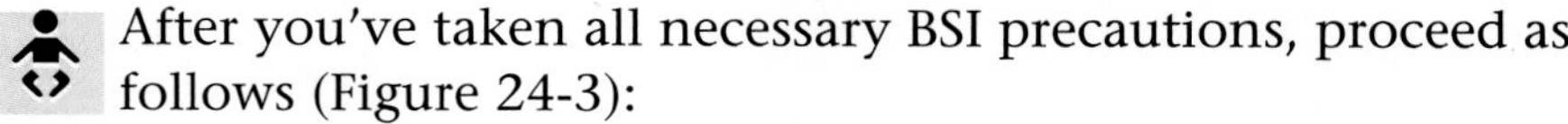

After you've taken all necessary BSI precautions, proceed as follows (Figure 24-3):

1. When the infant crowns, place the palm of your gloved hand on top of the baby's head. Apply very gentle pressure to prevent an explosive delivery.
2. If the amniotic sac hasn't broken, tear it open with your fingers. After the gush of fluid, push it away from the baby's head and mouth.
3. As the infant's head is being born, determine if the umbilical cord is wrapped around the baby's neck. If it is, attempt to slip the cord over the baby's shoulder. If unsuccessful, try to alleviate pressure on the cord.
4. After the infant's head delivers, support it.
5. Suction the baby's mouth and then the nostrils two or three times with a bulb syringe. Avoid contact with the back of the baby's mouth. If a bulb syringe isn't available, wipe the baby's mouth and then the nose with gauze or other clean fabric.
6. As the baby's torso is born, support the infant with both hands. Don't pull!
7. As the feet are delivered, grasp them firmly. Remember that babies are very slippery. Keep the infant at the level of the mother's vagina. You may place the infant on the mother's abdomen for warmth.
8. Continue to wipe blood and mucus from the baby's mouth and nose with sterile gauze. Suction the mouth and then the nose again with the bulb syringe.
9. Dry the infant. Then rub the baby's back or flick the soles of the baby's feet to stimulate breathing (Figure 24-4).
10. Keep the baby warm. Wrap him or her in a dry, warm blanket to conserve heat. Then place the baby on its side, head slightly lower than the trunk.
11. When the umbilical cord stops pulsating, tie it with gauze between the mother and the newborn. It should be placed at least six inches away from the baby. There's no need for you to cut the cord in a normal delivery. The EMTs will have the proper equipment to clamp and cut it when they arrive.

Normal Delivery

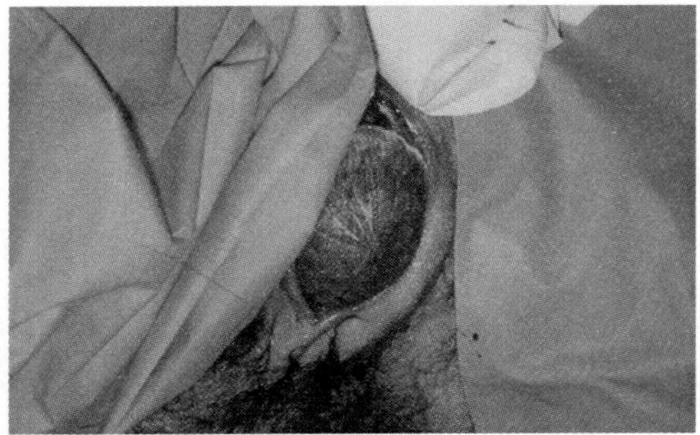

Figure 24-3a
Crowning.

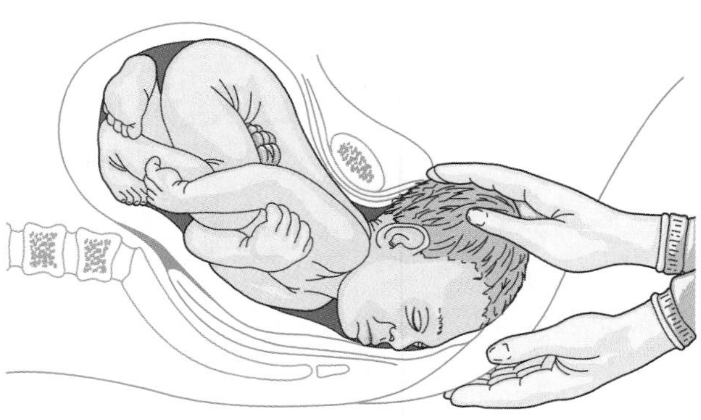

Figure 24-3b
Supporting the baby's head.

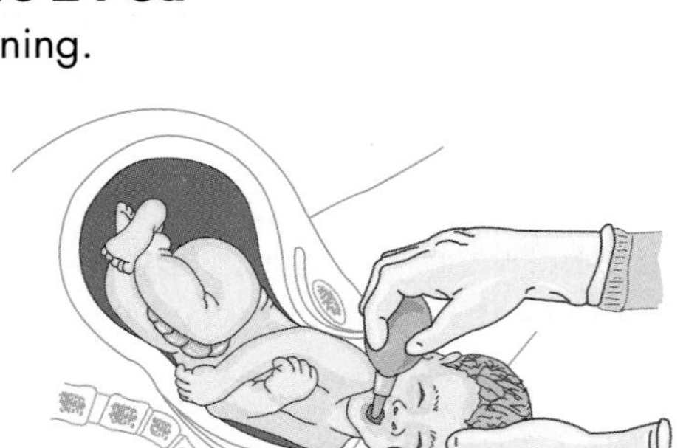

Figure 24-3c
Using a bulb syringe to suction the mouth and nose.

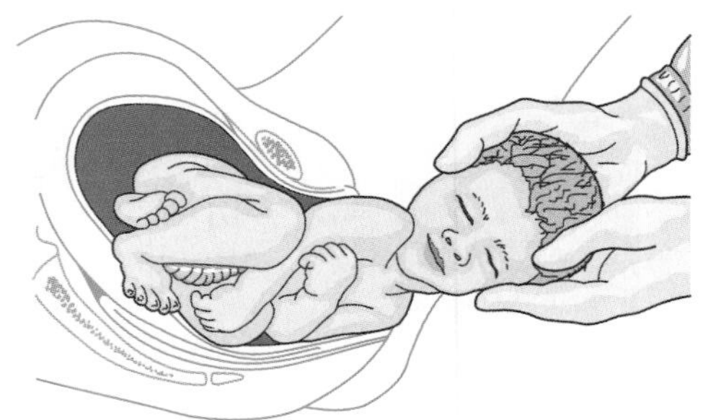

Figure 24-3d
Delivery of the upper shoulder.

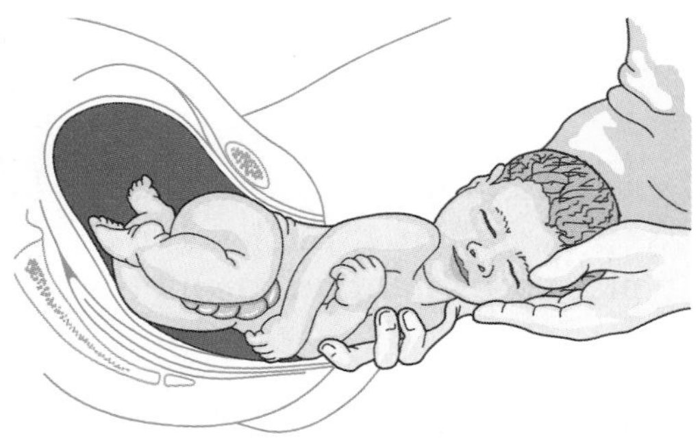

Figure 24-3e
Delivery of the lower shoulder.

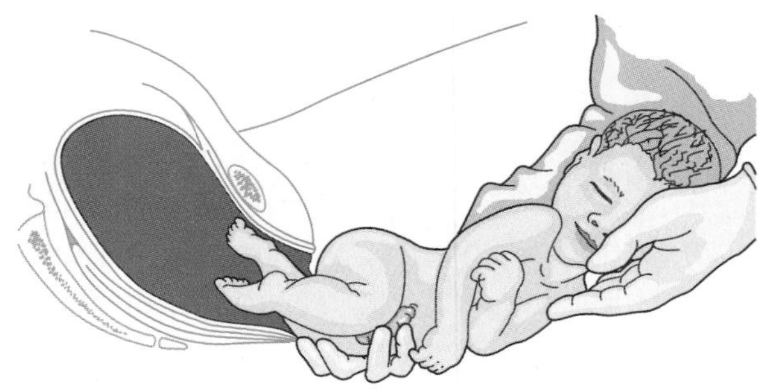

Figure 24-3f
Supporting the baby's body.

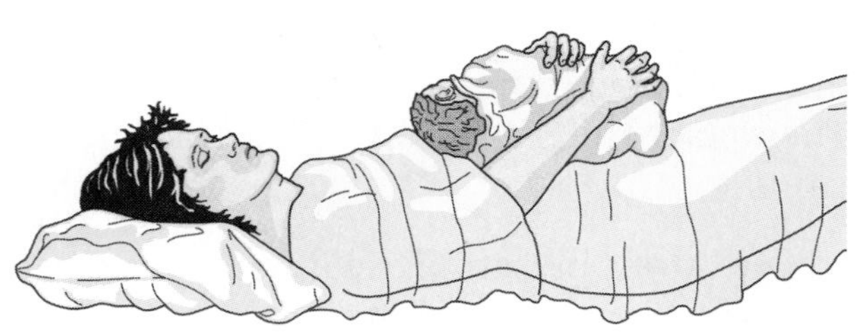

Figure 24-3g
Placing the newborn on the mother's abdomen.

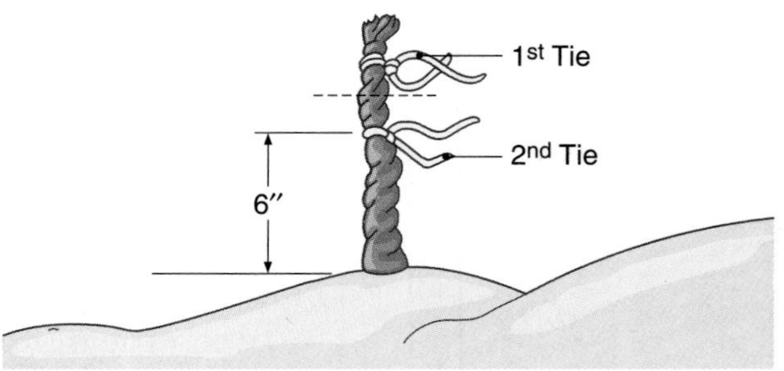

Figure 24-3h
Tying off the umbilical cord.

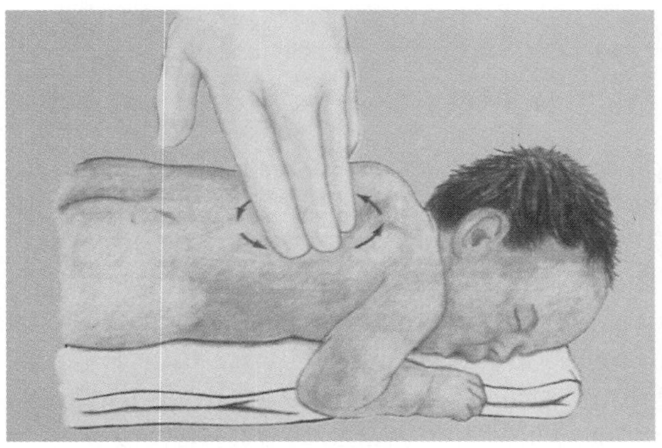

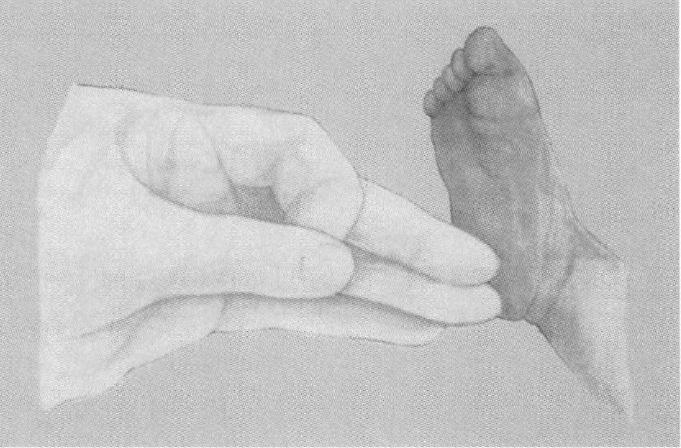

Figure 24-4
Stimulate the baby to breathe by rubbing the baby's back or tapping the baby's foot.

12. Record the time of the baby's delivery. If there's a chance of a multiple birth, prepare for a second delivery.

After delivery, make every effort to keep the mother and infant warm. If the infant is stable, encourage the mother to hold it. It's very important that you allow the mother to begin to bond with her baby.

DELIVERY OF THE PLACENTA

The placenta, or **afterbirth**, normally delivers about 20-30 minutes after the baby is born (Figure 24-5). Never try to pull it out. Don't delay transport of the patient for its delivery. Once the placenta is delivered, wrap it in a towel with about 75% of the umbilical cord. Place it in a plastic bag, and keep it at the level of the infant.

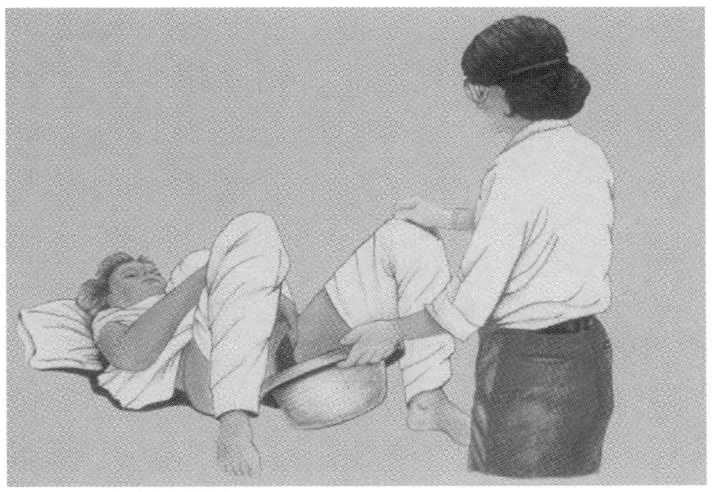

Figure 24-5
Collecting the placenta (afterbirth).

AFTER DELIVERY

MANAGEMENT OF THE MOTHER

After delivery of the placenta, place a sterile pad over the vaginal opening. Lower the mother's legs, and help her hold them together. Expect from 300-500 milliliters of blood loss (about two cups). Don't be alarmed by this. Don't alarm the mother. It's normal.

However, if the mother continues to bleed, then it may help to massage the abdomen over the uterus. With fingers fully extended, place the palm of your gloved hand on the mother's lower abdomen above the pubis. Massage the area in a kneading motion (Figure 24-6). This may help the uterus become firmer and reduce bleeding. If bleeding continues, check your massage technique.

If the mother has chosen to breast feed her baby, encourage her to start now. This stimulates the uterus to contract and helps to slow bleeding.

In general, keep contact with the mother throughout the process. Monitor respirations and pulse. Keep in mind that delivery is an exhausting procedure. Replace any blood-soaked sheets and blankets while awaiting transport.

MANAGEMENT OF THE NEWBORN

The key questions to ask yourself when you assess the newborn to determine the adequacy of the airway, breathing, and circulation are as follows:

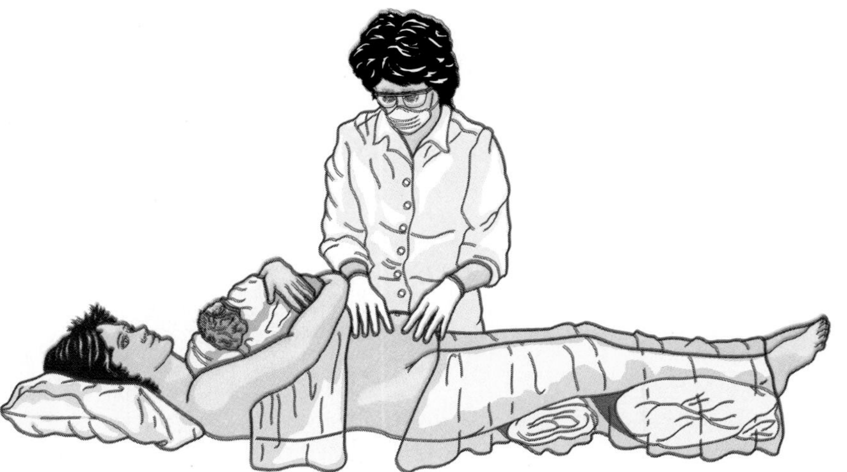

Figure 24-6
Massaging the area over the uterus to help reduce bleeding.

- Is the baby breathing regularly and rapidly, with a full cry?
- How fast is the baby's pulse? Is it above or below 100 beats per minute?
- What is the baby's color? Is there a pinkish glow or is the skin or mucous membranes blue?
- Is the baby moving and wiggling, or does the baby appear limp and floppy with poor muscle tone?

Within a minute after birth, most babies will be crying and wiggling. If this isn't so, then the baby may have a problem related to breathing. If there is a breathing problem or if the baby is sluggish or somewhat blue, then suction, dry, stimulate, and warm the baby vigorously. Then recheck vital signs. Heart rate should be above 100 beats per minute. Respirations should be above 40 per minute. If there's no improvement after one minute, then:

- Ensure an open and clear airway. Suction with the bulb syringe as needed.
- Ventilate at a rate of 40 breaths per minute with an infant-size BVM.
- After ventilating the infant for one minute, check the heart rate. If the heart rate is less than 80 beats per minute, begin chest compressions.

If the newborn's heart rate is above 100 beats per minute and he or she has adequate respirations but appears to be in respiratory distress, apply high flow oxygen by mask if you're equipped to do so. Signs of respiratory distress in the newborn include:

- Retractions (use of accessory muscles) at the base of the neck and between the ribs.
- "Seesaw" breathing between the chest and the belly.
- Nasal flaring.
- Respiratory rates above 80 breaths per minute.

The rule—rather than the exception—with newborns is that nearly all will perk up with suctioning, drying, stimulating, and warming. Rarely will you need to consider ventilation or CPR.

EMERGENCY CARE PLAN | CHILDBIRTH

■ PRIORITIES

Your top priorities for the patient in active labor are:

- Determining if there's time to transport or if the delivery must occur on scene.
- Assisting with the birth of the baby if the birth is imminent.
- Assessing and treating the newborn's airway, breathing, and circulation as needed, and preventing heat loss.
- Monitoring the mother for bleeding after delivery of the placenta.
- Continuous reassessment of the mother and baby.

■ PATIENT CARE APPROACH

Approach the pregnant patient in a calm and reassuring manner. Even though this may be your first time delivering a baby, you can reduce anxiety—your own as well as the patient's—by remaining calm. Understand that the pain of childbirth may be intense. Expect your patient to scream, moan, yell, or cry. Acknowledge this pain. Your patient will also show a variety of emotions during labor and delivery. Be nonjudgmental and supportive.

■ DANGER SIGNS

Spontaneous abortion, or miscarriage, is a complication that usually occurs early in pregnancy. The patient often has heavy vaginal bleeding, cramping pain in the lower abdomen, and may even have passage of tissue from the vagina. Treat the patient for shock as indicated and save any passed tissue or evidence of blood loss for hospital personnel.

In rare instances after a full term, normal pregnancy, the baby may not be in a head-down position in the birth canal. During labor, the baby may present an arm, leg, or shoulder instead of the head. This type of delivery should occur in a hospital if at all possible. So tell the mother not to push. Update responding EMS personnel. Do your best to calm and reassure the mother until they arrive. Never pull on a presenting limb, shoulder, or body part.

A normal pregnancy lasts about 280 days. If the birth occurs four weeks or more before the due date, the baby will be **premature**. Premature newborns often have respiratory problems. So be prepared to provide basic life support if needed.

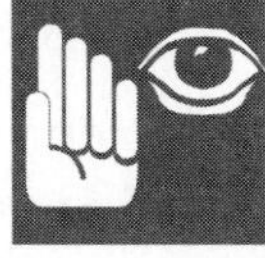

SCENE SIZE-UP

1. **ASSESS SCENE SAFETY.** Is it safe to enter? Remember that birth carries a high risk of infectious exposure, so take all necessary BSI precautions. Wear gloves, gown, mask, and eye protection if possible.

2. **DETERMINE NATURE OF ILLNESS.** What is the mother's chief complaint? Is she in active labor or is the pregnant patient simply ill or injured? Have contractions started? Activate the EMS system if you haven't already done so.

3. **TRIAGE THE PATIENT.** As you approach the patient, does it appear that birth is imminent?

4. **DETERMINE ACCESS AND EXTRICATION NEEDS.** Is there enough room to deliver the baby? Clear away enough space so that you can effectively assess the mother and assist with the birth.

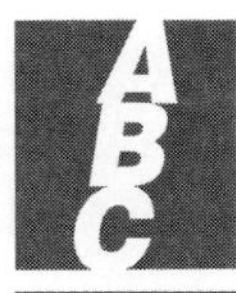

INITIAL ASSESSMENT AND TREATMENT

1. **FORM A GENERAL IMPRESSION.** What is the mother's approximate age? What is the mother's overall level of distress?

2. **CHECK MENTAL STATUS.** Is the mother awake and answering all questions appropriately? What does her emotional state appear to be? If she's showing signs of altered mental status, it may be due to hypoxia. Administer high flow oxygen as indicated.

3. **ASSESS THE ABCs.** Assure the mother's airway, breathing, and circulation. If she appears to be short of breath, apply oxygen if so equipped. If she's lying down and birth isn't imminent, make sure that she's lying on her left side. This will help to prevent her uterus from pressing against blood vessels and lowering her blood pressure.

4. **DETERMINE PRIORITY.** How far apart are contractions? Are contractions one to two minutes apart, lasting 45-90 seconds each? Is the mother having the urge to bear down? Is there a large, bloody show present? Is the mother telling you that the baby is coming? Is the baby crowning? If birth appears imminent, notify EMS dispatch and set up for delivery.

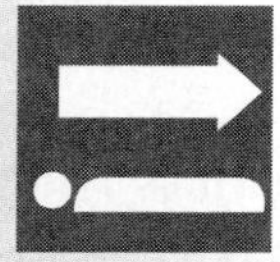

PHYSICAL EXAM AND TREATMENT

1. **GATHER A *SAMPLE* HISTORY.** If birth appears imminent, prepare to deliver the baby. Most of the SAMPLE history can wait. If birth doesn't appear imminent, proceed with the following:

   (S)igns and symptoms? Is the mother having contractions? Does she feel the urge to bear down or have a bowel movement? If this is the case, don't let the mother go to the toilet because birth is imminent.

   (A)llergies to medications?

   (M)edications? Does the patient take any medications that are related to the pregnancy? Does it appear that the mother has recently used illegal drugs that may affect the delivery of the infant or the infant's status? If so, expect to manage the infant's airway and breathing after delivery.

   (P)ertinent past history? How many weeks pregnant is she? Is there any chance of a multiple birth? If more than one baby is expected, request additional resources from EMS dispatch. Is this your patient's first baby? Has she delivered before? Does the mother have health problems that could be a factor in delivery? Does she or her doctor expect any complications?

(L)ast oral intake? How long ago has the patient eaten?

(E)vents leading to this point? When did the labor begin? Has it seemed to progress (contractions more forceful and closer together over time)? Has the amniotic sac ruptured ("water broken")?

2. **PERFORM A HEAD-TO-TOE EXAM.** Unless your patient has experienced trauma with this event, your physical exam need only include looking at the vaginal area to see if the baby is crowning. There's no need for any type of hands-on exam of the patient. Never touch the patient's vagina unless you're actually assisting with the delivery of the baby.

3. **TAKE VITAL SIGNS.** You should expect a mother in active labor to have vital signs that are a bit elevated. Careful monitoring of contractions is also important. You, another rescuer, or a member of the patient's family or friends should monitor them continuously. Time contractions from the beginning of one to the beginning of the next. They should become progressively stronger, closer together, and last longer as birth becomes more imminent. Remember that some women will progress to birth gradually, while others will progress very rapidly.

4. **PROVIDE TREATMENT AS NEEDED.**

   If the patient is still in labor: Allow her to assume any position that is most comfortable. Many women prefer to walk or stand while they are laboring. Others prefer to lie on their left side. Encourage the laboring patient to stay off her back. Observe the patient closely for signs that she may be preparing to deliver. Prepare an appropriate patient report for hand-off to incoming EMS personnel.

   If the patient is ready to give birth: Prepare for delivery. Most women want to deliver in a supine position. It helps to keep the patient's upper body supported at a slight angle rather than lying flat. Have another rescuer, family member, or friend stay by the patient's side while you prepare.

   While you assist with the delivery, be sure to talk to the patient. Encourage her. Let her know that you're there to help and that she's doing a good job. Do not encourage her to push. Do encourage her to breathe (she needs oxygen). Her body will take over and cause her to push when the time is right.

If the patient has delivered her own baby: First assess and treat the newborn. Suction, dry, stimulate, and warm the newborn. Do this aggressively if the newborn appears to be blue, sluggish, or in respiratory distress. If necessary, apply oxygen, ventilate, or begin CPR.

After you've assessed and treated the newborn, assess and treat the mother. Monitor her for signs of shock. Tie off the umbilical cord, and await delivery of the placenta. Keep her warm. Help the mother hold her newborn, if necessary, or help her put the newborn to her breast if she so desires. If the mother's bleeding appears to be excessive, massage the abdomen over the uterus.

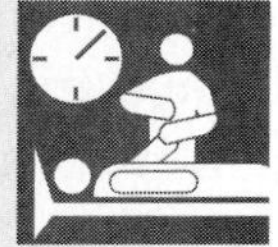

ONGOING ASSESSMENT AND TREATMENT

1. **REPEAT THE INITIAL ASSESSMENT.**

2. **REPEAT THE PHYSICAL EXAM.**

3. **PROVIDE REASSURANCE.**

CONCLUSION

It's preferable to get a patient in labor to a hospital where there's a more favorable environment and specially trained personnel. However, there'll always be those cases where it's better to prepare for delivery in the field. Most births occur without any hitches. When you're helping a laboring mother, you'll have the most positive impact on the delivery if you remember the priorities for both mother and newborn.

PATIENT HAND-OFF

1. **GIVE A PATIENT REPORT.** The following is an example of a patient history based on the scenario at the beginning of the chapter:

   This is Maria. Maria delivered her baby about five minutes ago. When I arrived, the baby was crowning. Delivery went smoothly and lasted only a few minutes. Her baby girl arrived pink, with good respirations, a full cry, strong fast pulse, and good muscle tone. I dried off the baby and wrapped her in this towel. Maria has lost about two cups of blood with the delivery. Both she and the baby appear stable with good vital signs. This is Maria's third child. Her pregnancy was normal and her baby is full term.

2. **CONDUCT THE TRANSFER OF CARE.** Make sure the mother is introduced to the EMS personnel who will be caring for her and her baby.

3. **ASSIST IN EXTRICATION AND TRANSPORT.** The mother and the baby should be extricated and transported together if possible. Be extremely careful. Take your time. Avoid having the mother walk. If you have to go down stairs, consider handing the newborn with the umbilical cord and placenta (if it has delivered) to another rescuer so that the mother doesn't have to worry about dropping the baby.

KEY TERMS

You may wish to use this list to review your understanding of key terms introduced in the chapter.

afterbirth the placenta, after it has been discharged from the body.

amniotic fluid the clear fluid that surrounds the fetus inside the amniotic sac.

amniotic sac the membrane that surrounds the fetus inside the uterus. *Also called* bag of waters.

birth canal the cervix and the vagina.

bloody show the mucus and blood that comes out of the vagina as labor begins.

cervix the neck or lowest part of the uterus.

crowning the bulging out of the vagina, caused by the fetus's head or other part pressing against it.

labor the process by which the fetus is expelled from the uterus into the vagina and then to the outside of the mother's body.

placenta the organ through which a developing fetus gets its nourishment and transports wastes.

premature delivery a birth that occurs four or more weeks before the due date.

spontaneous abortion delivery of the products of conception early in pregnancy. *Also called* miscarriage.

umbilical cord an extension of the placenta through which the fetus receives nourishment.

uterus a pear-shaped smooth muscle within which the fetus grows and develops. *Also called* womb.

APPLICATION QUESTIONS

You may wish to use these questions to review your understanding of the chapter. For answers with page references, see Appendix 2.

1. You've been called to assess a 34-year-old woman in active labor. The mother states that her water broke about two hours ago and that her due date is next week. You time the contractions and find them to be five minutes apart and lasting 20 seconds each. When you examine the vaginal area, you don't see signs of crowning. Do you think the patient should be transported to the hospital for delivery or should the delivery occur on scene? Explain your answer.

2. You're caring for a 27-year-old woman who is complaining of severe abdominal cramping and vaginal bleeding. The patient states that she's pregnant and isn't due for seven more months. What do you expect to be the problem?

CHAPTER 25 BEHAVIORAL EMERGENCIES

FIRST RESPONSE

Alex, a foreman at a new housing site, spots a man crawling out of the window of one of the houses under construction. "Hey, what's going on there?" Alex shouts. He can feel his anger as he chases after the man who is now rapidly walking away.

Alex catches up to him and says angrily, "Excuse me, but what were you doing in one of my houses?" The man turns to Alex, screeches an incomprehensible reply, and abruptly sits down on the sidewalk. He begins to wring his hands, mutter under his breath, and stare blankly at nothing in particular. Startled, Alex suddenly notices that the man appears to be wearing torn, dirty clothes.

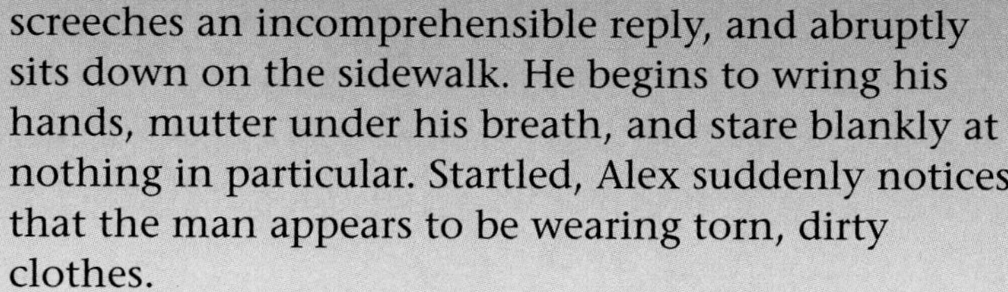

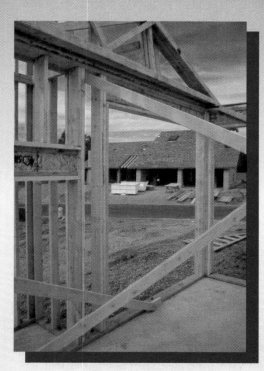

Alex takes a deep breath and collects himself. "Are you okay?" he asks. The man doesn't answer. Concerned, Alex asks a construction worker to call 9-1-1.

As a volunteer First Responder with the town's fire department, Alex has been trained to assess this type of patient from a distance. He begins. The man appears to be in no immediate physical distress. Though he tries to understand the man's muttering, Alex only hears a nonstop "word salad"—phrase after phrase of disjointed, unconnected language.

Alex breathes a sigh of relief when a car from the sheriff's office drives up. The officer nods at Alex and immediately recognizes the man. "Hey Bill, what's the matter?" the officer asks. The man turns to the officer and quickly turns away. "Old Bill here won't hurt you," the officer tells Alex. "He's a psychiatric patient at the board-and-care home on Kennedy Avenue. Sometimes Bill doesn't take his medications and wanders off. You did the right thing to keep your distance, though. If you had tried to grab him, he could've gotten out of control."

The officer makes a call to EMS dispatch and then gets Bill into the unit. He waves good-bye to Alex as he heads for the hospital where Bill can receive enough medication to stop his hallucinations.

LEARNING OBJECTIVES

Managing a patient who is having a behavioral emergency is seldom as straightforward as managing a medical or trauma call. These patients often are unpredictable and sometimes even dangerous. Often they require specific assessment and communication strategies.

By the end of the chapter, you should be able to:[†]

- 5-1.11 Identify the patient who presents with a specific medical complaint of behavioral change. (pp. 310-311)
- 5-1.12 Explain the steps in providing emergency medical care to a patient with a behavioral change. (pp. 312-315, 314-319)
- 5-1.13 Identify the patient who presents with a specific complaint of a psychological crisis. (p. 311)
- 5-1.14 Explain the steps in providing emergency medical care to a patient with a psychological crisis. (pp. 312-315, 314-319)

* Define a behavioral emergency. (p. 310)

* List common causes of behavioral emergencies. (p. 311)

CAUSES OF BEHAVIORAL EMERGENCIES

A **behavioral emergency** occurs when a patient exhibits abnormal behavior that's unacceptable or intolerable to the patient, family, or community. Causes include situational stress, illness or injury, mind-altering substances, mental illness, and psychological crises (Figure 25-1).

For example, think of how you'd feel if you arrived home from work to find your house burned to the ground or a loved one dead. You would be experiencing *situational stress*. Common reactions include crying, grief, disbelief, even rage. However, when these extreme emotions lead to violence or other inappropriate behavior, the patient may be having a behavioral emergency.

Illness and injury can cause a patient to have a behavioral emergency also. For example, common causes of combative or irrational behavior include:

[†]Numbered objectives are from the 1995 U.S. DOT "First Responder: National Standard Curriculum." Asterisks indicate supplemental material.

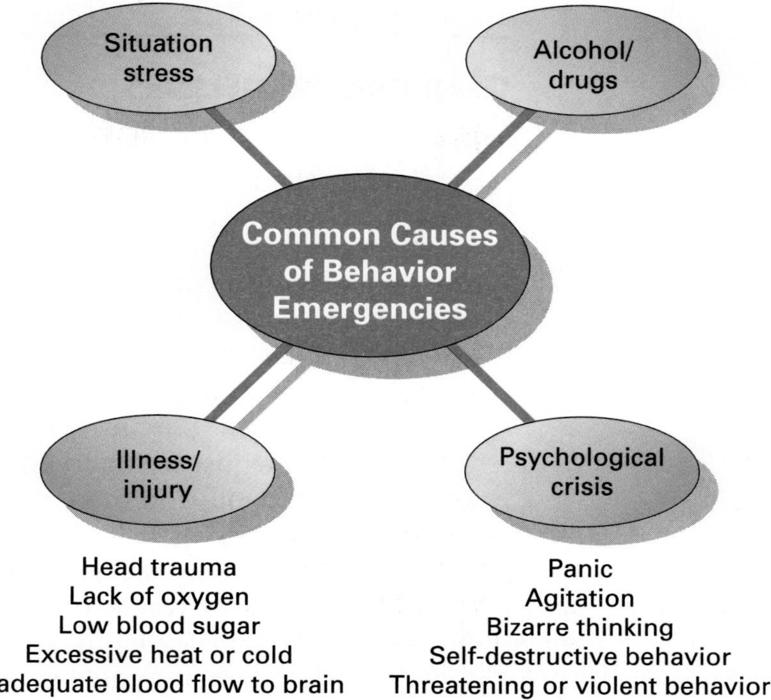

Figure 25-1
Common causes of behavioral emergencies.

- Low blood sugar (diabetes).
- Lack of oxygen (hypoxia).
- Inadequate blood flow to the brain (from shock, for example).
- Head trauma.
- Exposure to excessive heat or cold.
- Chronic conditions such as Alzheimer's disease.

In our society behavioral problems are very often due to mind-altering substances. Alcohol, for example, may cause violent behavior, uncontrolled weeping, even public sexual displays. Stimulants like cocaine or methamphetamines may cause signs of extreme **paranoia** or feelings of being all powerful. Hallucinogens such as LSD and psilocybin may cause the patient to hear or see things that aren't there.

Many patients with mental illness or in psychological crises may also have behavioral emergencies. Some may have **phobias** (abnormal fears), for example, or think and behave in bizarre ways. Some may suffer from **catatonia** (extreme withdrawal). Others may be depressed, suicidal, agitated, panicky, threatening, or violent.

MANAGING THE PATIENT

GENERAL GUIDELINES

There are some do's and don'ts of managing patients with behavior problems. The following is a brief example of some of the don'ts:

> You're managing a patient who is a bit drunk and sobbing uncontrollably. She's just learned that she has been fired from her job. You arrive at her side and immediately begin to assess her airway, breathing, and circulation. "Hey! What are you doing? Get away from me," she shrieks at you.
>
> "Ma'am, we're just trying to do our job. Why don't you just let me examine you, and then we can figure out how to help you."
>
> "If you want to help me, get me my job back."
>
> "Ma'am, I'm sorry you lost your job. I can't really do anything about that. Please let me make sure you're okay."
>
> "I'd be much better if you'd get out of my house. Get out. Now!"

As you can see, once you start battling with a patient, it's difficult to dig yourself out. So one of your goals must be to develop rapport. Remember the three questions that were posed in Chapter 7: What does my patient think and feel? What does my patient need? What do I need to get done as a First Responder? These questions can help you devise effective patient communication strategies.

Here are some additional suggestions to help keep you from falling into any major patient management holes (Figure 25-2):

- Tell the patient who you are and what you're going to do. You may need to explain this over and over again.

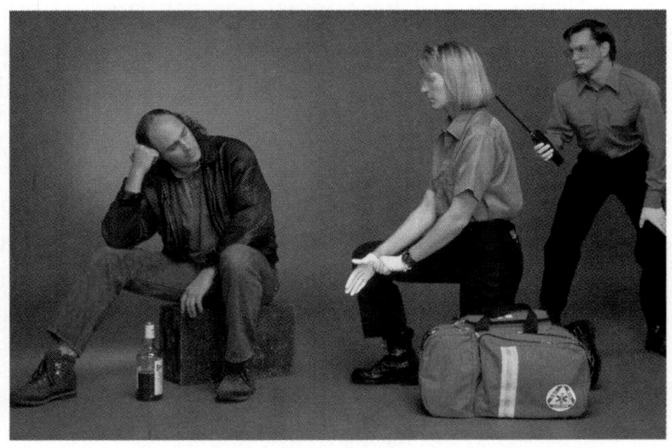

Figure 25-2
Start to build rapport with your patient by telling him who you are and what you're going to do.

- Follow a plan of action. It'll help make clear to the patient what will happen next.
- Identify one rescuer from your team as the primary contact with the patient. If more than one rescuer talks to the patient, the patient is likely to become confused or agitated.
- Be calm, and give the patient honest reassurance. Don't lie. If the patient is seeing or hearing things that aren't there, don't play along.
- Don't ask for more information than necessary.
- Without being judgmental, allow the patient to tell you what happened or what's wrong. Show the patient you're listening by repeating or by rephrasing the patient's words. Also use good eye contact.
- Acknowledge the patient's feelings, especially if the patient seems upset. Restate that you're there to help.
- If the patient tries to make you angry, don't take it personally. Don't threaten, challenge, or argue with the patient.
- Maintain a comfortable distance. Physical contact with an angry or threatening patient should be avoided. Even a hand on the shoulder could be seen as a threat.
- Don't make quick moves.
- Involve people the patient knows and trusts, such as family members or friends.
- Don't leave the patient alone. Accept the fact that the call may take a long time to complete.

Once you've built rapport with the patient, continue your assessments. Keep in mind that some behavioral emergencies are caused by physical problems. One of the most common is hypoxia, which you can treat with oxygen if you're so equipped.

RESTRAINING PATIENTS

Placing a patient in restraints should be avoided, unless the patient is a danger to himself or others. In general, guidelines for restraining patients include:

- If you must place a patient in restraints, have law enforcement present. Also get approval from medical oversight.
- Be sure that you have resources and assistance enough to restrain the patient safely.

- Never restrain a patient in a way that prevents accurate and timely assessment of airway, breathing, and circulation.
- Use only **reasonable force** to restrain a patient. In other words, use the force necessary to get the patient safely restrained and no more! Avoid injuring the patient in any way. Judge what would be reasonable by looking at the patient's size and strength, mental state, degree of abnormal behavior, and the method of restraint to be used.
- If you're attacked by any patient, you may use reasonable force to protect yourself.
- Be aware that after a period of combativeness and aggression, patients who seem calm may suddenly try to injure themselves or others.

EMERGENCY CARE PLAN | BEHAVIORAL EMERGENCIES

PRIORITIES

Your priorities in caring for a patient with a behavioral emergency are:

- Scene safety throughout the call.
- Early recognition and treatment of any life threats.
- Early recognition of the behavioral emergency.
- Establishing rapport with the patient, being calm, and listening to the patient's story.
- Completing an accurate physical exam of your patient.

PATIENT CARE APPROACH

Solid communication skills will go a long way toward easing your patient's fears. Use an empathetic, calm approach. Identify yourself, and let your patient know that you're there to help. Tell your patient what you're going to do before you do it. Build rapport. Use a calm, reassuring voice when asking questions. Allow

- Some patients may falsely accuse you of physical or sexual assault after you've restrained them. For this reason, carefully document all abnormal behavior exhibited by the patient. Have witnesses present during assessment and restraint of the patient, including rescuers of the same sex as the patient. The EMTs also may ask you to be a witness during transport.

PATIENTS WHO RESIST TREATMENT

Patients with a behavior emergency sometimes resist treatment. This can become a threatening or violent situation if you don't approach it cautiously. If you have a reasonable belief that the patient will harm himself or others, ask the police to assist you. If medical control agrees, the patient may be transported without consent.

your patient to tell his or her story, no matter how disjointed it may be.

DANGER SIGNS

Patients with behavioral problems have a greater likelihood of violence than others. So in addition to sizing up the scene, size up the patient. Watch your patient's body position and physical activity at all times. Be wary of patients who show signs of being suicidal. Remember that if they're willing to hurt or kill themselves, they may be willing to hurt you. Generally, any suicide threat no matter how casual should be taken seriously.

The bottom line is assume that any patient having a behavioral emergency may be violent. Most patients will pose no threat to you. However, it's better to be cautious than to trust someone you don't know. If you sense that your patient is a threat, stay away. Period. If your patient becomes threatening during assessment and treatment, pull back and call for the police. Your safety is never worth the risk!

Note that some patients also can pose a "flight risk." They may leave the scene or even launch themselves from the back of an ambulance.

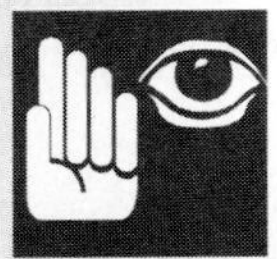

SCENE SIZE-UP

1. **ASSESS SCENE SAFETY.** Is the scene safe to enter? Take all necessary BSI precautions now. Check with the patient's family or bystanders to determine if the patient has a known history of aggression or combativeness. Look at the patient's posture. Is the patient sitting or standing in a threatening manner? Are the patient's muscles tense? Does the patient have quick, irregular movements? Are the patient's fists clenched? Is there any possibility that your patient is hiding a weapon in his or her hands? Is the patient within reach of anything that can be used as a weapon? Is your patient yelling or verbally threatening to harm himself or others? If the patient appears to be aggressive or combative, ask for police assistance.

2. **DETERMINE NATURE OF ILLNESS.** What is the patient's chief complaint? Determine if your patient has a behavioral emergency or if there's a behavioral component in a trauma or medical emergency. Activate the EMS system if you haven't done so already.

3. **TRIAGE THE PATIENT.** How much of a behavioral emergency does this appear to be? Do you need more help? Law enforcement?

4. **DETERMINE ACCESS AND EXTRICATION NEEDS.** Will there be any problems getting to the patient or getting the patient out? Does the patient need to be restrained? If so, do you have the proper and adequate equipment, training, and personnel?

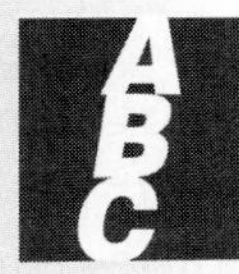

INITIAL ASSESSMENT AND TREATMENT

1. **FORM A GENERAL IMPRESSION.** What's the patient's sex and approximate age? What's the patient's level of distress? Be on the lookout for odd postures, repetitive movements, and disjointed language.

2. **CHECK MENTAL STATUS.** Many patients with behavioral emergencies have an altered mental status. Observe your patient's appearance, physical activity, speech patterns, and orientation to time (What day is it?), person (What's your name?), and place (Where are you?). Is your patient alert and answering all questions appropriately? If not, administer oxygen.

3. **ASSESS THE ABCs.**

   - **Airway.** Is the airway open and clear? If not, position the patient and open it.

   - **Breathing.** Is the patient's rate and depth of breathing adequate? Provide oxygen and ventilations as needed.

   - **Circulation.** Does the patient's skin condition seem to be normal? Is your patient's pulse weak or rapid? Treat the patient for shock, if necessary.

4. **DETERMINE PRIORITY.** Any patient with significant behavioral signs or symptoms, with altered mental status, or with airway, breathing, or circulation problems should be considered a high priority.

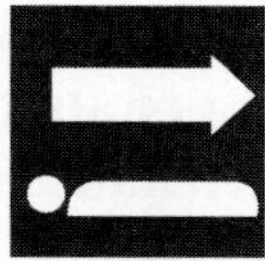

PHYSICAL EXAM AND TREATMENT

1. **GATHER A *SAMPLE* HISTORY.**

   (S)igns and symptoms? Is the patient showing any signs or symptoms of a medical or trauma condition? What is the patient's behavior?

   (A)llergies to medications?

   (M)edications? Does your patient take medications related to a behavioral problem? Has the patient been taking prescribed medications? Often patients with a psychiatric history will run out of, lose, or sell their medications, causing them to have a behavioral emergency. Common medications include the following: Stelazine®, Thorazine®, Mellaril®, Haldol® (for control of hallucinations);

Amitriptyline®, Nortriplyline®, Desyrel® (for control of depression).

(P)ertinent past history? Did the patient ever have this kind of episode in the past? When was the last time? What was done to treat the patient then?

(L)ast oral intake? How long ago did the patient eat? Was it anything unusual?

(E)vents leading to the problem? What initiated the call to 9-1-1?

2. **PERFORM A HEAD-TO-TOE EXAM.** In general, limit your hands-on exam with a patient who appears to be agitated. If your patient does allow an exam, focus on the following:

- **Head.** Is there any trauma to the head? Is there a smell of alcohol or other substance?
- **Neck.** Are there any signs of trauma? Are there signs of accessory muscle use with breathing? Is there a Medic Alert medallion?
- **Chest.** Are there any signs of trauma? Is there pain with palpation?
- **Abdomen.** Is the patient complaining of abdominal pain? Are there any signs of trauma? Is there nausea or vomiting? How hot or cold is the patient's skin?
- **Pelvis.** Are there any signs of incontinence?
- **Extremities.** Are there any signs of trauma? Are there any puncture wounds in the arms or legs ("needle tracks") indicating recent IV drug use?

3. **TAKE VITAL SIGNS.**

4. **PROVIDE TREATMENT AS NEEDED.** Aside from treating any other problems, your main goal should be to support and reassure your patient. Actively listen, and provide your patient with information as appropriate.

ONGOING ASSESSMENT AND TREATMENT

1. **REPEAT THE INITIAL ASSESSMENT.** Focus heavily on your patient's mood, emotional state, and whether or not your patient is still safe. Always be aware of your body position in relation to the patient's.

2. **REPEAT THE PHYSICAL EXAM.** Focus on the patient's chief complaint and, if possible, reconfirm important elements of the patient's SAMPLE history.

3. **PROVIDE REASSURANCE.**

PATIENT HAND-OFF

1. **GIVE A PATIENT REPORT.** The following is an example of a patient report based on the scenario at the beginning of the chapter:

   This patient is a male in his 40s. He seems to be experiencing a behavior problem. He is awake, muttering to himself, but won't interact with me. His airway, breathing, and circulation seem normal. I found him climbing out of one of the windows of an unoccupied house. He finally sat down after I chased him down. I haven't been able to gather any physical exam information. He won't answer my questions, and he won't allow me to perform a head-to-toe or take vital signs. He doesn't have any obvious injuries. His status hasn't changed since I first ran after him.

2. **CONDUCT THE TRANSFER OF CARE.** If the behavioral emergency is due to overdose, give the medications or drugs you find to the transporting EMTs.

3. **ASSIST IN EXTRICATION AND TRANSPORT.** Assist other rescuers as necessary.

CONCLUSION

Even in the short time you're with a patient with a behavioral emergency, you can help to reduce his or her crisis and keep it from spinning out of control. Approach the call with a structured plan:

- Ensure scene safety.
- Reassure the patient.
- Evaluate both physical and emotional complaints using a nonjudgmental approach.
- Provide supportive care until other rescuers with more training arrive.

KEY TERMS

You may wish to use this list to review your understanding of key terms introduced in the chapter.

behavioral emergency abnormal behavior in a patient that is unacceptable or intolerable to the patient, family, or community.

catatonia state of extreme withdrawal in which the patient is unresponsive; stupor.

paranoia extreme distrust and suspicion with no basis in reality; often includes resentment and anger which may lead to violence.

phobias persistent irrational fears of specific objects, activities, or situations.

reasonable force the force necessary to keep a patient from injuring himself or others.

APPLICATION QUESTIONS

You may wish to use these questions to review your understanding of the chapter. For answers with page references, see Appendix 2.

1. You've been called to care for a 30-year-old male who told his roommate that he wishes to kill himself. Upon assessing the patient, you note that he has two superficial cuts on his wrist and states that he tried to "end it all." The patient refuses to be transported to the hospital. Is he required to go anyway?

2. You've been called to care for a 25-year-old female who is reported to be "freaking out" by her roommate. When you arrive, you and your partner are the only rescuers on scene. You can hear screaming and yelling inside the home. Should you enter the residence to try to sort out the problem? Why or why not?

CHAPTER 26 OVERVIEW TO MANAGING TRAUMA PATIENTS

FIRST RESPONSE

Bev and Micah, experienced First Responders, are called to a head-on collision on Rte. 129. As they pull up to the scene, dispatch calls. "Rescue 18, reporting parties advise multiple victims with one possible fatality. Two additional units and two ambulances are en route. Medical helicopter is on standby."

Bev and Micah quickly pull equipment and move to the mangled wreckage. What they see sucks their breath away. Two sedans have impacted at high speed. There are two patients, one behind the wheel of each car. Both appear to be unresponsive. Micah moves to his patient, a woman in her 20s. She's wearing her seat belt, but it didn't help. The dashboard of her car has been wrenched from its mounts and now pins her against the seat. Micah can only see her neck and head above the crumpled dash. He feels for a pulse and finds none. She's dead, with no hope of resuscitation.

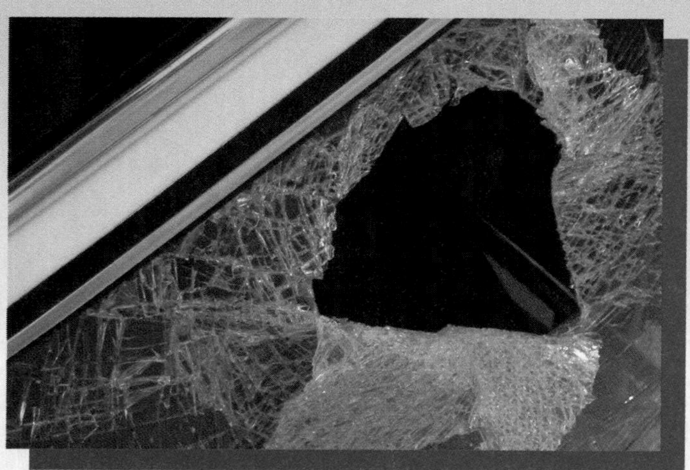

Micah moves to Bev and her patient. "Bev, my patient is dead. She's in cardiac arrest but pinned behind the wheel. There's no way we can get to her to do CPR. What have you got?"

Bev rattles off her priority report. "Twenty-year-old female, restrained with a lap and chest belt, awake but combative. She has head trauma and deep bruising to her chest and abdomen. She's pale, cool, and wet. I can't find a radial pulse. Let's get a collar on her, and then extricate her onto a backboard."

As they proceed with extrication, other rescue units arrive. They soon have the patient out of the wreck and in full spinal immobilization with high flow oxygen via nonrebreather. At one point another First Responder struggles to place a blood pressure cuff on the patient's arm. Micah turns to him, "There's no time for this. Let's get her loaded and off scene. Time is more important here!" In a matter of minutes the patient is loaded and en route to a trauma facility.

LEARNING OBJECTIVES

In the next four chapters you'll read about managing trauma patients in the field. You'll learn that whatever the trauma patient's problem, you should stick to the five-step plan you studied in Section 2 of this book.

In this chapter, you'll be introduced to a general emergency care plan with a focus on the high priority trauma patient. In Chapters 27 to 29, you'll learn how to manage specific trauma emergencies.

By the end of the chapter, you should be able to:[†]

* Identify the trauma patient. (p. 323)

* Explain the difference between low priority and high priority patients. (pp. 323, 328-329)

* List how the mechanism of injury, vital signs, and anatomic findings can be used to determine the priority of a trauma patient. (pp. 326, 328-329)

* Describe an emergency care plan for the overall assessment and treatment of trauma patients. (pp. 324-331)

WHAT IS A TRAUMA EMERGENCY?

In your career as a First Responder, you'll see many trauma patients. (Recall that the term *trauma* refers to any injury caused by an external force or violence.) Trauma is the number one killer of children and young adults in the USA. For every person killed by trauma, dozens more are permanently disabled.

Many trauma patients will be low priority patients, suffering from isolated injuries. Some, however, will be high priority with multiple injuries, mental status problems, and problems with airway, breathing, or circulation. In fact, critical trauma patients usually can't be stabilized in the field. They need definitive treatment in a hospital.

The **Golden Hour** refers to the time it takes from the moment of injury to the moment definitive care—often surgery—begins. The greater that time, the greater the likelihood of permanent disability and death. So, on the scene perform only those interventions necessary to maintain the patient's life. All other interventions should be performed en route to the hospital. Time is the enemy of critical trauma patients. Any delay can cost them their lives.

[†]Asterisks indicate material supplemental to the 1995 U.S. DOT "First Responder: National Standard Curriculum."

SPECIAL CONSIDERATIONS

Some patients—infants and children, elderly patients, and pregnant patients—need special consideration.

INFANTS AND CHILDREN

Infants and children are not small adults. Their physical differences affect how they respond to trauma and how they should be assessed and treated. Because they have proportionately larger heads, they're more prone to head injuries and more likely to land on their heads when they fall. In general their skeletons are more flexible and less protective. For example, while you're less likely to see broken bones in an infant or child, you're more likely to see internal injuries.

Infants and children are experts at hiding shock. They may look really well one minute and the next "crash" rapidly. If you see an infant or child that has suffered a significant mechanism of injury, treat him or her aggressively for shock, even if there are no signs of shock.

Also, remember that cold trauma patients do worse than warm trauma patients, and that infants and children lose heat rapidly. Keep them warm!

Finally, make sure that your immobilization equipment is designed to fit your patient. If it doesn't fit your patient, don't use it.

ELDERLY PATIENTS

Elderly patients are much more likely to suffer bone injuries. Even falls from a standing position can produce serious injuries to the skull, hips, pelvis, ribs, and spine. Because elderly patients

EMERGENCY CARE PLAN | TRAUMA PATIENTS

PRIORITIES

The First Responder's priorities when managing a trauma patient are as follows:

- Assuring scene safety.
- Performing a rapid assessment and treat life threats.

often have underlying heart or lung disease, their Golden Hour may be shortened.

Mental status may be difficult to determine in elderly patients. Determine what is normal for your patient before trying to assess problems.

Finally, many elderly patients suffer trauma following a medical emergency. For example, a car accident may be the result of a stroke or heart attack, a fall may be the result of fainting, and so on. Getting an accurate history from the patient and bystanders will help you get an accurate picture of the emergency.

PREGNANT PATIENTS

The number one cause of trauma-related fetal death is death of the mother. So, take care of mom and you'll be taking care of the baby.

Don't have patients who are pregnant more than 15-20 weeks lie flat on their backs. If they're supine, the weight of both the fetus and the uterus can press against blood vessels in the patient's abdomen, lowering blood pressure. If you must place a pregnant patient on a backboard, make sure you tilt it down slightly to the left. Otherwise, place the patient on her left side. Apply straps securely, but not tightly, across the pregnant patient's abdomen.

Women in the last few months of pregnancy have a much larger blood volume than normal. Some have as much as a 50% more. This additional blood may allow the mother to hide shock. It's also possible for her to look fine, even while the fetus is quite distressed. So, treat all pregnant patients aggressively if there's any chance that they have experienced a significant mechanism of injury.

- Identifing the critical trauma patient within the first minute or two.
- Preparing the patient for transport as quickly as possible.

Don't be distracted by minor or ugly wounds. They won't kill your patient. A closed airway, inadequate breathing, or a problem with circulation will.

■ PATIENT CARE APPROACH

Trauma patients are often in extreme pain. They'll be scared, and they'll feel out of control. Constantly reassure them. Help them to feel in control by informing them of every step you'll take before you take it.

■ DANGER SIGNS

Be on the lookout for mental status problems and problems with airway, breathing, and circulation. Watch for rapid changes. Look for early warning signs of shock—rapid pulse and poor skin condition, for example, and treat it aggressively.

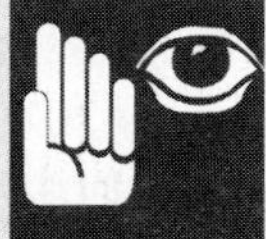

SCENE SIZE-UP

1. **ASSESS SCENE SAFETY.** Trauma calls potentially have countless scene hazards. Crash scenes may have downed power lines. Falls may have broken glass. There may even be an assailant who is still on scene with a loaded handgun. Be sure to take in the entire scene before entering (Figure 26-1). Also remember to take all necessary BSI precautions.

2. **DETERMINE MECHANISM OF INJURY.** What caused the trauma to occur? Be specific. Note how far the patient fell and onto what surface. See if the patient was wearing a seat

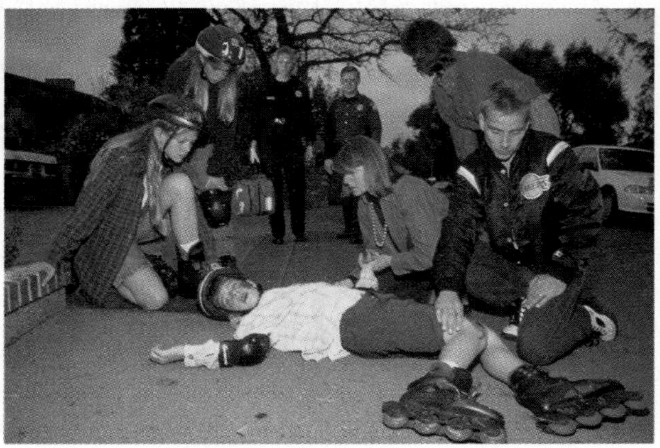

Figure 26-1
Take in the entire scene before entering.

belt when he crashed into the guardrail and how fast he was going. There'll be big differences in the injuries you find on the patient who didn't wear a seat belt in a car rollover and the patient who did. If the mechanism of injury suggests possible head or spinal injury, manually stabilize the patient's head and neck. Activate the EMS system, if you haven't already done so.

3. **TRIAGE THE PATIENT.** How many patients are there? How injured are your patients? Do you have enough personnel and resources on the way? Do you need to call for more?

4. **DETERMINE ACCESS AND EXTRICATION NEEDS.** Trauma calls often have access and extrication problems. Anticipate them. Call for specialized personnel and equipment as needed.

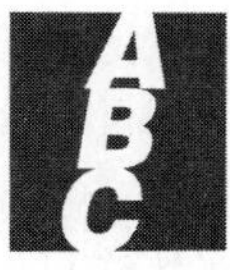

INITIAL ASSESSMENT AND TREATMENT

1. **FORM A GENERAL IMPRESSION.** Determine your patient's sex and approximate age. What's your patient's level of distress? What's his or her chief complaint?

   Remember *If the mechanism of injury is significant, tell your trauma patient to hold very still as soon as you make contact. Then manually stabilize the head and neck until the patient is properly immobilized.*

2. **CHECK MENTAL STATUS.** Use AVPU to help you determine your patient's mental status. Note that altered mental status in a trauma patient may indicate a head injury or shock.

3. **ASSESS THE ABCs.**

   - **Airway.** Is the airway open? If not, use the jaw-thrust maneuver to open the airway. Maintain manual stabilization of the head and neck (Figure 26-2).

   - **Breathing.** Is your patient breathing? Is breathing adequate? The number one cause of cardiac arrest among trauma patients is hypoxia. So if your patient is showing any sign of respiratory problems or if the patient has sig-

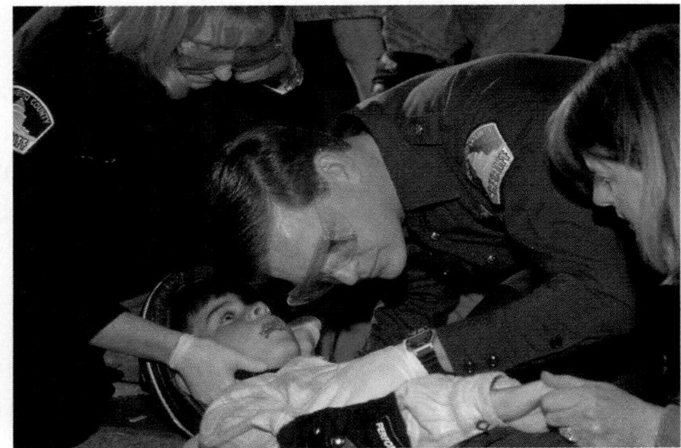

Figure 26-2
Maintain manual stabilization of the head and neck until the patient can be properly immobilized.

nificant injuries, apply high flow oxygen immediately. Ventilate if necessary.

- **Circulation.** Does your patient have a pulse? If so, is it weak or rapid? What's your patient's skin condition? Are there any signs of major bleeding? Treat for shock and control major bleeding at this time.

4. **DETERMINE PRIORITY.** Identify the high priority trauma patient within the first one or two minutes of assessment. Don't forget the Golden Hour. Rapid identification is critical if you want to give the patient a fighting chance.

   Your trauma patient is a high priority patient if he or she has any problem with mental status, airway, breathing, or circulation. Also, rapidly look and feel for major **blunt injury** (a blow to the body that doesn't break through its surface) or **penetrating injury** (an injury that does break through the surface). If the patient has either, consider him or her a high priority.

   Any significant mechanism of injury such as those listed below also call for you to classify your patient as a high priority:

- Ejection of a patient from a vehicle.
- Car rollover when the patient isn't wearing a seat belt.
- Death of another occupant in a car crash.
- Major intrusion into the passenger space.
- Gunshot or stab wound.

- Falls of greater than 15 feet.

- Auto-pedestrian impacts of greater than 15 mph.

Remember *Don't be afraid to use your "gut instinct" when you assess a trauma patient. While he or she may not match up perfectly with the criteria listed here, the patient may still be a high priority. Always err on the side of the patient.*

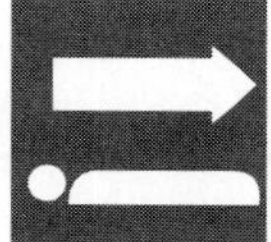

PHYSICAL EXAM AND TREATMENT

1. GATHER A *SAMPLE* HISTORY.

(S)igns and symptoms? Use the PQRST mnemonic as a way to describe any pain.

(A)llergies to medications?

(M)edications? This information will help you better understand your patient's medical history.

(P)ertinent past history? This information is particularly helpful when you're managing an elderly patient.

(L)ast oral intake?

(E)vents leading to the injury or illness? Gather an accurate picture of how the trauma occurred. Try to determine if a medical emergency occurred before or after the trauma call.

Figure 26-3
Look and feel much more carefully for injuries.

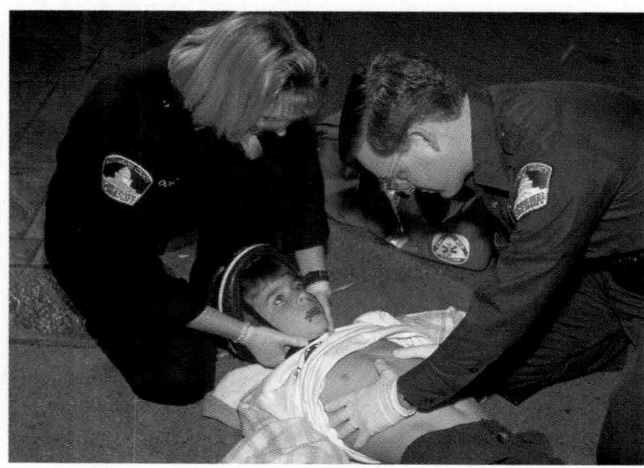

2. PERFORM A HEAD-TO-TOE EXAM. Look and feel much more carefully for any injuries to the head, neck, chest, abdomen, pelvis, back, and extremities (Figure 26-3). Use DOTS (deformities, open injuries, tenderness, swelling) to help you.

3. TAKE VITAL SIGNS. Assess all vital signs as appropriate. Blood pressure is less important than the other vital signs for determining the presence of shock.

4. **PROVIDE TREATMENT AS NEEDED.** If you're still waiting for transport, now is the time to complete any bandaging, splinting, or other low priority interventions. Keep your patient warm. Give nothing by mouth. Maintain manual stabilization of the patient's head and neck until the patient is properly immobilized.

ONGOING ASSESSMENT AND TREATMENT

1. **REPEAT THE INITIAL ASSESSMENT.** High priority trauma patients should have their ABCs assessed every five minutes. Remember that mental status is a good indicator of whether or not your patient is getting enough oxygen. Watch and treat for signs of shock.

2. **REPEAT THE PHYSICAL EXAM.** Focus on the patient's chief complaint, major injuries, and vital signs (Figure 26-4). Check all interventions to be sure they're still effective.

3. **PROVIDE REASSURANCE.**

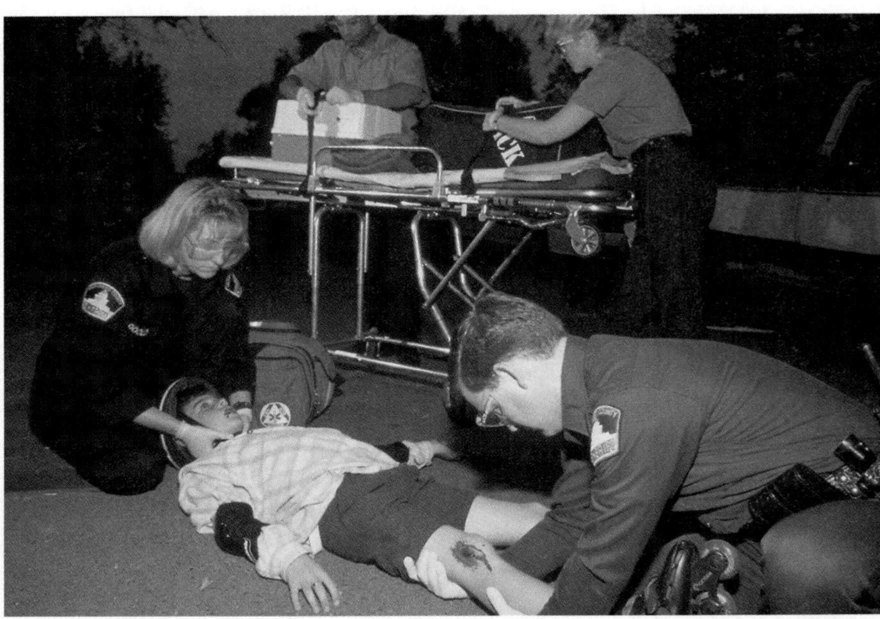

Figure 26-4
Repeat the initial assessment and physical exam during ongoing assessment.

PATIENT HAND-OFF

1. **GIVE A PATIENT REPORT.** The following is an example of a patient report based on the scenario at the beginning of the chapter:

   Our patient is a 20-year-old lap-and-chest restrained female who hit another vehicle head on at freeway speed. The patient in the other car is dead. Our patient is complaining of pain to her head, chest, and abdomen. She's alert and slightly combative, with a clear airway, labored respirations, and no radial pulse. Her skin is pale, cool, and moist. She's a high priority trauma patient. We're unable to determine a SAMPLE history as she's too combative. We've found bruising to her head, chest, and abdomen. Her vital signs are: respirations 32 and labored, pulse 120. We're manually stabilizing her spine. We're administering high flow oxygen. We've seen no changes in the patient in the past five minutes.

2. **CONDUCT THE TRANSFER OF CARE** (Figure 26-5).

3. **ASSIST IN EXTRICATION AND TRANSPORT.**

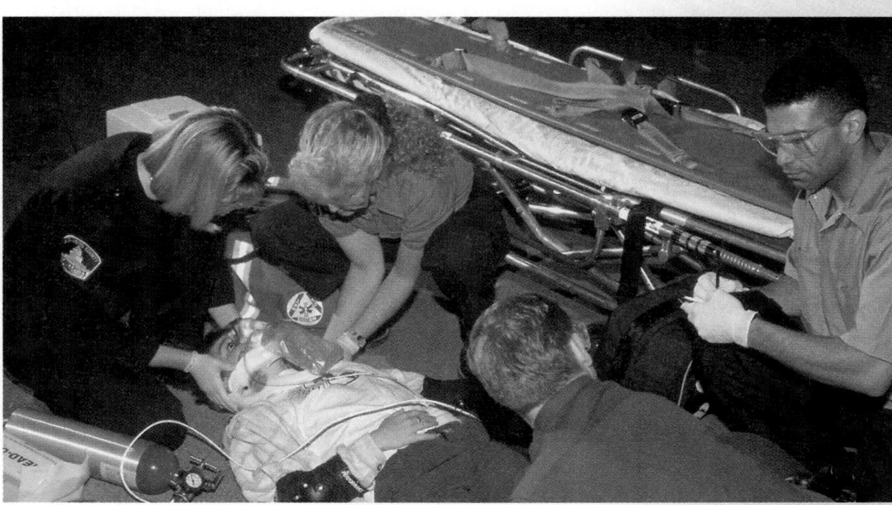

Figure 26-5
Conduct the transfer of care.

CONCLUSION

Trauma patients need an organized approach that allows you to determine quickly if they're high or low priority. High priority trauma patients need aggressive airway, breathing, and circulation support. They also need rapid transport to a hospital. Most treatment should occur en route because time is always more important. As with all patients, trauma patients should be assessed for injuries, treated, and then reassessed to determine if interventions have been effective.

KEY TERMS

You may wish to use this list to review your understanding of key terms introduced in the chapter.

blunt injury an injury caused by a blow to the body that doesn't break through the body's surface.

Golden Hour refers to the time it takes from the moment of injury to the moment of definitive care, which is often surgery. The greater that time, the greater the likelihood of permanent disability and death.

penetrating injury an injury caused by a force that breaks through the body's surface.

APPLICATION QUESTIONS

You may wish to use these questions to review your understanding of the chapter. For answers with page references, see Appendix 2.

1. You're managing a 24-year-old patient who fell from a roof. He appears to have injuries to the extremities and is obviously in shock. Another rescuer arrives and begins to splint the patient's legs. What is your response to this?
2. You've completed an initial assessment of your trauma patient and she appears to be a low priority. What should you do next?
3. Explain the concept of the Golden Hour.

CHAPTER 27 INJURIES TO THE HEAD AND SPINE

FIRST RESPONSE

Jaime is uneasy today. The undertow at the beach is particularly strong. As he sits in his lifeguard tower, he spots some Army servicemen trying to outdo each other at body surfing. Finally, one of them gets it wrong. Running full tilt into the surf, the soldier tries an ugly dive below the waves and ends up pinwheeling several times in a shower of salt spray. The young man's friends applaud the gymnastics, laugh, and cheer.

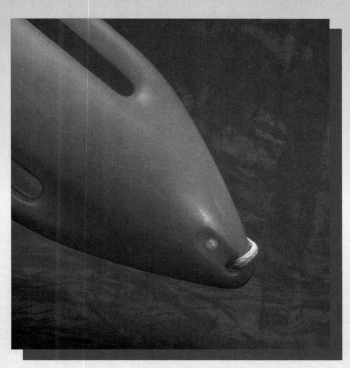

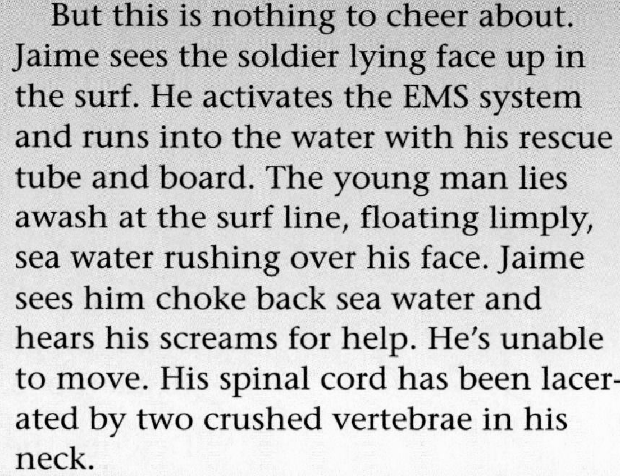

But this is nothing to cheer about. Jaime sees the soldier lying face up in the surf. He activates the EMS system and runs into the water with his rescue tube and board. The young man lies awash at the surf line, floating limply, sea water rushing over his face. Jaime sees him choke back sea water and hears his screams for help. He's unable to move. His spinal cord has been lacerated by two crushed vertebrae in his neck.

"Hold on," Jaime tells him. "I'm going to float you to shore." He places his rescue board beneath the patient. Soon he's joined by additional lifeguards. "We need to hold his head and neck completely still," Jaime tells them. One of the lifeguards maintains manual stabilization of the patient's head and neck, while all work together to get the patient safely to shore.

During Jaime's initial assessment, he finds that his patient, Phil, is having difficulty breathing. At Jaime's request, one of the other lifeguards applies high flow oxygen.

The paramedics arrive only minutes after Jaime's call. They immobilize the patient's spine as Jaime gives them a patient report. Throughout all of this, Phil remains alert. He calls out to his friends, now at his side, sobered and quiet except to offer encouragement. Soon Phil is loaded into the ambulance, bound for the regional trauma center.

LEARNING OBJECTIVES

Both head and spine injuries can devastate a patient's life. Think for a moment about spending your life in a wheel chair or on a ventilator, unable to care for yourself or your loved ones. The physical trauma of such injuries is surpassed only by the emotional catastrophe that may result.

As a First Responder, your management of the head- or spine-injured patient can directly affect the patient's outcome. Early recognition of a possible head or spine injury can help to reduce permanent disability and even prevent death. Failing to suspect either of them can have devastating, even lethal consequences.

By the end of the chapter, you should be able to:†

- 5-3.4 Relate mechanism of injury to potential injuries of the head and spine. (p. 335)
- 5-3.5 State the signs and symptoms of potential spine injury. (pp. 336-337)
- 5-3.6 Describe the method of determining if a responsive patient may have a spine injury. (pp. 335-337, 339)
- 5-3.7 List the signs and symptoms of injury to the head. (pp. 335-336)
- 5-3.8 Describe the emergency medical care for injuries to the head. (pp. 338-347, 348-352)

* Describe the emergency medical care of injuries to the spine. (pp. 338-347, 348-352)

RECOGNIZING POSSIBLE HEAD AND SPINE INJURIES

Head and spine injuries often occur together. For example, a blow to the head may cause damage to the scalp, skull, and even the brain. But the force or energy of that blow doesn't have to stop there. If it's great enough, it can injure the spinal cord.

So whenever you suspect injury to the head, always suspect injury to the spine.

†Numbered objectives are from the 1995 U.S. DOT "First Responder: National Standard Curriculum." Asterisks indicate supplemental material.

MECHANISMS OF INJURY

Both the head and spine may be injured by blunt or penetrating trauma. Common mechanisms of injury include:

- Car crashes.
- Motorcycle crashes.
- Pedestrian-vehicle crashes.
- Falls.
- Diving accidents.
- Assaults, particularly if the patient is beaten with a heavy object.
- Hangings (spinal injury only).
- Gunshot wounds to the head, neck, chest, abdomen, or pelvis.

When assessing a mechanism of injury, ask questions that will help you understand the forces involved in the trauma. The picture you draw from this information will suggest how severely your patient may be injured. For example, if your patient is a victim of a fall, find out the distance he fell and the surface he fell on. If your patient is in a crash, look for a shattered windshield or a dented helmet.

It's critical that you respect the mechanism of injury even when there are no signs or symptoms of trauma. It's possible for a patient to suffer a broken vertebrae or damage to the spinal cord, for example, and still feel no pain, particularly if alcohol is involved.

Remember *If the mechanism of injury suggests it, suspect spine injury, even if there are no signs or symptoms.*

SIGNS AND SYMPTOMS

HEAD INJURIES

Head injuries may be open or closed injuries to the scalp, skull, or brain. Open injuries may expose the bones of the skull or even brain matter. They're also likely to bleed (scalp injuries usually bleed profusely). A closed head injury may present with swelling or a dent in the skull. The brain may be injured in either open or closed head injuries. Injuries to the brain range from "getting your bell rung"—a jarring of the brain known as *concussion*—to various types of bleeding, bruising, and laceration injuries.

In head trauma, internal bleeding and swelling can cause pressure to build up inside the skull. The brain is extremely sensitive to this. If there's no relief, that pressure can lead to further brain damage and death. The brain will respond to an increase in pressure with mental status changes. So watch the patient's mental status carefully.

In general, signs and symptoms of head injury include the following:

- Altered mental status.
- Irregular or abnormal breathing patterns.
- Slow, bounding pulse.
- Bruises, cuts, and swelling to the scalp.
- Dents or depressions in the skull.
- Penetrating injury.
- Blood or fluid draining from the nose or ears.
- Bruising around the eyes and behind the ears.
- Nausea, vomiting.
- Visual disturbances.
- Headache.
- Seizures.

Again, the number one sign of significant head injury is altered mental status. The head-injured patient may ask repetitive questions. He or she may be confused, combative, or even unresponsive. If your patient doesn't remember the cause of injury, assume he or she has lost consciousness at least briefly. Consider this to be serious.

> **Remember** *Whenever you suspect injury to the head, always suspect injury to the spine.*

Spine Injuries

Spine injuries include injury to the spinal cord as well as injury to any of the 33 bones that make up the spinal column. The most devastating spine injury occurs in the area of the neck, or cervical spine. Signs and symptoms of a possible spine injury may include the following:

- Tenderness in the area of injury.
- Pain with movement. (Don't have the patient move to confirm this!)
- Pain along the spine or down the legs. This pain may come and go.
- Bruises, cuts, or swelling along the spinal column.
- Significant trauma to the head, neck, shoulders, back, abdomen, or lower extremities.
- Numbness, weakness, or tingling of the arms or legs.
- Lack of sensation or paralysis below the suspected injury site.
- Paralysis of the arms or legs.
- Breathing difficulty.
- Incontinence.
- Unresponsiveness.

Remember *Always suspect spine injury in any unresponsive trauma patient, as well as when the mechanism of injury suggests it.*

PATIENTS MOST AT RISK

Patients at high risk for head injuries include elderly patients and patients who abuse alcohol. Both are more likely to fall. Elderly patients have bones that are more brittle, which make them more likely to experience broken bones, even bones of the head. Alcohol abusers often have blood clotting problems that make them more likely to have bleeding inside the skull.

Patients most at risk for spine injuries are those who are unrestrained or restrained improperly in vehicle collisions. The elderly also are at risk as the result of significant falls.

Infants and children also are at risk for head injuries. Their heads are larger in proportion to their bodies. So not only are they more likely to fall, they're also more likely to fall on and injure their heads.

PROTECTING THE PATIENT'S SPINE

MANUAL STABILIZATION

Whenever you suspect spine injury, tell your patient to hold very still as soon as you make contact. Then manually stabilize the cervical spine. That is, hold it firmly and steadily in a neutral, in-line position. (*Neutral* means that the head shouldn't be pushed forward or pulled back. *In-line* means that the patient's nose should be in line with his or her navel.) Hold that position until the patient is properly immobilized.

You may begin simply by saying something like "Ma'am, I'm going to hold your head to remind you to keep it very still while we find out where your injuries are." If your patient's head isn't already in a neutral, in-line position, gently guide it there. If the patient complains of pain or if you feel resistance, stop immediately. Then maintain the patient's head in the position in which you found it.

Stabilizing the cervical spine is always a top priority. In fact, it's as important as assessing and treating your patient's ABCs. If possible, have another rescuer perform this task while you keep your hands free to perform assessments and treatment.

If you don't have spinal immobilization equipment, continue to manually stabilize the patient's head and neck until other EMS rescuers with more training arrive. If you're allowed, complete spinal immobilization using the techniques outlined below.

SPINAL IMMOBILIZATION

Many EMS systems allow First Responders to use spinal immobilization equipment. If you're not in one of these systems, the following information will help you when you're called to assist other EMS rescuers. Be sure to follow all local protocols.

Spinal immobilization is the process by which the spine is made immovable. It should keep your patient's spine—from the neck to the pelvis—in a neutral, in-line position, even if the patient is tipped sideways or angled up or down. It requires the use of a stiff **cervical collar** and a **backboard**. It also requires a device that anchors the head to the backboard and straps to anchor the rest of the patient's body.

As you can imagine, proper immobilization covers up a good deal of your patient's body, especially the back. The straps also make it difficult to expose the patient's chest, abdomen, and pelvis. Anticipate this. Complete a careful visual assessment before applying spinal immobilization equipment.

In addition, before and after spinal immobilization, it's critical that you assess circulation, sensation, and movement in your patient's extremities. Do this as follows:

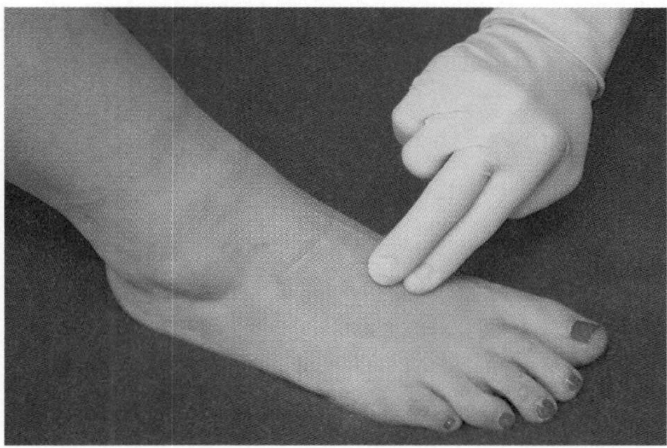

Figure 27-1
Assessing the pedal pulse.

- *Assess circulation in all extremities.* Does the patient have a radial pulse in both arms? Does the patient have pulses (**pedal pulses**) in both feet (Figure 27-1)?
- *Assess sensation in all extremities.* As you touch the tips of the patient's fingers and then the toes, ask: "Can you feel me touching you?" (See Figure 27-2.)
- *Assess movement in all extremities.* Ask the patient, "Can you move your hands and feet?" The patient should be able to "wave" each one (Figure 27-3).

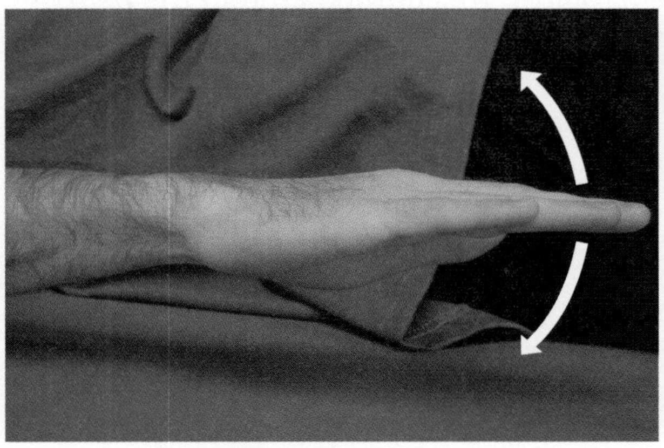

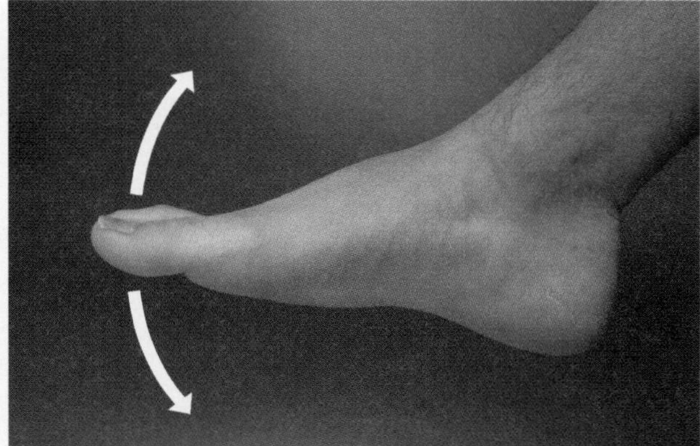

Figure 27-2
Can the patient move his or her hands and feet?

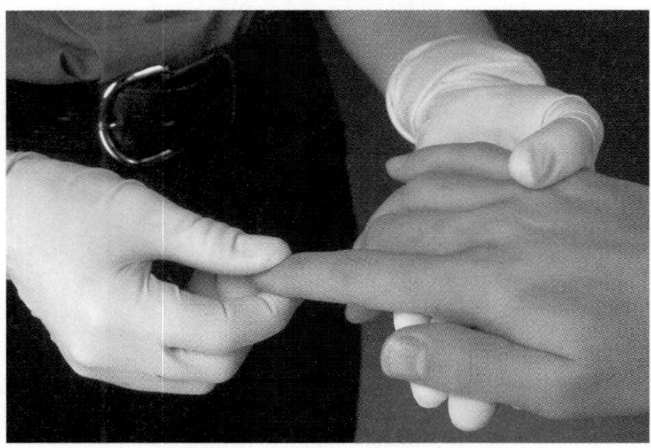

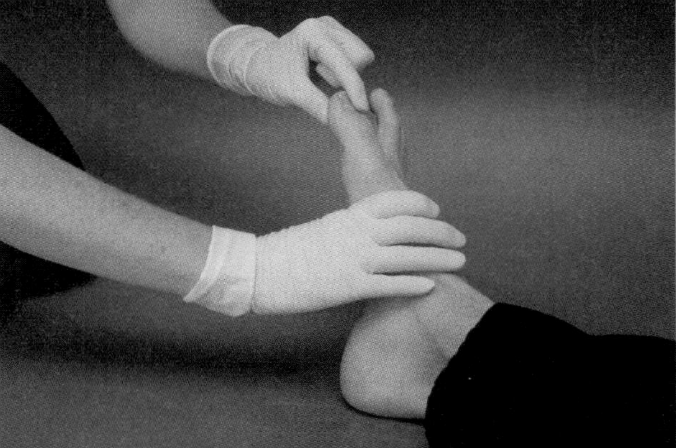

Figure 27-3
Can the patient feel you touch his or her fingers and toes?

Assess, intervene, and reassess. If at any time you find that pulse, sensation, or movement is absent or compromised in an extremity, document your findings. Then be absolutely certain to report them to the EMS rescuers who take over care.

CERVICAL COLLARS

Officially called *rigid cervical spinal immobilization devices*, cervical collars help to reduce neck movement (Figure 27-4). We say *reduce* because even the best collar doesn't prevent movement. So stress to your patients that the collar is meant to remind them to keep the head still.

A poorly fitting cervical collar will do more harm than good (Figure 27-5). Too small, and it's likely to cause problems with the airway. Too big, and it's likely to extend the head. Either way, it won't stabilize the patient's neck properly. If you can't find a collar to fit your patient, place a rolled towel around the patient's

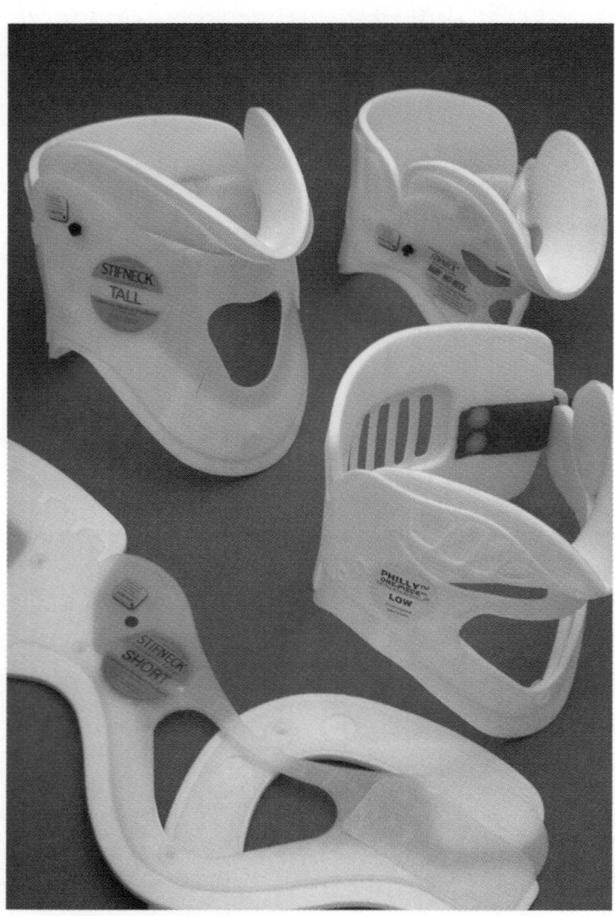

Figure 27-4
Examples of rigid cervical immobilization devices, or cervical collars.

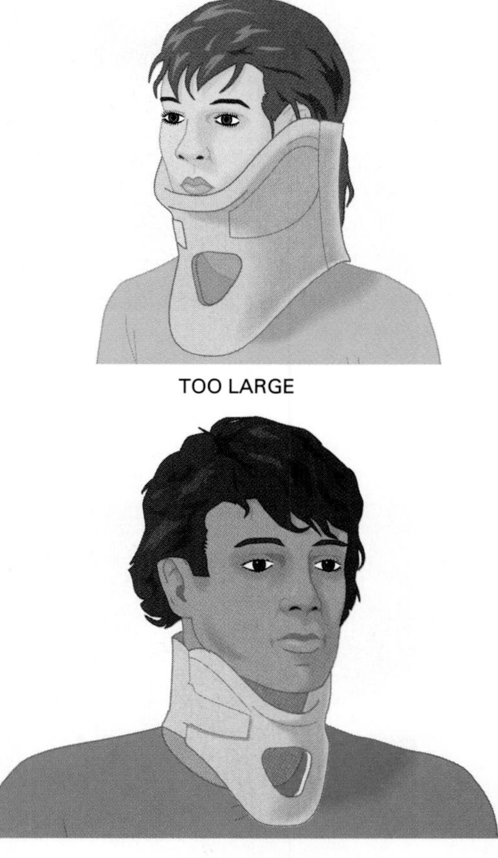

Figure 27-5
If a cervical collar is too small or too big, it won't stabilize the patient's neck properly.

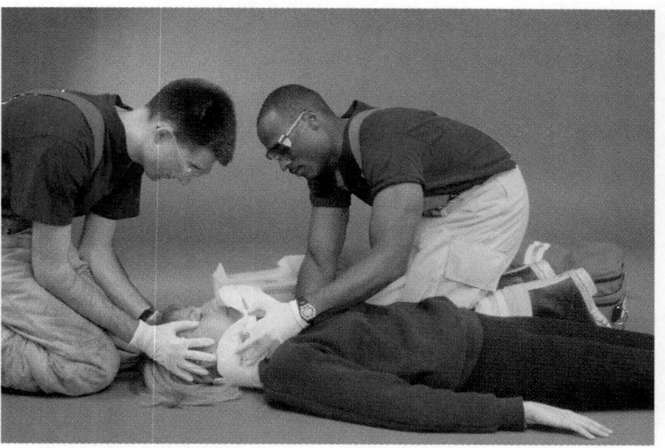

Figure 27-6a
While holding manual stabilization, position the collar.

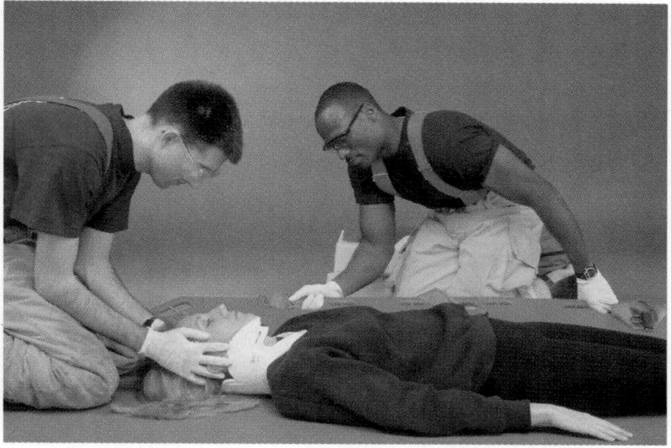

Figure 27-6b
Continue to hold manual stabilization after the collar is applied.

neck. Tape it to the backboard, and hold manual stabilization until the patient is properly immobilized.

There are various types of rigid cervical collars. Stifneck™, Philadelphia™, and Nec-Loc™ are a few. Sizing is based on the specific design of the device, so follow the manufacturer's directions. Always use the stiffest collar you can find. Stay away from soft foam collars. They're for decoration only.

To apply a rigid cervical collar to a patient, take BSI precautions and follow the manufacturer's directions. Usually, this requires two rescuers (Figure 27-6). In general, one rescuer should manually stabilize the patient's head and neck. The other should assess the cervical spine, as well as pulses, sensation, and movement in all four extremities. After the collar is applied, maintain manual stabilization until the patient is completely immobilized on a long backboard.

Short Backboard Immobilization

The short backboard is available in vest or rigid styles. It's used to immobilize noncritical patients found in a sitting position. The vest-type backboard seems to support the patient better, and it slides around much less. It also has extra support straps for a snug fit and handholds to assist with vertical extrication (out of the roof of a car, for example).

To apply a short backboard to a noncritical patient in a sitting position, take BSI precautions and follow these steps (Figure 27-7):

1. Manually stabilize the patient's cervical spine.
2. Apply a cervical collar.

Applying a Short Backboard to a Sitting Patient

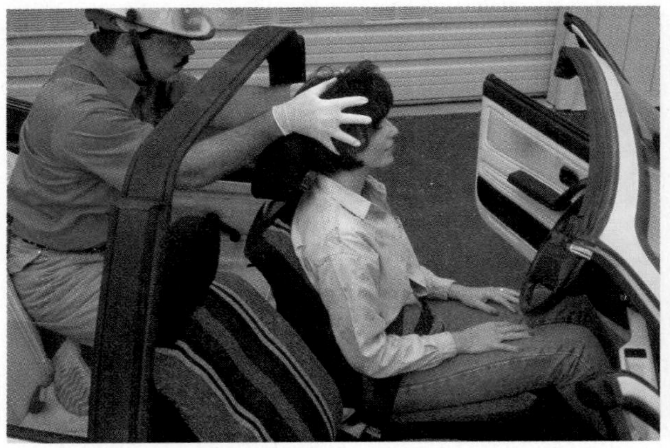

Figure 27-7a
Manually stabilize the head and neck.

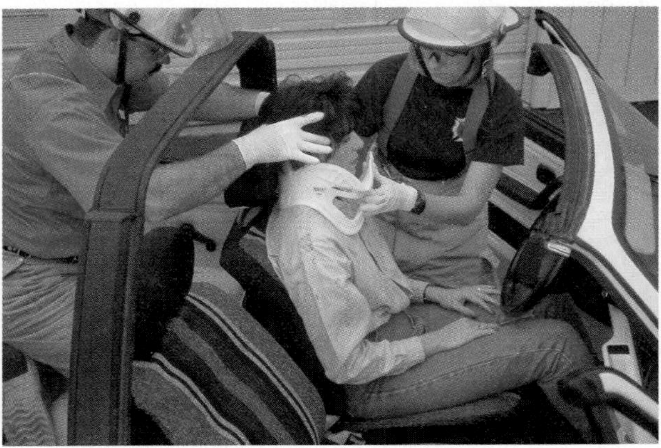

Figure 27-7b
Apply a cervical collar.

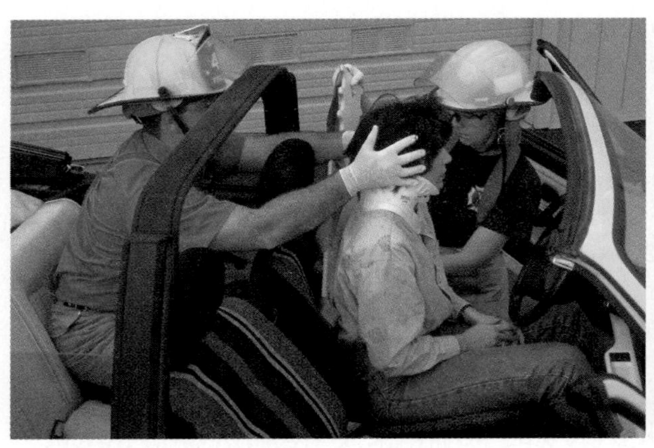

Figure 27-7c
Position the short backboard behind the patient.

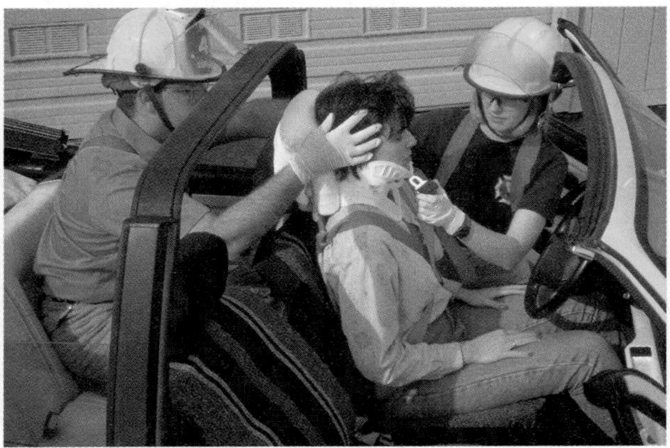

Figure 27-7d
Secure the device to the patient's torso.

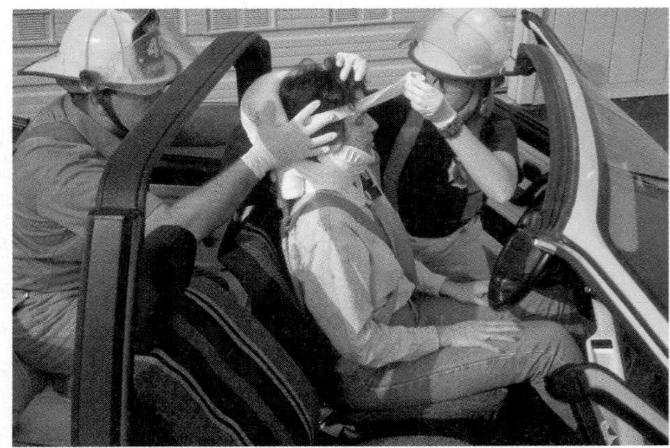

Figure 27-7e
Pad as necessary, and secure the patient's head.

3. Position the short backboard behind the patient.

4. Secure the patient's torso. Then check to see that the straps aren't too tight or too loose. They should be snug, but they shouldn't cause discomfort. Avoid jostling or moving the patient while doing this.

5. If needed, pad behind the patient's head to maintain a neutral, in-line position. Then secure the patient's head to the short backboard.

Once the patient is secure to the short backboard, he or she must be lifted or rotated onto a long backboard. Position the long backboard under the patient's buttocks. Rotate and lower the patient onto it. Slide him into place. Then secure him. Reassess pulses, sensation, and movement in all four extremities.

> ***Warning*** *Any short backboard will add minutes to immobilization. So don't use one if you have to move a patient with a life-threatening condition. See "Rapid Extrication" later in this chapter for directions.*

Long Backboard Immobilization

The long backboard is used to immobilize the suspected spine-injured patient from head to toe. Here are a few points to remember:

- Never release manual stabilization of the patient's cervical spine until he or she is completely immobilized on a long backboard.

- Because a backboard is straight and a patient's back is curved, immobilization may be uncomfortable. To maintain a neutral position use rolled towels or blankets to fill the voids.

- Patients who are immobilized can't keep their airways clear if they vomit. Constantly monitor them. If they do vomit, quickly turn them to the side and suction if necessary.

Some patients will resist your best attempts to immobilize their spines. The combative intoxicated patient is one good example. Use your common sense in these situations. If the patient is fighting you or if he's trying to corkscrew himself inside your equipment, he may be better off left alone to lie still.

However, if an adult refuses spinal protection, you must inform him or her of all the consequences. These include the possibility of permanent paralysis and, in the case of neck injury, possibly death. Carefully document any call where the patient refuses spinal immobilization. Make sure other rescuers witness this refusal, and call your medical director as appropriate.

For infants and children, use immobilization devices made especially for them, such as the Pedi-Pak™. Also, when an infant or child is in a supine position, their proportionately larger heads may actually be flexed (the chin forced toward the chest). To help reduce this problem, establish a neutral position and place a small pad under the shoulders.

Supine Patient If you find the suspected spine-injured patient in a supine position, secure him or her directly to a long backboard. You'll need at least two rescuers. Three or more are preferable. Remember that one rescuer should maintain manual stabilization until the patient is completely immobilized. At that time, reassess pulses, sensation, and movement in all four extremities.

To immobilize a supine patient on a long backboard, follow these steps (Figure 27-8):

1. Position the long backboard beside the patient.
2. Begin a log roll of the patient.
3. When you've rolled the patient to your chest, have another rescuer position the board under the patient. Quickly inspect the patient's back if you haven't already done so.
4. Then, at the command of the rescuer at the head, roll the patient onto the board.
5. Pad the voids between the patient and the board. Avoid jostling or any unnecessary movement of the patient.
6. Immobilize the torso to the backboard first.
7. Then immobilize the patient's head.
8. Finally, secure the patient's legs.

Standing Patient If the patient is found in a standing position, you'll need three or four rescuers to immobilize him on a long backboard. Follow these steps (Figure 27-9):

1. Have the first rescuer stand in front of the patient to manually stabilize the cervical spine. Then apply a cervical collar.

Applying a Long Backboard to a Supine Patient

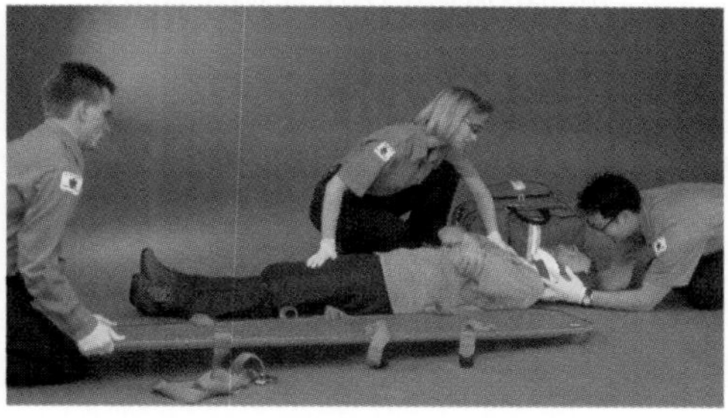

Figure 27-8a
Position the long backboard.

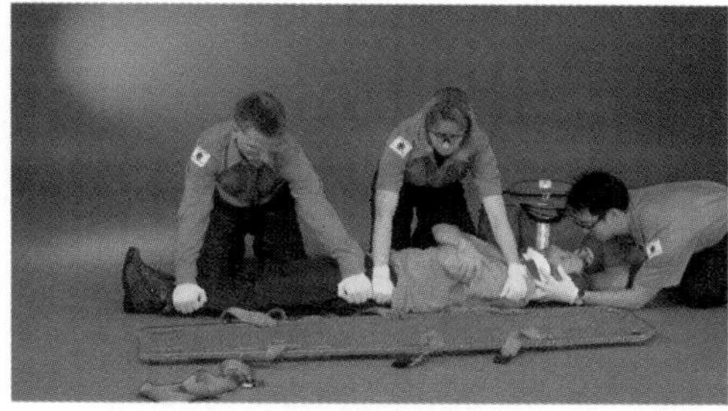

Figure 27-8b
Get in position for a log roll.

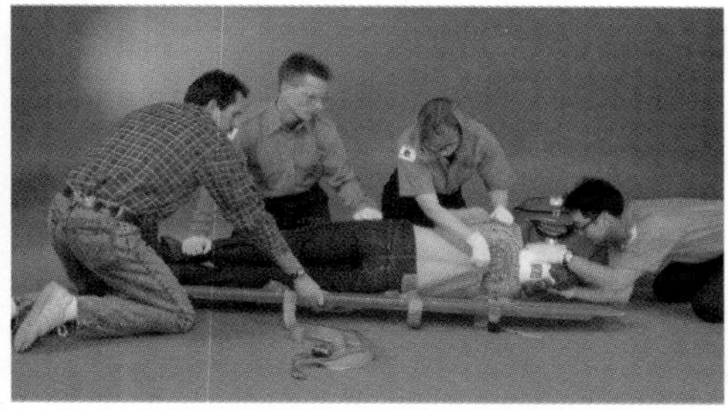

Figure 27-8c
Slide the board under the patient.

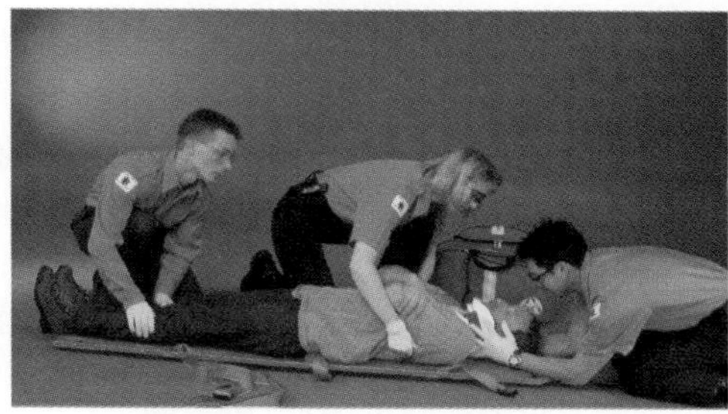

Figure 27-8d
Roll the patient onto the long backboard.

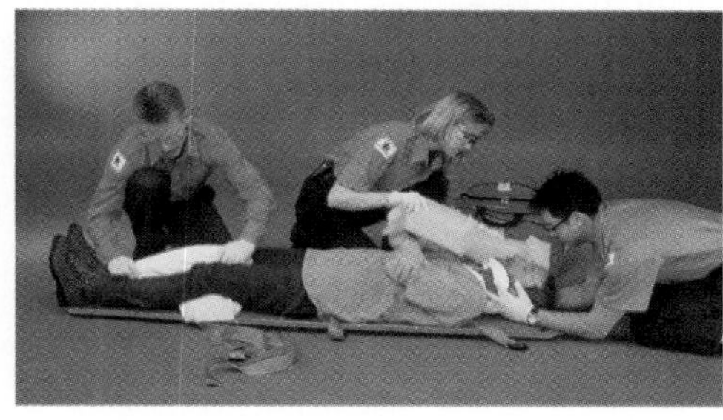

Figure 27-8e
Pad the voids.

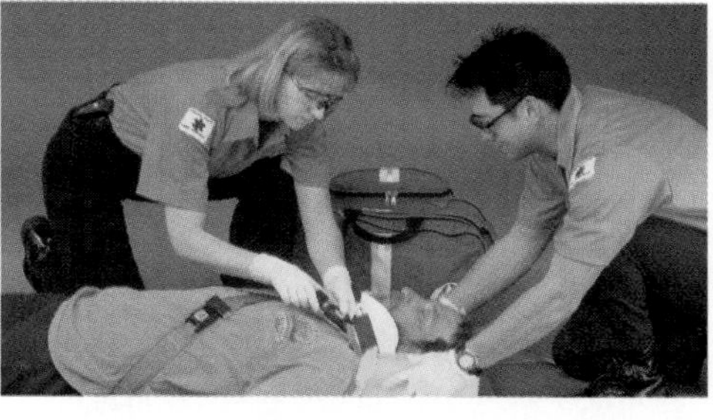

Figure 27-8f
Secure the patient's torso first.

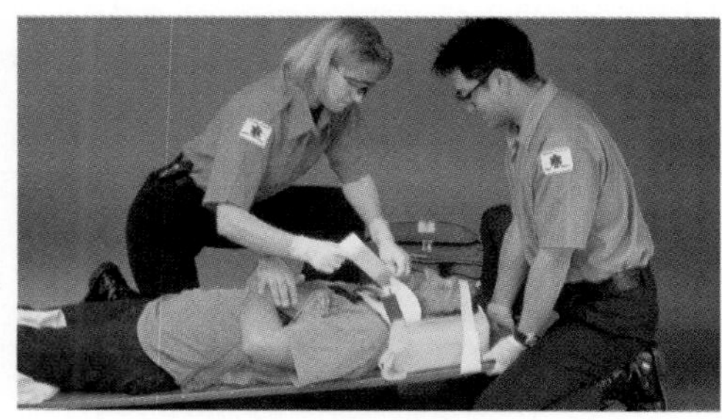

Figure 27-8g
Then secure the patient's head.

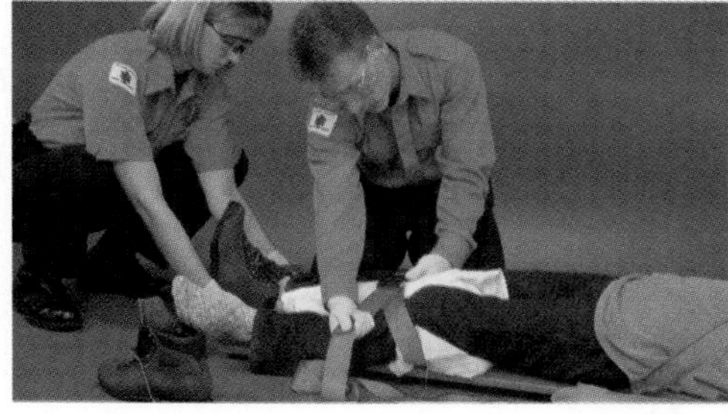

Figure 27-8h
Finally, secure the patient's legs.

Applying a Long Backboard to a Standing Patient

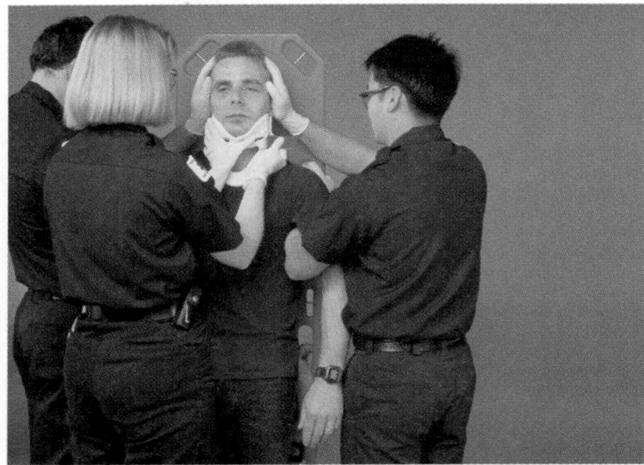

Figure 27-9a
Secure the patient's head, and reach under the patient's arms to secure the board.

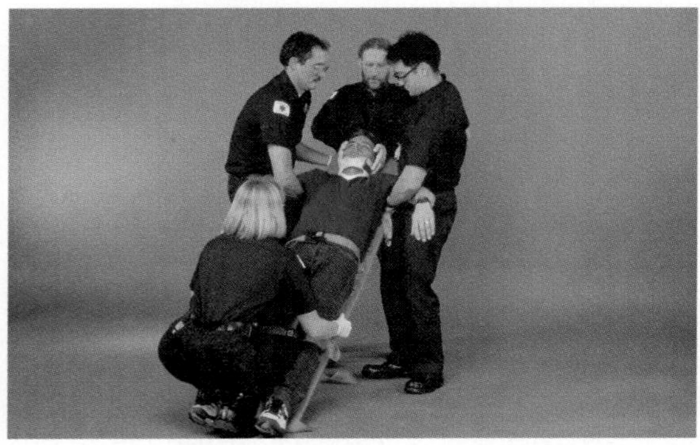

Figure 27-9b
Tip the board back.

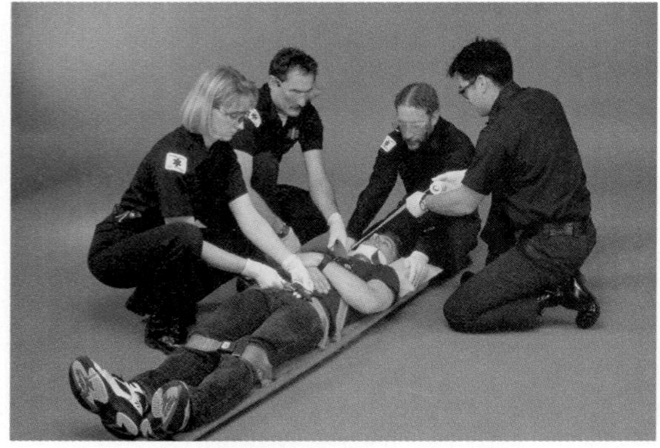

Figure 27-9c
Keep the patient from sliding until the board is horizontal.

2. The second and third rescuers should stand at the sides of the patient. With the hand closest to the patient, each reaches under the patient's arm and grasps the board. With the hand farthest from the patient, they should secure the patient's head.
3. The second and third rescuers place the leg closest to the patient behind the board. Then they begin to tip the top of the board backward.
4. As the board tips back, all three (or four) rescuers must keep the patient and the board from sliding until the patient is in a level horizontal position.

Rapid Extrication In an urgent move of a suspected spine-injured patient, you won't have time to use a short backboard. Instead, three or four rescuers can perform what is called a "rapid extrication." To perform a rapid extrication of a sitting patient, take BSI precautions and follow these steps (Figure 27-10):

1. Get behind the patient to manually stabilize the cervical spine.
2. Apply a cervical collar.
3. If necessary, support the patient's body while another rescuer frees the patient's legs.
4. Then rotate the patient in short coordinated moves.
5. When the patient's back and buttocks are in position, place the long backboard by the patient.
6. Lower the patient onto the long backboard.
7. Then slide the patient in position on the board in short coordinated moves.
8. Secure and extricate the patient.

Note that a sitting patient may be extricated without a short backboard, even when it's not necessary to perform an urgent move.

Rapid Extrication

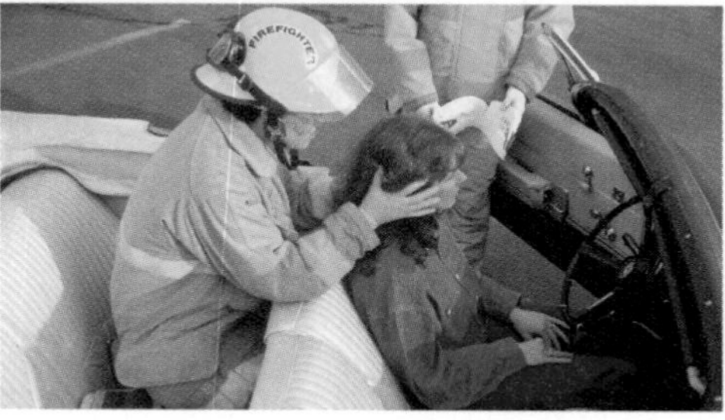

Figure 27-10a
Manually stabilize the head and neck.

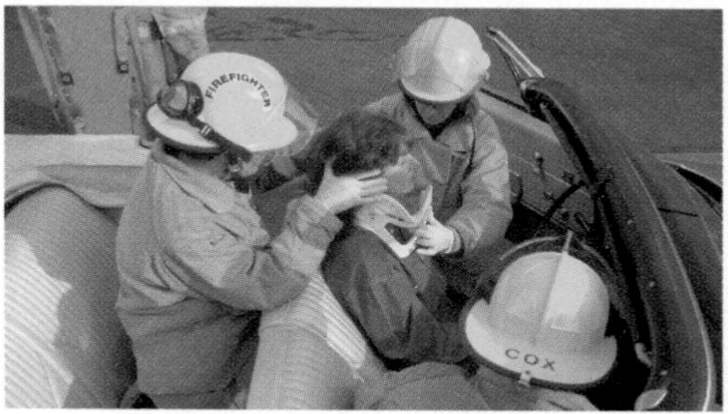

Figure 27-10b
Apply a cervical collar.

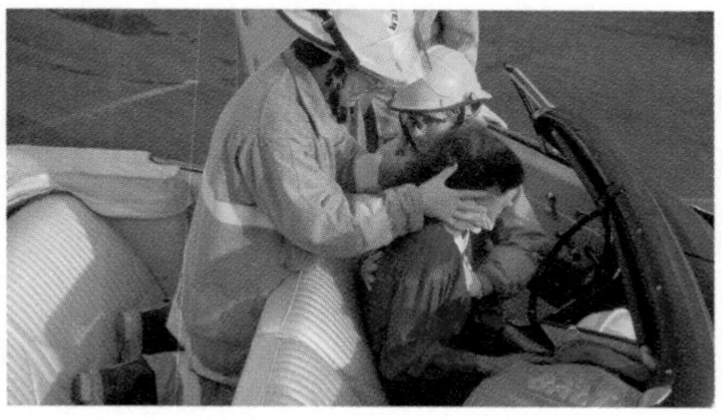

Figure 27-10c
Support the torso as you free the legs.

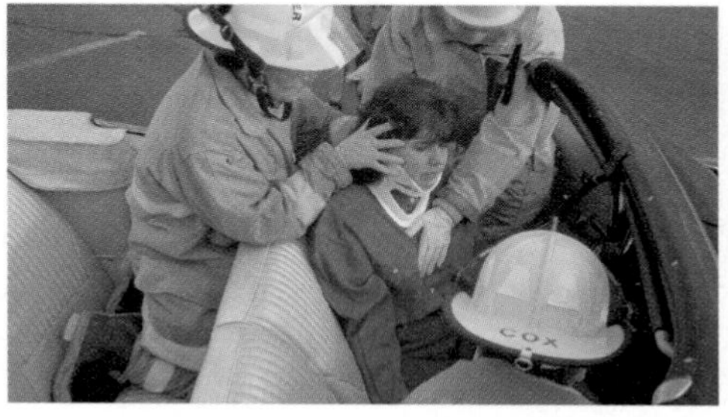

Figure 27-10d
Rotate the patient in short coordinated moves.

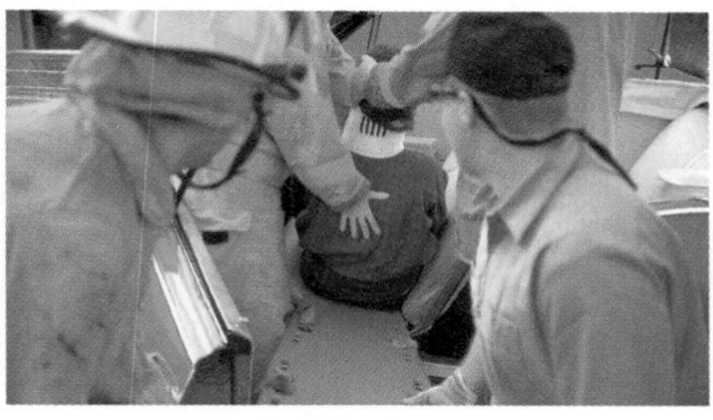

Figure 27-10e
Position the patient—back in the doorway, feet and buttocks on the seat.

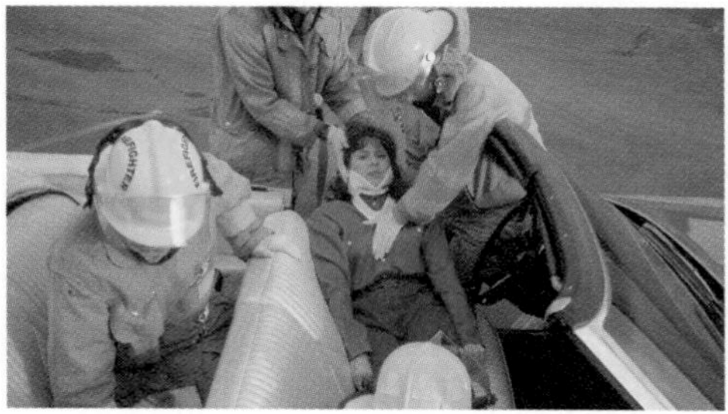

Figure 27-10f
Lower the patient onto the long backboard.

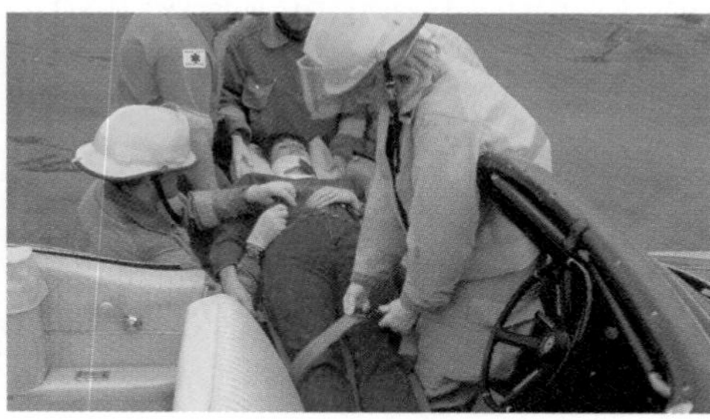

Figure 27-10g
Slide the patient in position in short coordinated moves.

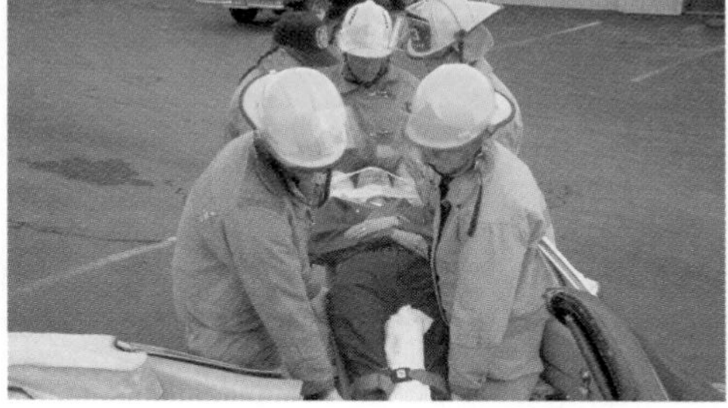

Figure 27-10h
Secure and extricate the patient.

EMERGENCY CARE PLAN | PATIENTS WITH HEAD OR SPINE INJURIES

PRIORITIES

Your priorities for a patient with suspected head or spine injury include:

- Early recognition of the potential for head or spine injury. (Remember the patient's Golden Hour.)
- Immediate manual stabilization of the patient's cervical spine.
- Aggressive support of the patient's airway, breathing, and circulation while maintaining the patient in a neutral, in-line position.
- An accurate physical exam that identifies all major signs and symptoms.
- Constant reassessment of the patient's status.

PATIENT CARE APPROACH

You'll take care of many patients with varying degrees of head and spine injuries. Reassure them, but don't make any false claims. Patients who can't move at first may very well recover. Patients who can move initially still may have damage to the brain or spinal cord. If your patient has suffered a head injury, know that he or she may be combative or irrational. Communicate clearly, and be patient.

DANGER SIGNS

Watch for any sudden change in your patient's mental status. A sudden decrease may indicate that a head injury is getting worse. Be on the lookout for any airway, breathing, or circulation problems.

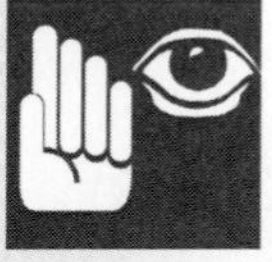

SCENE SIZE-UP

1. **ASSESS SCENE SAFETY.** Is the scene safe to enter? Trauma scenes often involve hazards, including broken glass, blood, jagged metal, and so on. Take all BSI precautions and wear the appropriate personal protective equipment.

2. **DETERMINE MECHANISM OF INJURY.** What happened? How was your patient injured? Be specific about finding out impact speeds, whether or not the patient was wearing a seat belt, how your patient landed after the fall, and so on. Activate the EMS system if you haven't already done so.

3. **TRIAGE THE PATIENT.** How many patient's are there? How badly are they hurt? Do you have enough personnel and resources on the way? Do you need to call for more?

4. **DETERMINE ACCESS AND EXTRICATION NEEDS.** Are you able to get to your patient? If specialized personnel are working to extricate your patient, maintain manual stabilization and the patient's ABCs as long as necessary.

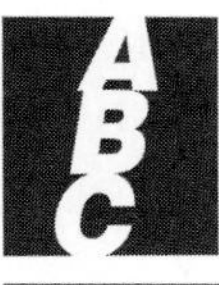

INITIAL ASSESSMENT AND TREATMENT

1. **FORM A GENERAL IMPRESSION.** Determine your patient's sex and approximate age. What's your patient's level of distress? What's his or her chief complaint?

   Remember *If the mechanism of injury is significant, tell your trauma patient to hold very still as soon as you make contact. Then manually stabilize the head and neck until the patient is properly immobilized.*

2. **CHECK MENTAL STATUS.** Remember a head-injured patient may be confused, combative, or have no memory of the trauma incident. Be on the lookout for alcohol abuse. If your patient has an altered mental status, apply high flow oxygen, if you're equipped to do so.

3. **ASSESS THE ABCs.**

   - **Airway.** Is the airway open? If not, use the jaw-thrust maneuver. Maintain manual stabilization of the cervical spine.

Warning *If you're unable to establish or maintain an open airway with the jaw-thrust maneuver, you may need to use a head-tilt/chin-lift maneuver. Remember, an uninjured cervical spine means nothing if your patient dies from a blocked airway or inadequate ventilations. Follow all local protocols.*

- **Breathing**. Is your patient breathing? Is breathing adequate? If your patient is showing any signs of breathing problems, apply high flow oxygen if you're so equipped. Ventilate if necessary.

- **Circulation**. Does your patient have a pulse? If so, is it weak or rapid? Slow and bounding? What's your patient's skin condition? Are there any signs of major bleeding from the head, neck, or back? Control major bleeding, and treat for shock at this time. However, don't use the shock position. Maintain the patient in a supine position or, if necessary, in the position in which the patient was found.

4. **DETERMINE PRIORITY.** Your head- or spine-injured patient is a high priority if you observe any of the following:

   - Problems with mental status, airway, breathing, or circulation.

   - Significant blunt or penetrating trauma to the head, neck, shoulders, back, or abdomen.

   - Any problems with the pulses, sensation, or movement in any one of the patient's four extremities.

   - Any major mechanism of injury, such as ejection from a vehicle, a car rollover, the death of an occupant in a car crash, major intrusion in the passenger space, gunshot or stab wounds, falls of greater than 15 feet, or auto-pedestrian impacts greater than 15 mph.

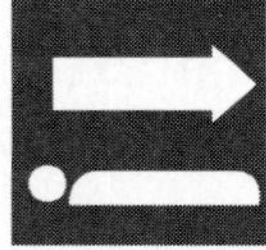

PHYSICAL EXAM AND TREATMENT

1. **GATHER A *SAMPLE* HISTORY.** Remind the patient not to move while you ask questions.

   (S)igns and symptoms? Are there any signs of trauma to the head or back? Is there any pain to the head, neck, or back? Are there any problems with vision? Is there vomiting? Changes in mental status? Numbness or tingling in the extremities? Use the PQRST mnemonic to help you describe the patient's pain.

   (A)llergies to medications?

   (M)edications?

   (P)ertinent past history?

   (L)ast oral intake?

   (E)vents leading to the injury or illness? Gather an accurate picture of how the trauma event occurred. If the patient is unresponsive, obtain information from others at the scene to determine the mechanism of injury and the patient's mental status before you arrived.

2. **PERFORM A HEAD-TO-TOE EXAM.** Look and feel carefully for any injuries to the patient's head, neck, chest, abdomen, pelvis, back, and extremities. Check for signs of incontinence. Assess pulses, sensation, and movement in the extremities.

3. **TAKE VITAL SIGNS.** Assess all vital signs as appropriate. An accurate assessment of mental status is critical.

4. **PROVIDE TREATMENT AS NEEDED.** Complete emergency care of any external wounds, including head injuries.

Use the proper equipment to immobilize the patient now. If you're not allowed, then maintain manual stabilization of the patient's cervical spine until EMS workers with more training take over.

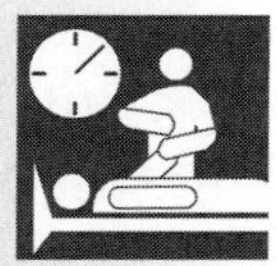

ONGOING ASSESSMENT AND TREATMENT

1. **REPEAT THE INITIAL ASSESSMENT.** Remember that head-injured patients in particular may experience very rapid changes in mental status that can affect airway and breathing. So reassess every five minutes.

2. **REPEAT THE PHYSICAL EXAM.** Focus on the patient's chief complaint, major injuries, and vital signs. Reassess pulses, sensation, and movement in the extremities. Check all interventions to be sure they are still effective.

3. **PROVIDE REASSURANCE.**

CONCLUSION

Both head and spine injuries can devastate a patient's life. As a First Responder, your management of these patients can directly affect how well they will do. With your head- and spine-injury patients, as with all your patients, remember the Golden Hour and:

- *Assess* your patient's responsiveness, airway, breathing, and circulation.
- *Intervene* by treating life threats and by protecting the patient's spine from further injury.

PATIENT HAND-OFF

1. **GIVE A PATIENT REPORT.** The following is an example of a patient report based on the scenario at the beginning of the chapter:

   This is Phil. He's 23 years old. A short while ago he ran into the surf, dove under a wave, and hit his head on the bottom. When he reached the surface, he was unable to move his arms or legs and needed a surf rescue to get him to shore. He can't feel anything below his neck at this time. Phil is alert. His airway is open, but he's having difficulty breathing. His pulses are strong and regular. He's a high priority patient. We found no other signs of major trauma. We haven't completed a SAMPLE history. At this time we've manually stabilized his cervical spine and have applied high flow oxygen. There have been no changes in his status in the past five minutes or so.

2. **CONDUCT THE TRANSFER OF CARE.**

3. **ASSIST IN EXTRICATION AND TRANSPORT.** Assist other rescuers with extrication as necessary.

- *Reassess* the patient to see if your interventions are working or if the patient's status has changed.

KEY TERMS

You may wish to use this list to review your understanding of key terms introduced in the chapter.

backboard a rigid, flat device that is used to immobilize a patient's spine.

cervical collar a rigid device used to reduce the movement of the cervical spine.

pedal pulses pulse points found in the ankle and foot; usually, at the dorsalis pedis artery.

APPLICATION QUESTIONS

You may wish to use these questions to review your understanding of the chapter. For answers with page references, see Appendix 2.

1. You and your partner are managing a patient who has suffered massive head injuries after being thrown from his bicycle. The two of you find that the jaw-thrust isn't working even after numerous attempts. You decide to perform a head-tilt/chin-lift, but your partner says, "Hey, what about this guy's spine? You can't do that!" What is your response to him?

2. You've responded to a male in his 20s who has walked away from a vehicle rollover. He has a large bruise above his left eye. He also says that his neck feels a bit stiff. He's had two or three beers in the past hour. You tell him that you need to stabilize his head and neck, and he says, "Hey, look, I'm fine. I can feel all ten fingers and toes. I don't think my neck is broken. So lay off and leave me alone!" What is your response to him?

CHAPTER 28 MUSCLE AND BONE INJURIES

FIRST RESPONSE

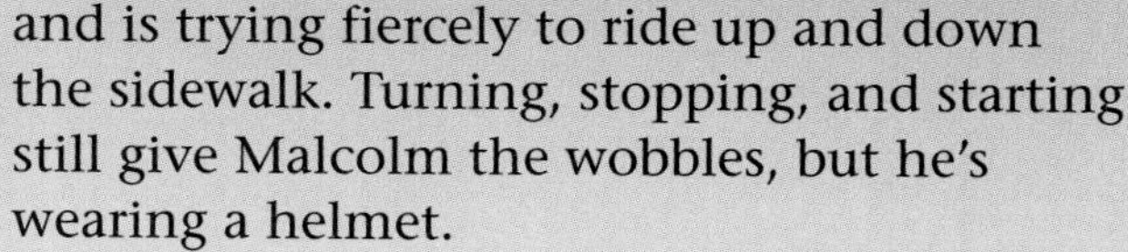

Jennie is an experienced First Responder. She's run many trauma calls in her years with the state search and rescue team. Today Jennie will need to draw on her experience to handle a trauma call closer to home.

Jennie's son—six-year-old Malcolm—is riding his bike in front of the house. Malcolm has recently graduated to a two-wheeler and is trying fiercely to ride up and down the sidewalk. Turning, stopping, and starting still give Malcolm the wobbles, but he's wearing a helmet.

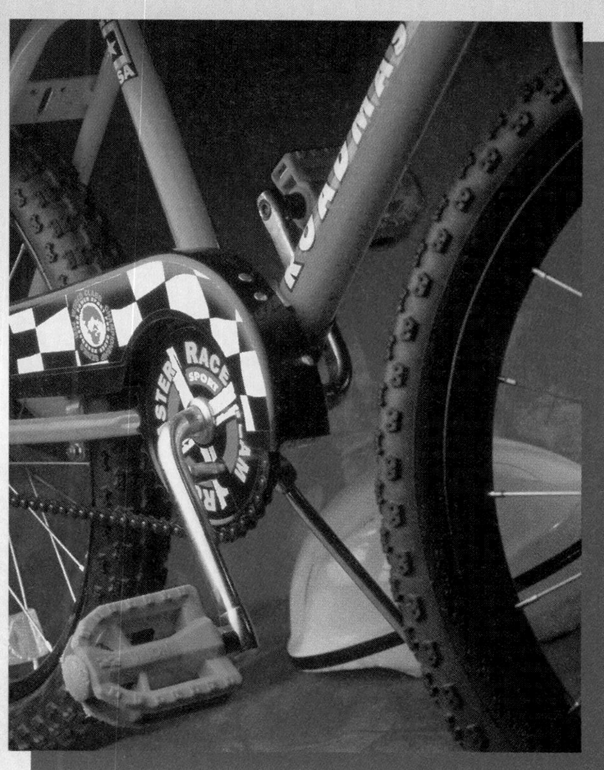

Without warning, Malcolm's two-wheeler teeters off balance. The barely controlled wobble turns into a spastic lurch. In the blink of an eye Malcolm is thrown from his bike into a brick retaining wall. On impact he lets out a shriek. His upper arm and collarbone have snapped.

Jennie sees it all, rushes to his side, and yells to a neighbor to call 9-1-1. With trembling hands she completes an initial assessment of her son. He's awake and alert, complaining of pain to his arm and shoulder. Malcolm has no neck or back pain, but Jennie has him remain supine. Malcolm's face streams with tears as the pain in his arm and shoulder grows more intense.

Jennie quickly examines her son and sees obvious deformities to his upper arm and collarbone. She shows Malcolm how to cradle his fractured arm in his good one. She knows that this will reduce the pain and stabilize the fractures. She completes a physical exam on Malcolm just as the volunteer fire department and ambulance corps arrive.

When Malcolm is fully immobilized, Jennie helps to load him into the back of the ambulance. Then she hops in for the ride to the hospital. She allows herself to breathe a sign of relief. It could have been worse, much worse.

LEARNING OBJECTIVES

Muscle and bone injuries are common in EMS. For patients they can be extremely painful and scary. In certain instances, they can be life-threatening. In this chapter, you'll learn about assessing and treating common muscle and bone injuries, except those to the head and spine, which were covered in Chapter 27.

By the end of the chapter, you should be able to: †

- 5-3.1 Describe the function of the musculoskeletal system. (p. 356)
- 5-3.2 Differentiate between an open and a closed painful, swollen, deformed extremity. (p. 358)
- 5-3.3 List the emergency medical care for a patient with a painful, swollen, deformed extremity. (pp. 360-363, 368-372)

* Relate mechanism of injury to muscle and bone injuries. (pp. 356-357)

* Describe the signs and symptoms of muscle and bone injuries. (pp. 357-359)

* Explain the basic concepts behind effective splinting. (pp. 361-367)

THE MUSCULOSKELETAL SYSTEM

Before you begin this chapter, go back to Chapter 4 to review both the anatomy and function of the musculoskeletal system. You also may wish to study the names of the major bones in the human body (see anatomical illustrations in Chapter 4). Knowing the proper names—*sternum* instead of breastbone or *femur* instead of thigh bone, for example—can only help you to communicate more effectively with other EMS workers.

RECOGNIZING MUSCLE AND BONE INJURIES

MECHANISMS OF INJURY

Common mechanisms of musculoskeletal injury include **direct force**, **indirect force**, and **twisting force**. *Direct force* refers to the damage done immediately upon impact of a blow to the

†Numbered objectives are from the 1995 U.S. DOT "First Responder: National Standard Curriculum." Asterisks indicate supplemental material.

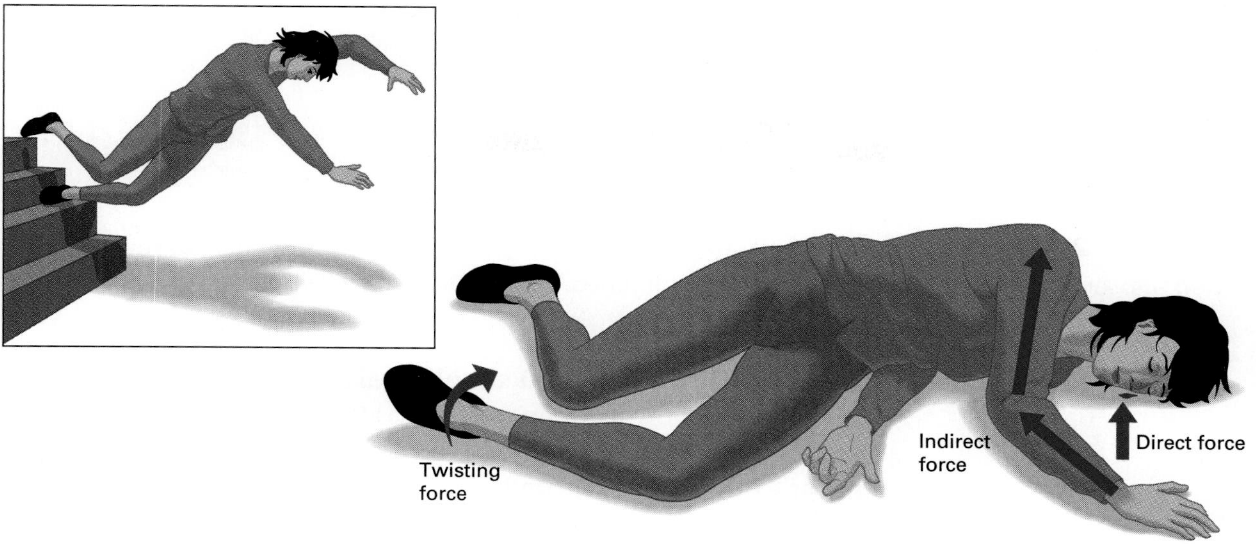

Figure 28-1
Examples of direct force, indirect force, and twisting force.

body. *Indirect force* refers to the damage that continues to be done in the body until the energy of a blow is spent. *Twisting force* refers to damage done when a part of the body turns one way and a connecting part is forced to turn another.

For example, let's say a person catches her foot on a rug or a step (Figure 28-1). She immediately reaches out an arm to try to break her fall. When her hand hits the ground, the energy of the blow travels up her arm, resulting in a dislocated shoulder. (This injury was caused by indirect force.) When her head hits the floor, she incurs cuts and bruises to her forehead. (These are caused by direct force). In addition, when her foot was caught, it remained stationary as the rest of her body turned to fall (a twisting force), which resulted in a sprained ankle.

When you determine the mechanism of injury, always consider the forces involved. An obvious injury to muscle and bone may actually be an indication of more serious injuries elsewhere in the patient.

SIGNS AND SYMPTOMS

In days past EMS workers had to know the difference between a **fracture** (a break in a bone) and a **dislocation** (displacement of a bone in a joint) or a **sprain** (stretching or tearing of ligaments) and a **strain** (pulling or tearing of muscles). However, in the field these distinctions are not important, because field treatment is same.

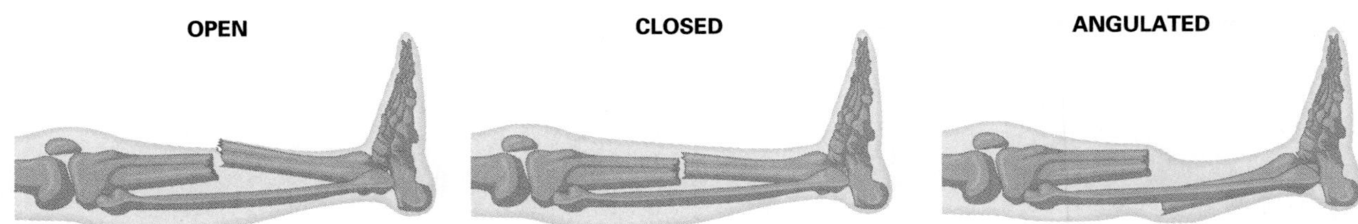

Figure 28-2
Open, closed, and angulated musculoskeletal injuries.

There is a distinction you should make, however. That's the difference between an open and a closed injury. An open bone or joint injury is characterized by a break in the skin. This can happen, for example, when the jagged ends of a broken bone pierce the skin. A closed bone or joint injury has no break in the skin. A musculoskeletal injury also can be deformed, or **angulated** (Figures 28-2 and 28-3).

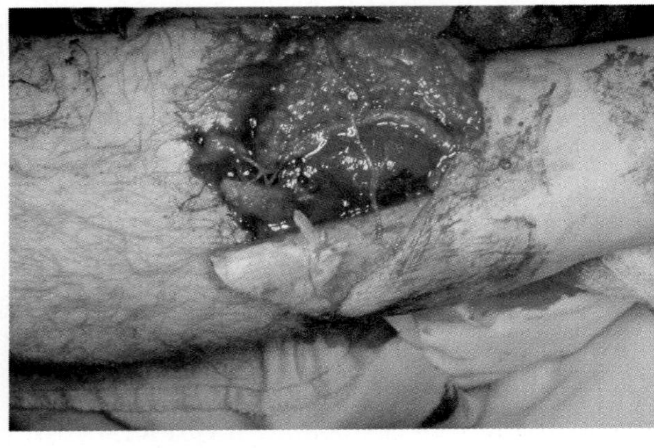

Figure 28-3a
Open fracture.

The signs and symptoms of muscle and bone injuries include the following:

- Pain and tenderness. (An injury is said to be tender when touching it causes pain.)
- Swelling.
- Deformity.
- Bruising.
- Grating of bone ends (this is called *crepitus*).
- Exposed bones.

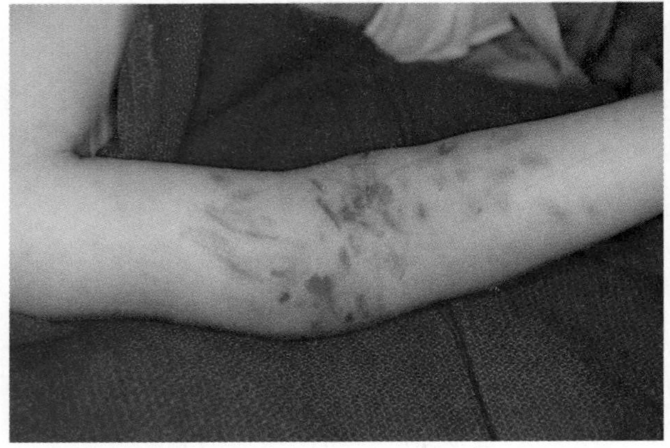

Figure 28-3b
Closed fracture.

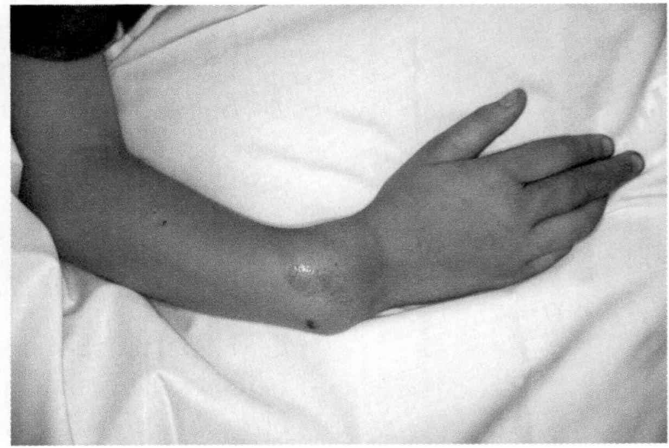

Figure 28-3c
Angulated fracture.

- Reduced ability to move the injured extremity.
- A joint locked in position.

Signs and symptoms of muscle and bone injuries often are so similar that when an injury occurs to an extremity, it's simply called a **PSD** (painful, swollen, deformed) **extremity**.

ASSESSMENT CONSIDERATIONS

Muscle and bone injuries present a unique assessment problem. They often get all the press, because they can look so awful, even when they're not life-threatening. In fact they can keep you from noticing injuries that do pose a life threat. When you assess a trauma patient, always be concerned about the patient's ABCs. Don't let a painful, swollen, deformed leg, for instance, make you lose sight of the fact that your patient may be slipping into shock.

Injuries to the extremities should always be assessed after treating the patient for any life threats and after checking for injuries to the rest of the body. Extremity injuries are fairly easy to spot. It may not be as easy to determine injuries to the pelvis or the ribs. So in general, when assessing a patient for muscle or bone injuries:

1. *Ask* the patient where he or she hurts.
2. *Look* for signs of injuries.
3. *Feel* for signs of injuries.

This three-step method helps you to locate injuries rapidly. By asking the patient's help, you can keep from causing extra pain unnecessarily. When you do palpate (feel) for injuries, your touch should be firm and focused. Avoid rapid-fire head-to-toe exams that don't allow the patient to respond. Stay away from "granny pats," those light pats that fail to elicit pain even if an injury exists.

A few more tips on muscle and bone injuries:

- Bone injuries involving the pelvis and the femur can lead to severe internal bleeding and shock. Never forget to assess your patient for life threats.
- Rib injuries often can be identified by having your patient take a deep breath. Pain with breathing is one of the most reliable indicators.
- Patients with pelvic fractures may or may not be able to walk. However, they often will complain of pain to the groin in addition to pelvic pain with palpation.

- Consider both direct and indirect forces when you assess a trauma patient. It takes such a tremendous force to break a thigh bone (femur), for example, that you have to suspect other injuries to your patient's body as well.

It may be difficult to determine if a pre-verbal child has been injured. One of the best ways to determine injury is to watch how the baby uses the suspected limb. Does the baby move it? Does he or she bear weight on the suspected leg? Does the baby reach and grab objects with the suspected arm? Usually, you'll see reduced movement of the injured limb.

PATIENT MANAGEMENT

GENERAL TREATMENT

After taking BSI precautions, provide emergency care for a painful, swollen, deformed extremity as follows:

1. Treat all life threats. Administer high flow oxygen if you're so equipped.
2. Allow the patient to remain in a position of comfort, unless of course you suspect spine injury.
3. Manually stabilize the extremity above and below the injury site (Figure 28-4). That is, place one gloved hand above and one gloved hand below the injury to keep it from moving. Don't try to pull the bones to realign them. Don't try to replace protruding bones.
4. Cover open wounds with sterile dressings.
5. Help reduce pain and swelling by applying a cold pack to the injury site. Be sure dressings or a towel is between the injury and the cold pack.

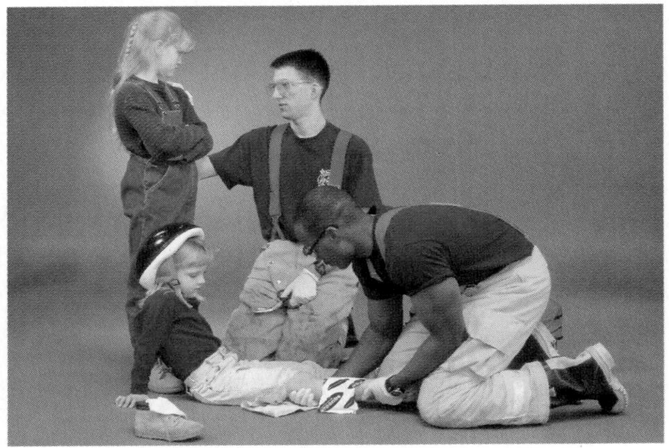

Figure 28-4
Manual stabilization of a painful, swollen, deformed extremity.

6. Assess the area below the injury site for pulse, sensation, and movement. Document your findings.
7. Place padding under the extremity to help the patient feel more comfortable.

Manually stabilize the injured extremity until a splint can be applied. Make sure the extremity is well supported, particularly if it becomes necessary to move the patient. Reassess pulses, sensation, and movement and document your findings. Report them to the EMS crew who takes over patient care.

Emergency care for injuries to the ribs, pelvis, and other bones in the trunk of the body includes the following. Support the patient's airway, breathing, and circulation. Control all major bleeding, and treat for shock. Dress open wounds. Note that activation of the EMS system is very important. Major injuries to the trunk of the body often lead to respiratory distress or shock.

SPLINTING

Many First Responders are trained and equipped to splint injured extremities. Used to immobilize bones and joints, splinting helps to prevent further muscle and bone injury and reduces bleeding and pain. Some general guidelines for splinting are as follows:

- Assess and treat life threats first. Splinting an extremity should never take priority.
- If the patient has signs of shock or other life threats, prepare immediately for transport. Don't delay by trying to splint individual injuries. Instead, guide the patient's body into a neutral, in-line position and immobilize him from head to toe on a long backboard. The backboard will serve to "splint" the injured extremities until the patient can get to a hospital.
- Keep splinting simple. Most splints must be removed at the hospital.
- Make sure that the splint you use fits the patient. Poorly fitted splints allow movement, and you don't want that. Even a properly sized splint, when applied incorrectly, can cause nerve, blood vessel, and tissue damage. Applied too tightly, it can cut off circulation to an extremity.
- Pad splints before applying them.
- Assess below the injury site for the patient's pulse, sensation, and movement before and after splinting. This can be done by checking the patient's fingers and toes. So leave them exposed.

Applying a Splint

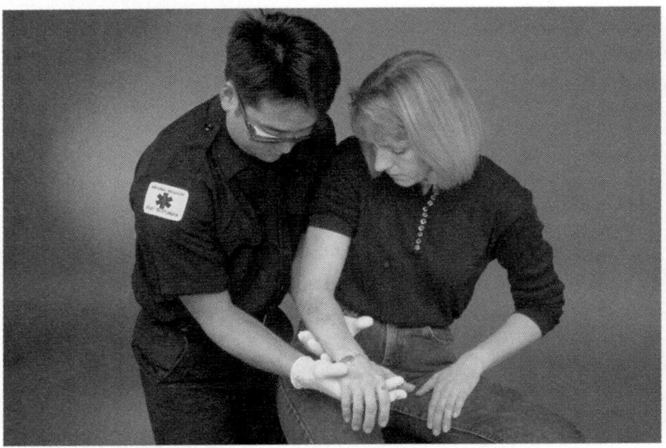

Figure 28-5a
Apply manual stabilization.

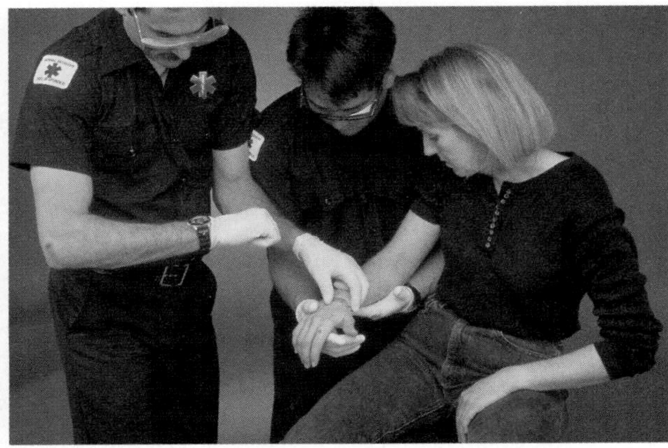

Figure 28-5b
Assess pulse, sensation, and movement below the injury site.

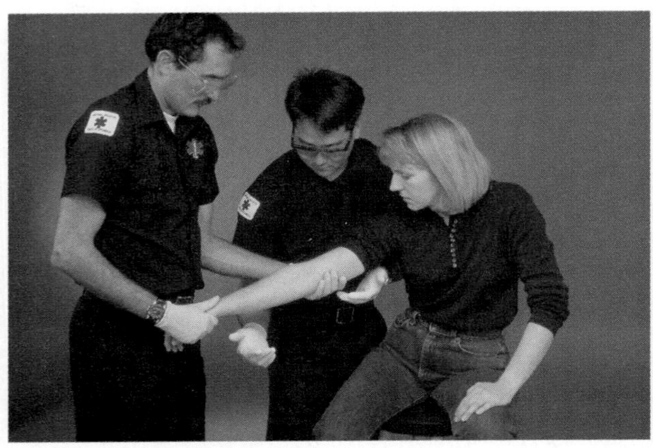

Figure 28-5c
If there's deformity and there's cyanosis or pulselessness below the injury site, then apply gentle traction.

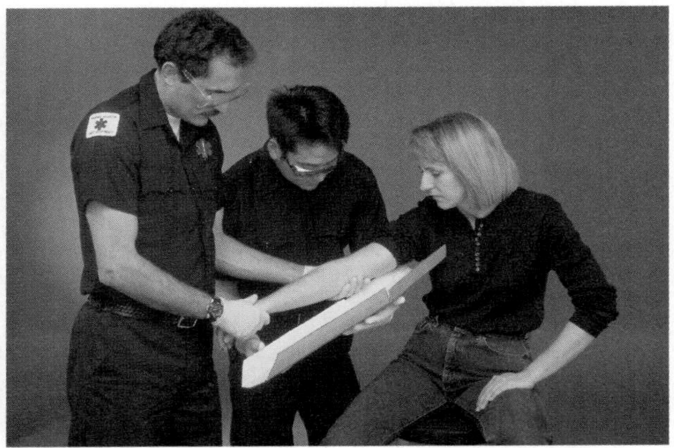

Figure 28-5d
Measure and pad the splint.

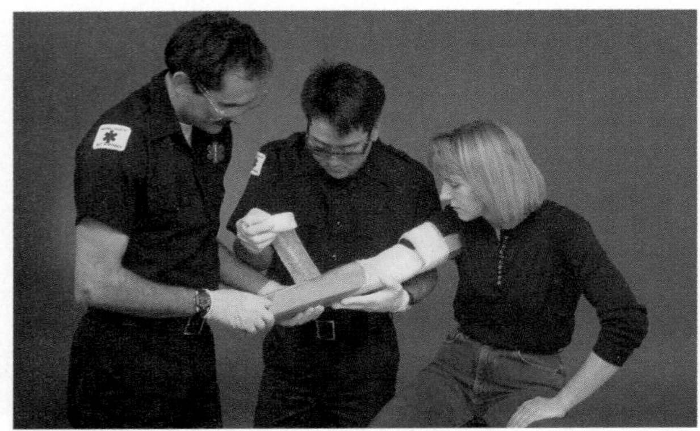

Figure 28-5e
Apply the splint.

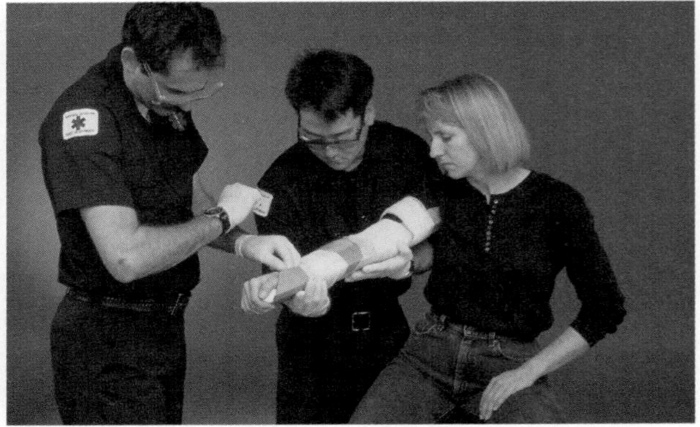

Figure 28-5f
Reassess pulse, sensation, and movement.

- If possible, splint an injured extremity before moving a patient.

To splint an injured extremity, first take BSI precautions. Then remove or cut away the patient's clothing from the injury site. Cover open wounds with sterile dressings. Then splint as follows (Figure 28-5):

1. Apply manual stabilization. Don't release it until the injured extremity is properly immobilized.
2. Assess pulse, sensation, and movement below the injury site.
3. If there's deformity and if the extremity below the injury is cyanotic (bluish) or has no pulse, then align the extremity with gentle traction (pulling). However, if the injury site is at a joint, stop traction immediately if you feel any resistance at all.
4. Measure the splint, and pad it appropriately.
5. To immobilize long-bone injuries, apply the splint so that the joint above and below the injury site is immobilized too. To immobilize a joint, apply the splint so that the bones above and below it are immobilized (Figure 28-6).
6. Reassess pulse, sensation, and movement in the extremity. Document your findings, and report them to the EMS crew when they take over care.

TYPES OF SPLINTS

There are several types of splints available. There are air splints (Figure 28-7), vacuum splints (Figure 28-8), cardboard splints, various rigid splints, and improvised splints such as pillows. A sling and swathe, made from two triangular bandages, works well

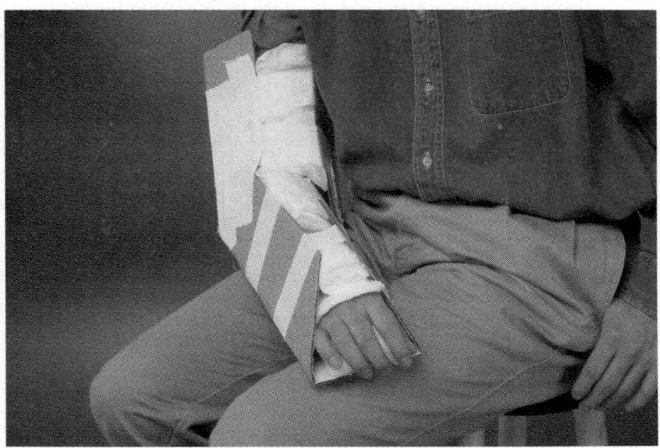

Figure 28-6
A splinted joint.

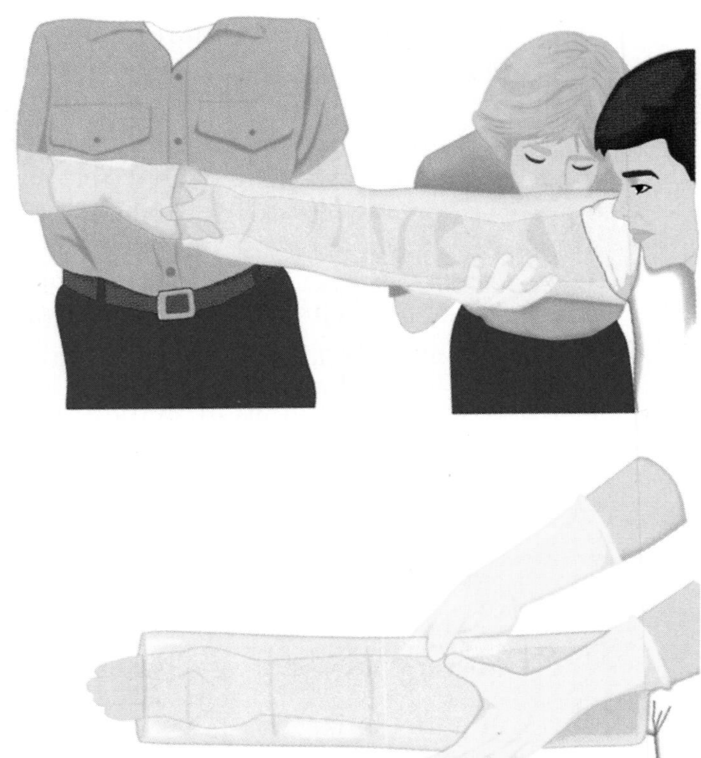

Figure 28-7
Applying an air splint.

to immobilize a shoulder joint (Figure 28-9). A tongue depressor is effective on a finger injury (Figure 28-10). Don't be afraid to be creative. A pillow or blanket wrapped around an injured limb and secured with tape makes an excellent splint (Figure 28-11).

One of the best splints is the patient's own body. The patient can immobilize an injured shoulder and arm by cradling the injured arm against the body with the uninjured arm. Also, there will be times when you won't want to cause more pain by trying to fit an injured limb in a splint. In these cases propping the patient's injured limb up on a pillow, for example, may cause less pain.

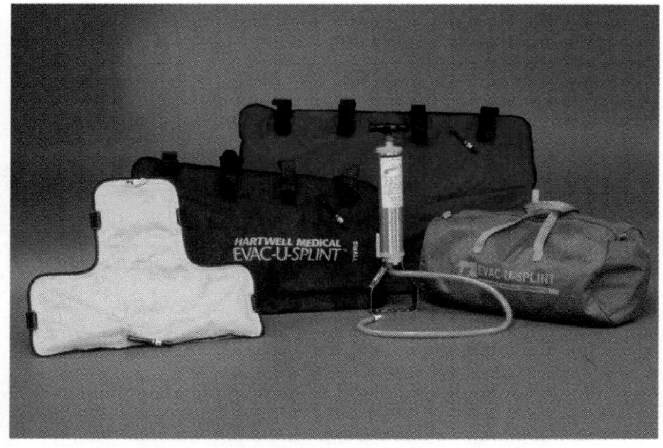

Figure 28-8
A vacuum splint kit.

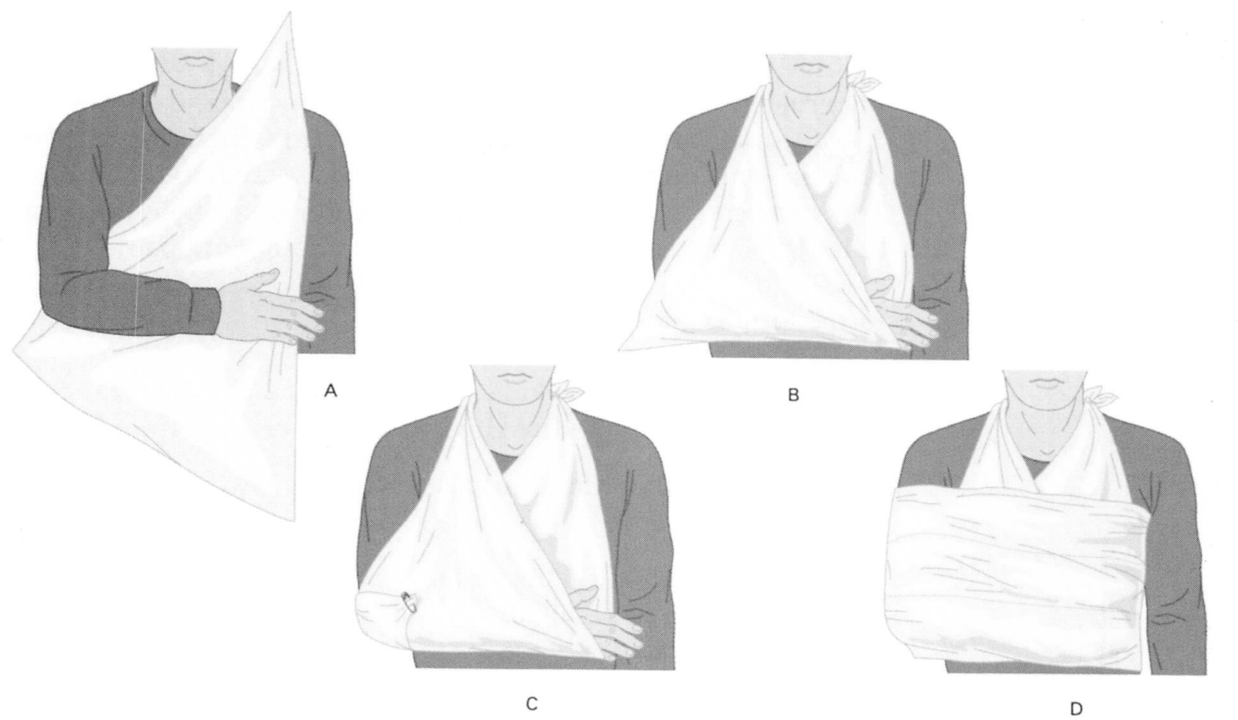

Figure 28-9
Sling and swathe.

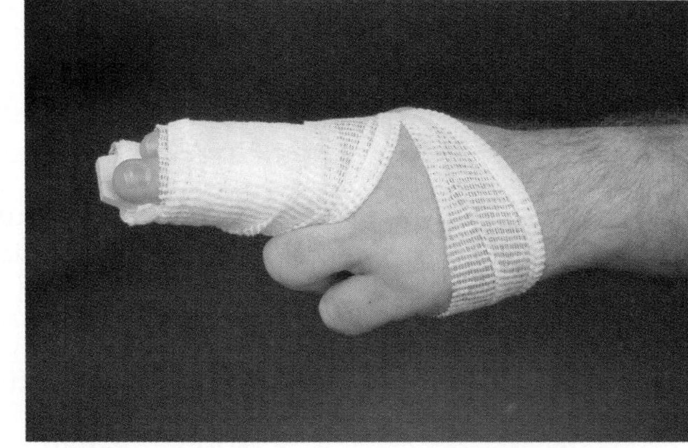

Figure 28-10
Tongue depressor as a splint.

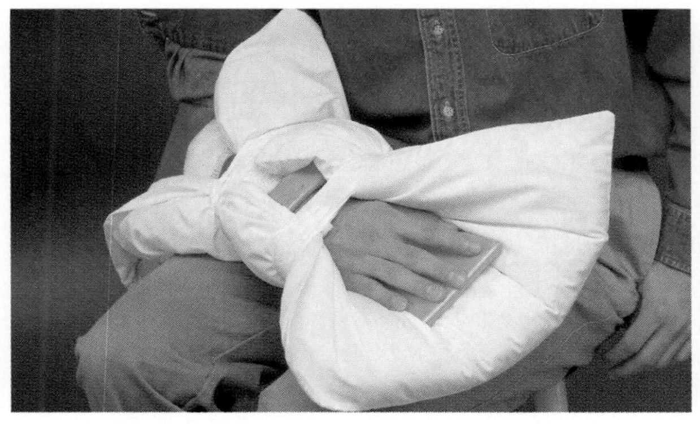

Figure 28-11a
Pillow splint.

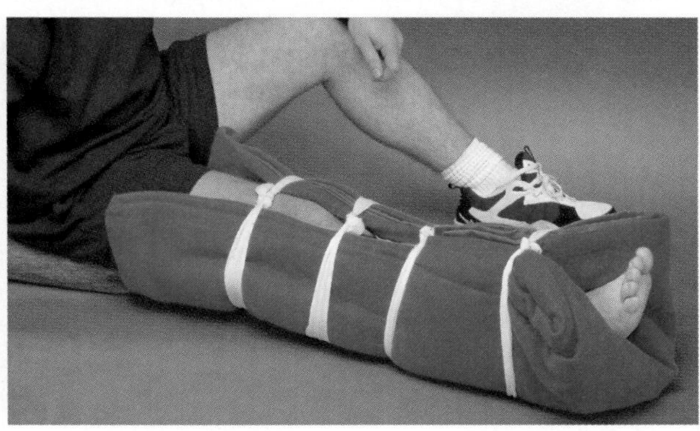

Figure 28-11b
Blanket splint.

A special type of splint you should be aware of is the **traction splint**. It applies a pulling force to a broken femur. When the upper leg is injured, the thigh muscle can spasm and contract. These muscles are very strong. By contracting, they can cause the broken bone ends to damage tissue, blood vessels, and nerves. This can be extremely painful. The traction splint helps to immobilize the bone ends and prevent further injury and pain.

Use a traction splint only for a closed painful, swollen, deformed injury of the mid-thigh.

- Don't use it when the knee of the injured leg is also injured, the injury is close to the knee, or the lower leg is injured.
- Don't use it for a hip injury, pelvis injury, lower-leg injury, or ankle injury.
- Don't use it when the lower leg is partially amputated (connected only by a small amount of tissue). Traction would risk complete separation.

Several types of traction splint are available. Apply them according to manufacturer directions. Remember to assess pulses, sensation, and movement before and after splinting. In general, you can apply a traction splint by following these steps (Figure 28-12):

1. After manually stabilizing the injured leg, apply manual traction. Don't release it until the leg is completely immobilized.
2. Prepare and adjust the splint to the proper length. Then place it under the patient's leg.
3. Fasten the ischial strap.
4. Apply and secure the ankle hitch.
5. Apply mechanical traction.
6. Position and secure the support straps on the patient's leg.

After application, check both the ischial strap and the mechanical traction device to make sure they fit properly. Secure the patient's torso to a long backboard to immobilize the hip. Then secure the traction splint to the long backboard to prevent movement.

Applying a Traction Splint

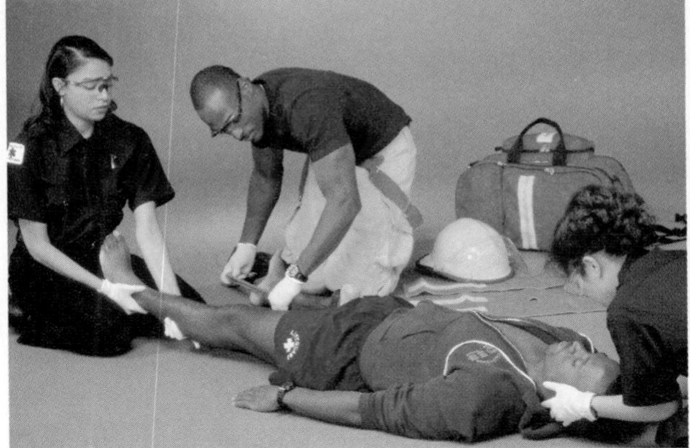

Figure 28-12a
After manually stabilizing the injured leg, apply manual traction.

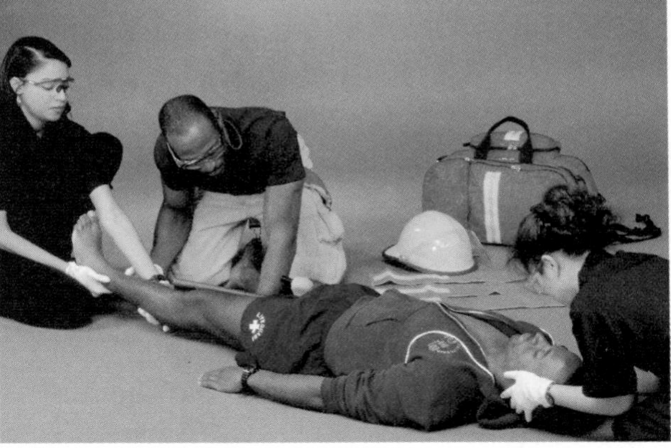

Figure 28-12b
Prepare and adjust the splint to the proper length and place it under the patient's leg.

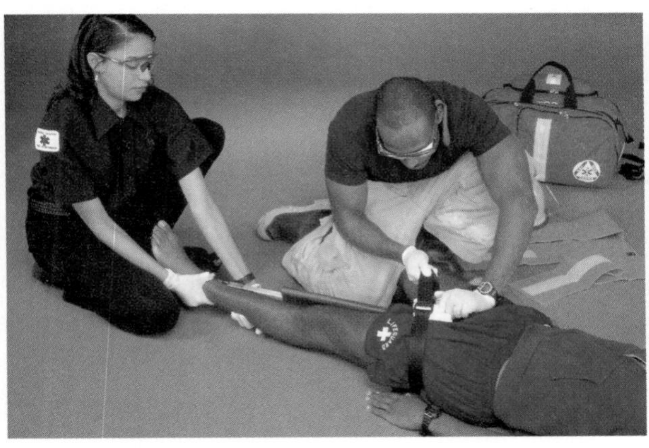

Figure 28-12c
Fasten the ischial strap.

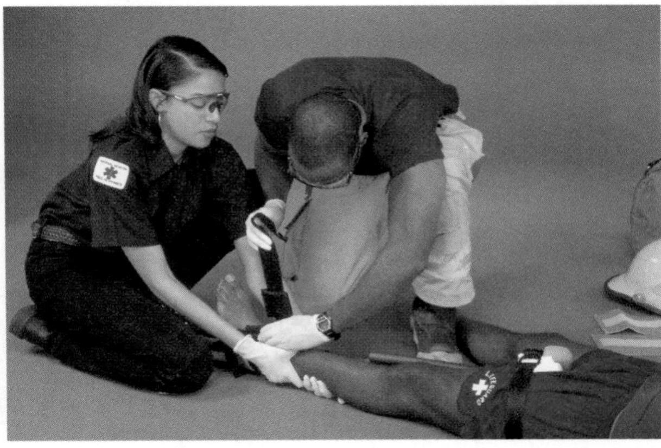

Figure 28-12d
Apply and secure the ankle hitch.

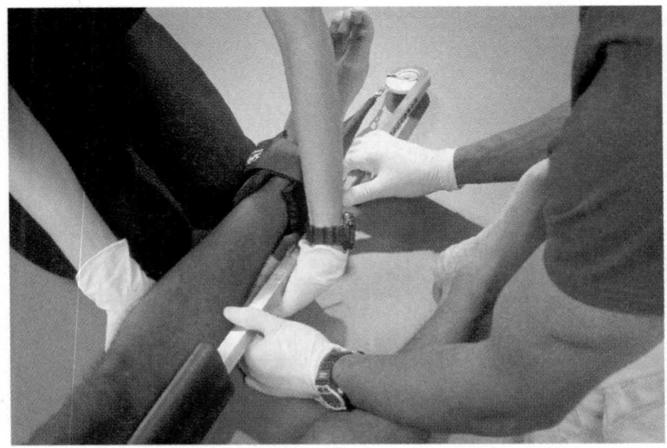

Figure 28-12e
Apply mechanical traction.

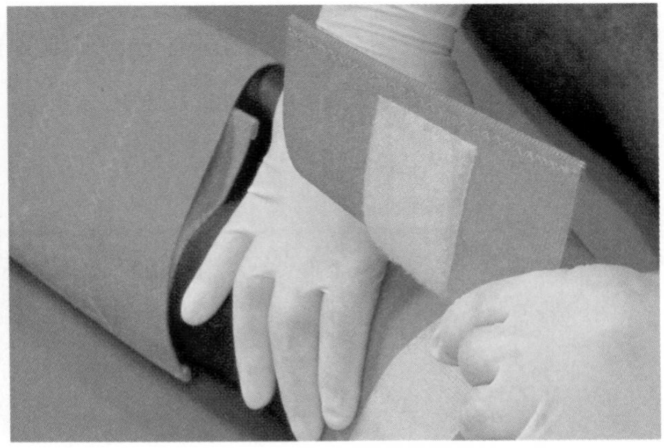

Figure 28-12f
Position and secure the support straps on the patient's leg.

EMERGENCY CARE PLAN | PATIENTS WITH MUSCLE AND BONE INJURIES

■ PRIORITIES

Your priorities for a patient with injuries to muscles and bones are:

- Determine the mechanism of injury, so you can prepare for your patient's injuries.
- Keep the ABCs a top priority, along with spinal immobilization when appropriate. Remember that significant muscle and bone injuries can cause shock.
- Manually stabilize an injured extremity until it's immobilized. Splint the injured limb before moving the patient, if possible.
- Assess pulse, sensation, and movement below the injury site of an injured limb before and after splinting.

■ PATIENT CARE APPROACH

Musculoskeletal injuries can be extremely painful. Your patients may be scared, especially if their injuries have caused gross deformity of an arm or leg. Communicate clearly with them. Explain all the steps of assessment and treatment. Inform them that immobilization of a limb will probably hurt.

■ DANGER SIGNS

Be on the lookout for any problems with airway, breathing, and circulation. Watch for signs of shock.

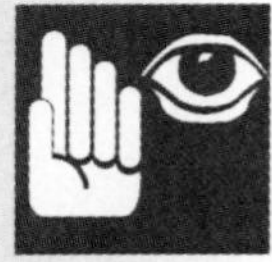

SCENE SIZE-UP

1. **ASSESS SCENE SAFETY.** Is the scene safe? Does the patient's mechanism of injury pose a threat to you? Take all BSI precautions now.

2. **DETERMINE THE MECHANISM OF INJURY.** What caused the injury? Consider the forces that impacted the patient.

Try to accurately identify the height of the fall, the speed of the car, and so on.

3. **TRIAGE THE PATIENT.** Is there more than one patient on scene? Do you have enough resources to handle the call? It may take a lot of hands to immobilize a patient's injured leg and then extricate him or her. Activate the EMS system if it hasn't been activated already.

4. **DETERMINE ACCESS AND EXTRICATION NEEDS.** Clear a space around the patient to allow you to assess and immobilize the injury. You'll need to make enough room for all the rescuers necessary to carry the patient during extrication.

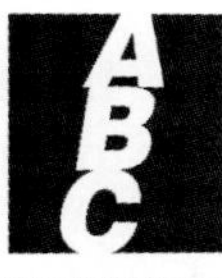

INITIAL ASSESSMENT AND TREATMENT

1. **FORM A GENERAL IMPRESSION.** What is the patient's sex and approximate age? What's the patient's level of distress? Don't let your patient's response to a painful extremity injury distract you from problems with the airway, breathing, or circulation.

2. **CHECK MENTAL STATUS.** Did your patient lose consciousness? If your patient has an altered mental status, apply high flow oxygen, if you're so equipped.

3. **ASSESS THE ABCs.** Treat airway, breathing, and circulation problems as necessary.

4. **DETERMINE PRIORITY.** If your patient has multiple extremity injuries, has sustained a significant mechanism of injury, or has airway, breathing, or circulation problems, consider your patient a high priority.

   If your patient's extremity injury is very unstable, consider manual stabilization at this time.

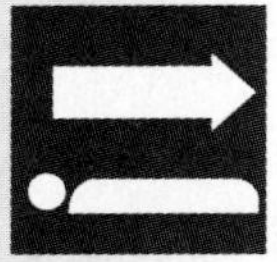

PHYSICAL EXAM AND TREATMENT

1. **GATHER A *SAMPLE* HISTORY.**

   (S)igns and symptoms? Is the patient in pain? Are there signs of injury? Is there any impairment of a limb? Is the patient unable to bear weight on the limb? Recall DOTS (deformities, open injuries, tenderness, swelling) to help you look and feel for injuries.

   (A)llergies to medications?

   (M)edications?

   (P)ertinent past history? Does the patient have a history of falls? Have there been previous injuries to the same site?

   (L)ast oral intake?

   (E)vents leading to the injury or illness? Gather an accurate history of these events. They will tell you a lot about the patient's pattern of injuries.

2. **PERFORM A HEAD-TO-TOE EXAM.** Look for DOTS (deformities, open injuries, tenderness, swelling) to the head, neck, chest, abdomen, pelvis, and extremities.

3. **TAKE VITAL SIGNS.**

4. **PROVIDE TREATMENT AS NEEDED.** Manually stabilize an extremity injury or immobilize it with a splint as appropriate. Remember that ice packs may be able to provide your patient with some relief from pain and swelling.

ONGOING ASSESSMENT AND TREATMENT

1. **REPEAT THE INITIAL ASSESSMENT.**

2. **REPEAT THE PHYSICAL EXAM.** Reassess the patient's pain and injuries. Be sure to reassess pulse, sensation, and movement below the injury site.

3. **PROVIDE REASSURANCE.**

PATIENT HAND-OFF

1. **GIVE A PATIENT REPORT.** The following is an example of a patient report based on the scenario at the beginning of this chapter:

   This is my son, Malcolm. He was riding his bike with his helmet on when he was thrown into a retaining wall, striking his left arm and shoulder. He had no loss of consciousness. He's awake and alert with normal airway, breathing, and circulation. He has pain, swelling, and deformity in his left collar bone and upper arm. He has no neck or back pain, but I've had him remain in a supine position. He has no drug allergies, takes no medications, and has no previous medical history. He last ate about two hours ago. At this time he's calm and immobilizing his left arm and shoulder against his body with his right arm.

2. **CONDUCT THE TRANSFER OF CARE.**

3. **ASSIST IN EXTRICATION AND TRANSPORT.** Patients with musculoskeletal injuries should be carried if these injuries are significant.

CONCLUSION

Muscle and bone injuries are common in EMS. For patients they can be very painful, scary, and in certain cases life-threatening. So whether or not you are trained and equipped to splint a painful, swollen, deformed extremity, you should:

- *Assess* your patient's responsiveness, airway, breathing, and circulation.
- *Intervene* by treating life threats and by protecting the patient from further injury.
- *Reassess* the patient to see if your interventions are working or if the patient's status has changed.

KEY TERMS

You may wish to use this list to review your understanding of key terms introduced in the chapter.

dislocation displacement of a bone in a joint.
fracture a break in a bone.
PSD extremity a painful, swollen, deformed extremity.
sprain stretching or tearing of the ligaments that connect bones.
strain pulling or tearing of muscles.

APPLICATION QUESTIONS

You may wish to use these questions to review your understanding of the chapter. For answers with page references, see Appendix 2.

1. You're managing a 37-year-old male who was hit by a car traveling 45 miles per hour. He has an altered mental status, as well as multiple fractures to his ribs, pelvis, and legs. The ambulance has arrived, and you assist the EMTs with patient packaging. What would be the best way to manage this patient's extremity injuries?
2. As you're managing a patient who has fractured his collarbone (clavicle), your partner is trying to fit the patient's arm with a sling and swathe. This procedure is causing the patient a lot of pain. Do you have any suggestions?

CHAPTER 29 SOFT-TISSUE INJURIES

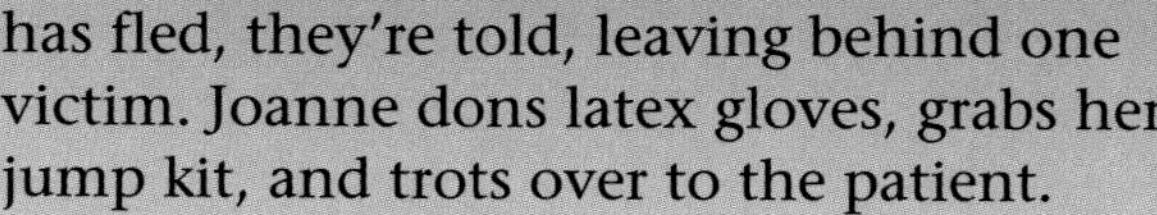

FIRST RESPONSE

Joanne is a community service officer with the police department. She's riding with Officer Marta van Dyke to gain more experience in law enforcement. Their shift begins quietly enough with a few routine traffic stops. It ends with a call to an assault.

When they arrive at the address, dispatch informs them that the scene has been secured by two police officers. The assailant has fled, they're told, leaving behind one victim. Joanne dons latex gloves, grabs her jump kit, and trots over to the patient.

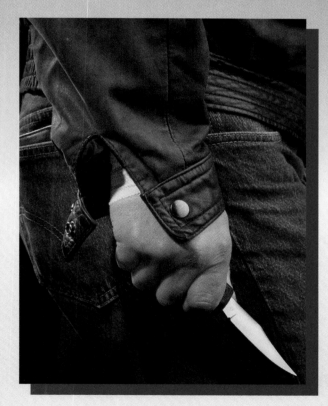

The patient, Mitch, is a male in his early 20s. He's been stabbed with an oversized butcher knife. Joanne catches her breath as she sees that the knife is still embedded in his abdomen. He's fighting to grab it, but the officers on scene pin him down. "Watch out," they tell Joanne and Marta. "This guy bites! He's half whacked on beer and speed and feeling no pain."

While Marta verifies that an ambulance is on the way, Joanne quickly completes an initial assessment. She confirms that Mitch is in shock, but he's too violent to place on oxygen. Joanne's concerned, but she doesn't want her hands near his snapping jaws. Instead, she calls out for bulky dressings to stabilize the knife. "Shouldn't we just pull it out?" asks one of the officers.

"No," Joanne explains, "it could be pressing against a blood vessel. If we take it out, we could cause some serious bleeding." As Joanne stabilizes the blade, Mitch falls silent. Joanne repeats her initial assessment. She finds that Mitch's shock signs have worsened.

The transporting EMTs arrive and rush over. It isn't long before Mitch is loaded into the idling ambulance and on the way to the hospital. Later Joanne learns that he went into cardiac arrest in the ER. He was pronounced dead with the knife still in his abdomen.

LEARNING OBJECTIVES

Soft-tissue injuries are among the most common injuries you'll manage as a First Responder. They range from superficial cuts and scrapes to life-threatening penetrating injuries. Your priorities will include bleeding control, treatment for shock, and preventing further injury and contamination.

By the end of the chapter, you should be able to: [†]

- 5-2.6 Establish the relationship between body substance isolation (BSI) and soft-tissue injuries. (p. 376)
- 5-2.7 State the types of open soft-tissue injuries. (p. 375)
- 5-2.8 Describe the emergency medical care of the patient with a soft-tissue injury. (pp. 376, 384-389)
- 5-2.9 Discuss the emergency medical care considerations for a patient with a penetrating chest injury. (p. 379)
- 5-2.10 State the emergency medical care considerations for a patient with an open wound to the abdomen. (p. 380)
- 5-2.11 Describe the emergency medical care for an impaled object. (p. 379)
- 5-2.12 State the emergency medical care for an amputation. (p. 381)
- 5-2.13 Describe the emergency medical care for burns. (pp. 381-383)
- 5-2.14 List the functions of dressing and bandaging. (p. 376)

* Describe the principals for correctly dressing and bandaging soft-tissue injuries. (pp. 376-378)

RECOGNIZING SOFT-TISSUE INJURIES

WHAT IS SOFT TISSUE?

The term **soft tissue** in this chapter refers primarily to the skin and the underlying fatty layer. The skin itself is a two-layered organ. The **epidermis** is the outer, protective layer. It's made up of cells that are constantly wearing away and regenerating. The

[†]Numbered objectives are from the 1995 U.S. DOT "First Responder: National Standard Curriculum." Asterisks indicate supplemental material.

dermis lies beneath the epidermis. It includes capillaries, nerves, and sweat glands.

Skin is one of the main gatekeepers of the body. It works to keep harmful bacteria out, prevents too much water loss, and helps to regulate body temperature. It also contains sense organs for touch, pressure, temperature, and pain.

Sandwiched between the skin and muscles is a layer of **subcutaneous fat.** This layer anchors skin to muscle. It also insulates the body from cold.

TYPES OF SOFT-TISSUE INJURIES

Soft-tissue injuries include three types of open wounds: **abrasions, lacerations**, and **puncture wounds** (Figures 29-1 and 29-2). An abrasion is an injury to the top layer of skin. It occurs when skin is scraped against a rough surface. Skinned knees and rug burns are common examples. A popular term is "road rash," which is caused by scraping along hardtop after a tumble off a skateboard, bike, or motorcycle. The biggest problem with an abrasion is that it often becomes infected.

A laceration is any break or cut in the skin. It's usually caused by the forceful impact of a sharp object. Lacerations vary in depth. Deep ones can cut through nerves, tendons, and ligaments down to the bone. Bleeding from a laceration may be severe, especially if an artery or vein has been severed.

A puncture wound, or penetrating injury, is caused by a sharp, pointed object thrust through the skin. External bleeding is usually minor. However, internal bleeding and tissue damage may be severe. Infection is very common. An example of a high severity puncture wound is a gunshot or stab wound. Gunshot wounds often have both entry and exit wounds.

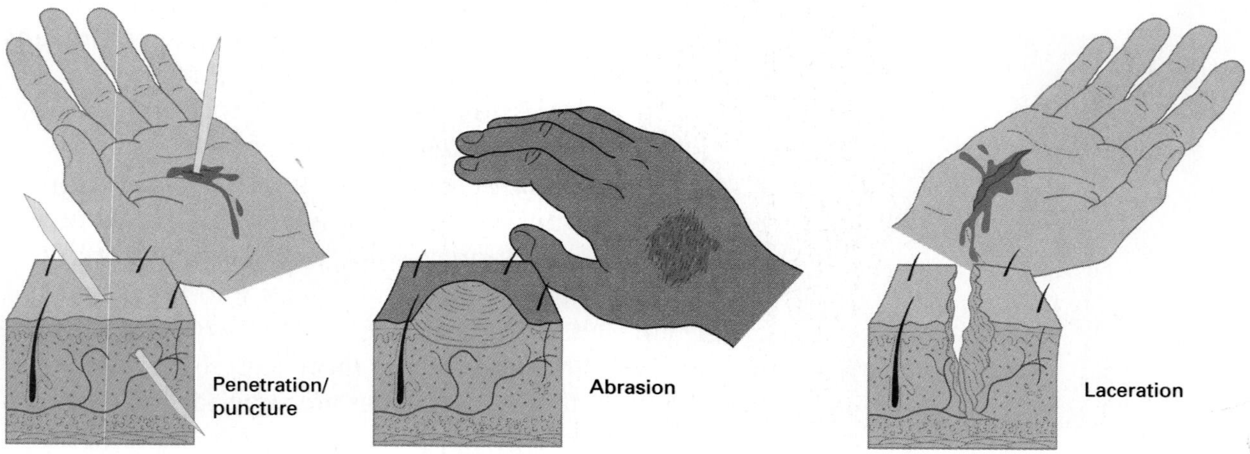

Figure 29-1
Soft-tissue injuries may be classified in three categories.

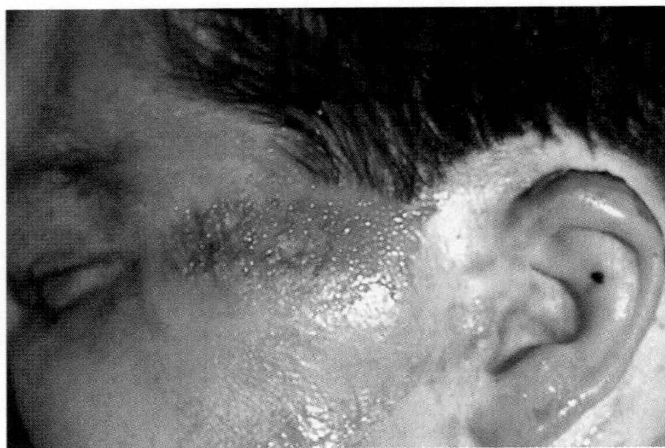

Figure 29-2a
Abrasion.

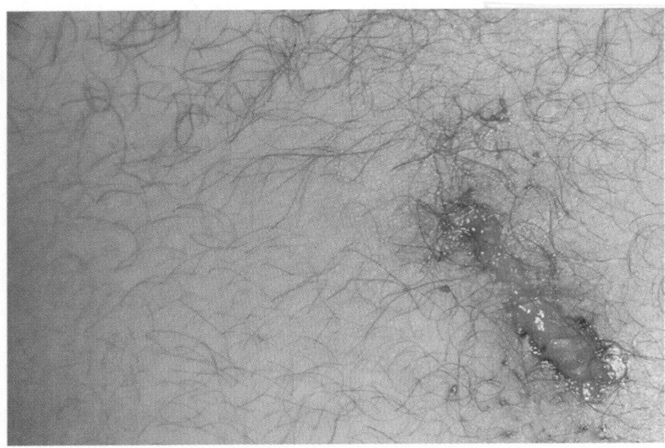

Figure 29-2b
Puncture wound, or penetrating injury.

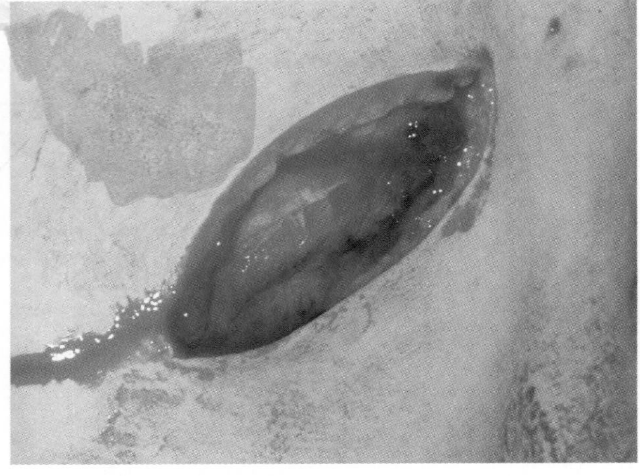

Figure 29-2c
Laceration.

PATIENT MANAGEMENT

GENERAL MANAGEMENT TECHNIQUES

In general, manage any type of soft-tissue injury by following these steps:

1. *Observe BSI precautions.* Lacerations with arterial bleeding may require a full BSI response: gloves, gown, mask, and eye protection.
2. *Control bleeding.* Assess the wound and bleeding point. Intervene by using direct pressure, elevation, and pressure points. Reassess the bleeding to determine if your bleeding control methods are effective.
3. *Apply a sterile dressing, and bandage securely in place.* Don't try to clean out wounds, significant or not. They need to be cleaned by hospital personnel.

DRESSING AND BANDAGING

Dressings and bandages are used to stop bleeding and to protect soft-tissue injuries from further damage, contamination, and infection (Figure 29-3). A **dressing** is any cloth or paper material that is applied directly to a wound. A **bandage** is any material that holds a dressing in place. In a pinch any clean material can be used as either one.

Dressings come in all shapes and sizes—2" × 2" gauze pads to towel-size trauma dressings. A special type of dressing is an **occlusive dressing**, which is made to be airtight. Bandages range from a traditional triangular bandage to gauze and tape to self-adhering bandages like Kerlix® and Kling®. Although they're more expensive, self-adhering bandages are superior to all other types of bandages. They make bandaging quick and easy, even around the bumpiest elbow and knobbiest knee.

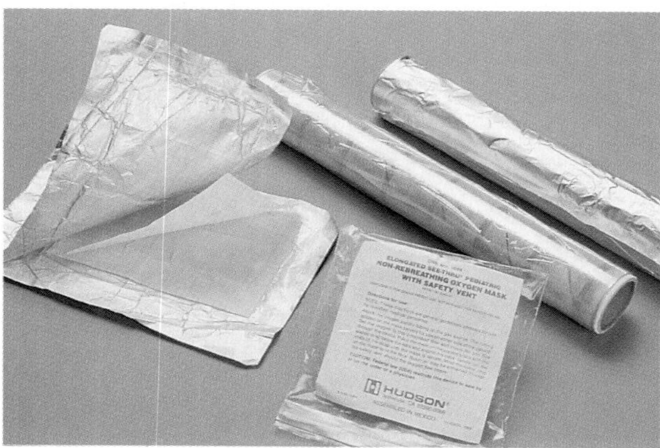

Figure 29-3a
Occlusive dressing.

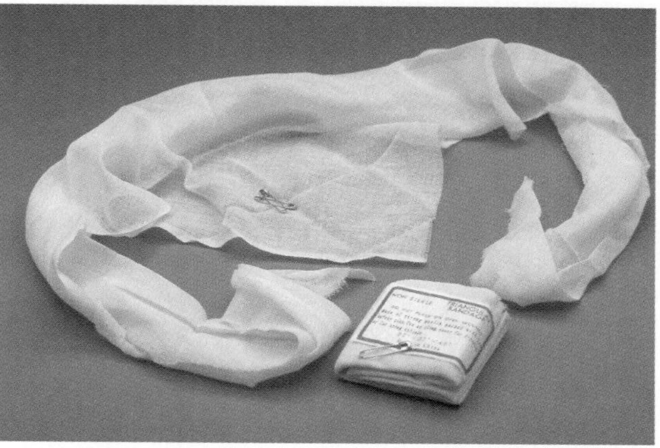

Figure 29-3b
Triangular bandage.

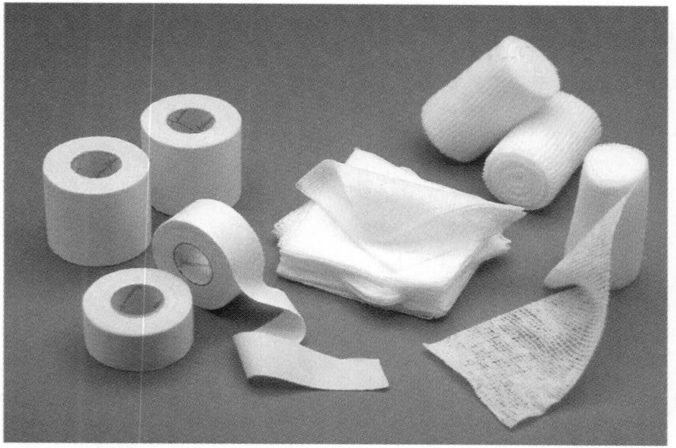

Figure 29-3c
Roller bandage, and adhesive tape.

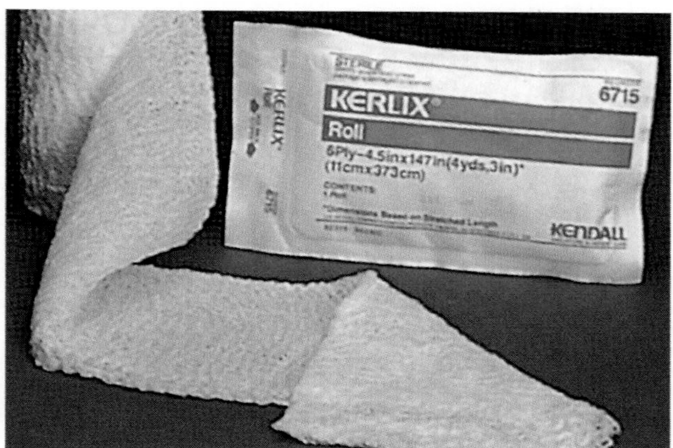

Figure 29-3d
Self-adhering bandages.

Bandages should be snug (Figure 29-4). Apply one a bit more tightly, and it can help to control bleeding. (This is called a "pressure bandage.") However, never cause additional injury and never impair your patient's breathing or circulation. Be careful when wrapping an arm or leg, especially at a joint. Blood vessels and nerves run close to the surface of the skin behind the knee, for example. Too much pressure can cause problems. So assess pulse, sensation, and movement below the wound before and after bandaging. Loosen the bandage on an extremity if the limb appears to be cold, bluish, or numb.

Good bandaging is effective and simple. Does your bandage stop the bleeding and protect the wound without taking a month of Sundays to apply? If it does, then your bandaging method is probably good. And remember, no matter how pretty a bandaging job is, it's all coming off at the hospital.

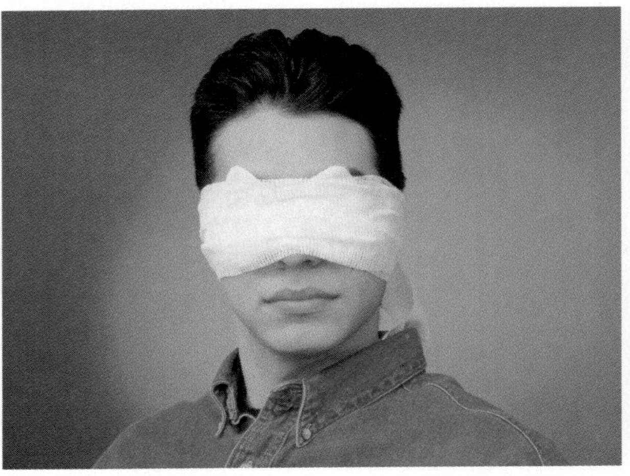

Figure 29-4a
Bandaging for eyes.

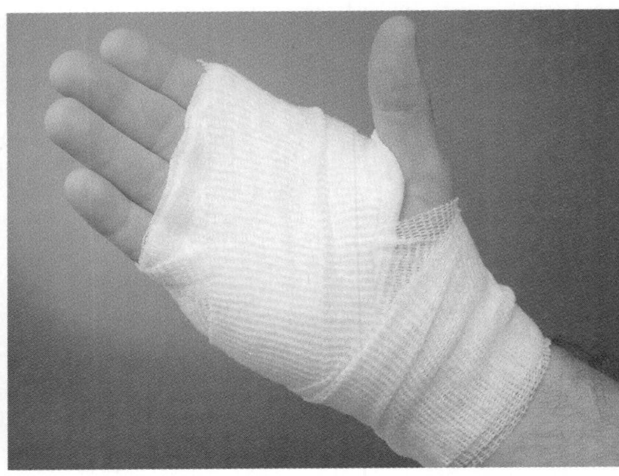

Figure 29-4b
Bandaging for hands.

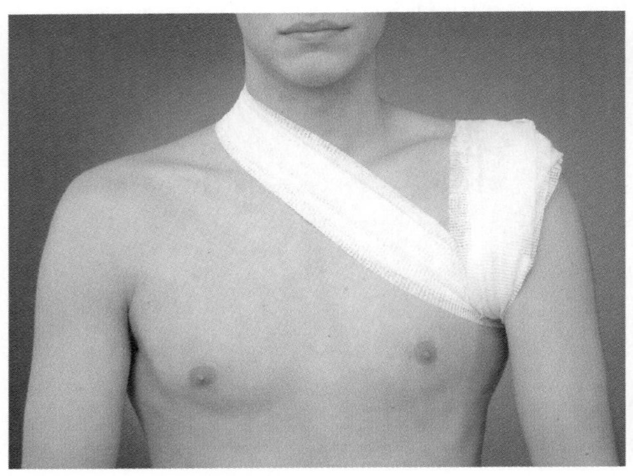

Figure 29-4c
Bandaging for shoulders.

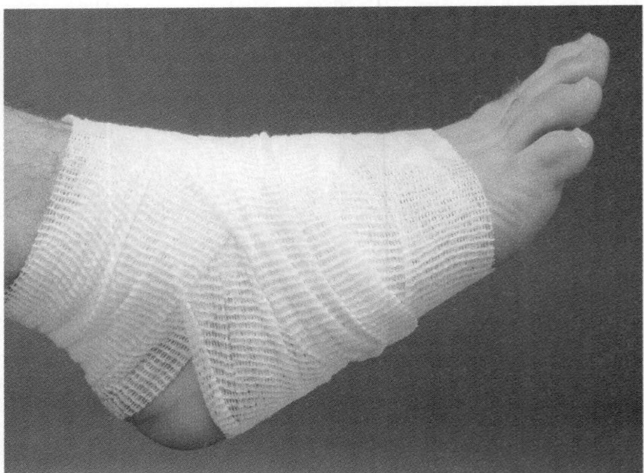

Figure 29-4d
Bandaging for ankles or feet.

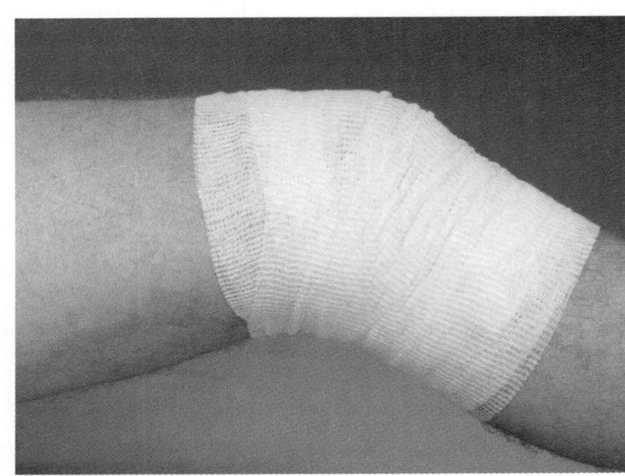

Figure 29-4e
Bandaging for knees.

CARE OF SPECIFIC INJURIES

Neck Injuries

Soft-tissue injuries to the neck can bleed significantly. Deep injuries can allow air in the blood as an *air embolism* or underneath the skin as *subcutaneous emphysema*. Seal all significant soft-tissue injuries to the neck with an occlusive (airtight) dressing.

Chest Injuries

Significant soft-tissue injuries to the chest also can allow air to flow where it shouldn't. This can severely compromise your patient's breathing. Apply an occlusive (airtight) dressing to all open chest wounds (Figure 29-5). Seal the dressing on three sides. The open side will act as a one-way valve. This will allow air out of—but not into—the chest cavity. If no spinal injury is suspected, place the patient in a position of comfort.

Impaled Objects

The general rule is don't remove an impaled object. Leave it in the patient, because it could be controlling bleeding. Manually secure the object. Expose the wound area, and control any bleeding. Then use bulky dressings to stabilize the object in place (Figure 29-6).

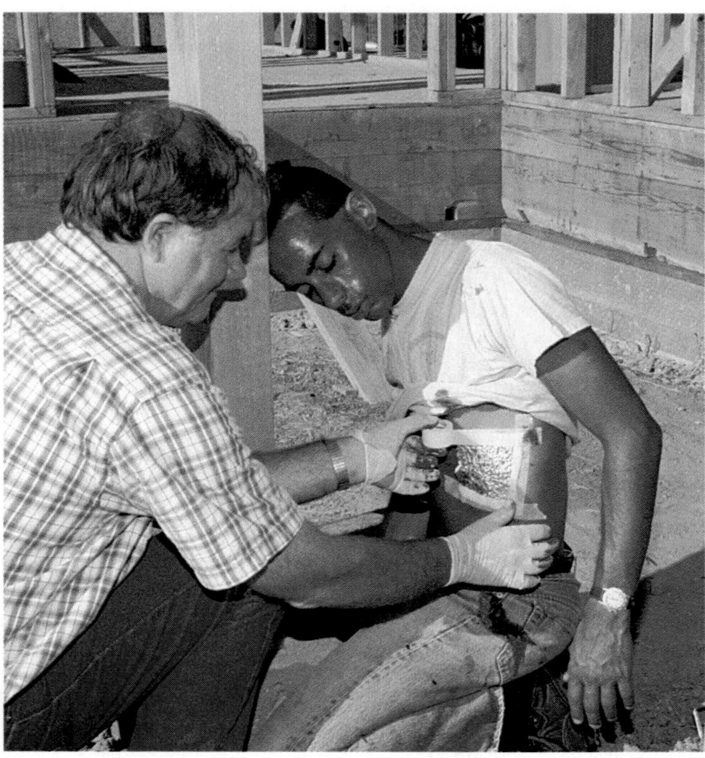

Figure 29-5
Bandaging a chest injury.

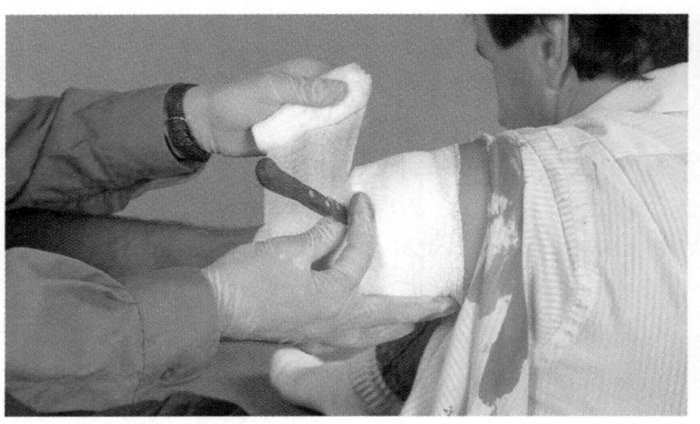

Figure 29-6
Stabilizing an impaled object.

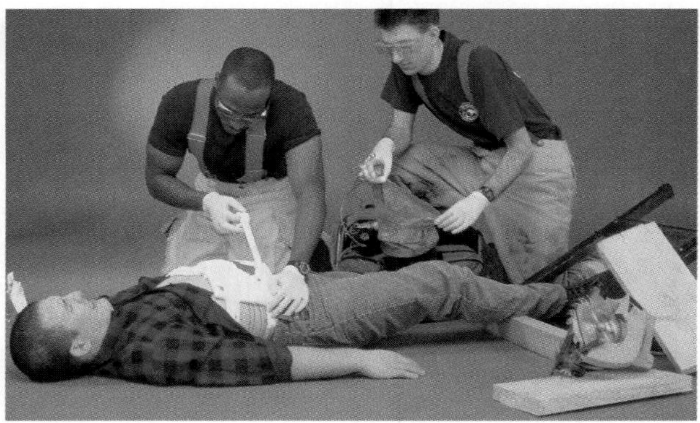

Figure 29-7
Dressing an abdominal evisceration.

There are exceptions to this rule. You may remove an impaled object from your patient's cheek. You may also remove any object that interferes with airway management or CPR. If you do, control bleeding as needed.

Eviscerations

An **evisceration** is an injury that exposes internal organs. An injury to the abdomen that exposes a patient's intestines is the most common type. To care for an evisceration, don't try to replace the exposed organs. Instead, cover them with a thick, moist dressing (Figure 29-7).

Eye Injuries

Blunt or penetrating injuries to the eye are quite common. Handled incorrectly, they can lead to permanent vision loss. Since a person's eyes track *conjugately*, or together as a pair, always cover both eyes. This will help stop the good eye from moving and the injured eye from further injury as it tracks with it. Cover your patient's eyes lightly with a dressing and bandage. Avoid applying any pressure.

Injuries to the Hands and Feet

When bandaging hands or feet, leave the fingertips or toes exposed. This will allow you to monitor circulation in the limb. Remove any jewelry that might pinch off circulation should swelling occur. Make sure that fingertips or toes maintain good color and temperature.

Bandage a hand so that it maintains the natural curl of the fingers. It helps to place a gauze roll in the palm of the patient's hand before bandaging. This is called "bandaging in the position of function."

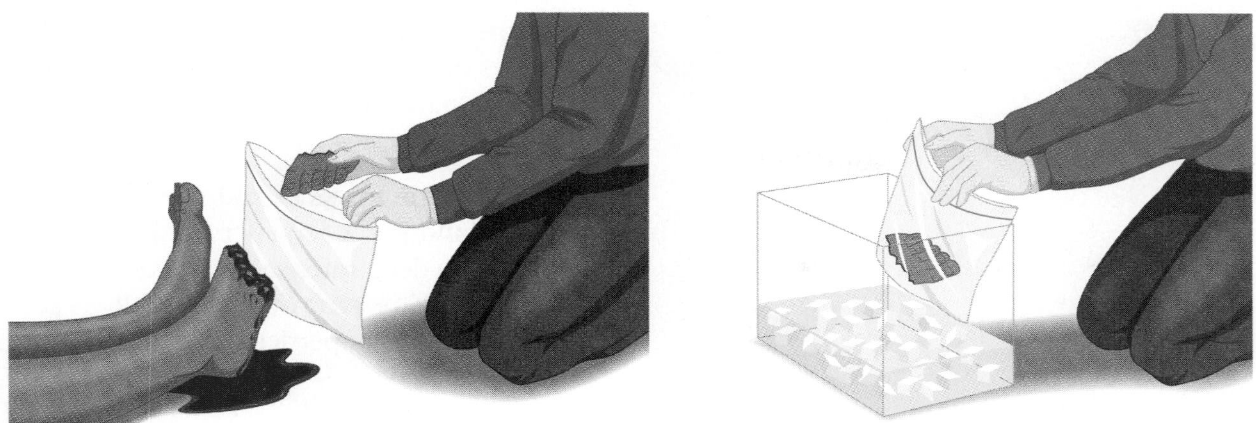

Figure 29-8
Caring for an amputated body part.

Amputations

An **amputation** is a complete separation of tissue, usually involving the extremities. Control bleeding, which may be minimal or severe, as you would any other open injury. If you can, locate the amputated part for possible reimplantation. Keep it dry by putting it in a water-tight plastic bag. Place the sealed bag into a container filled with a mixture of ice and water (Figure 29-8). Don't use ice alone. Never use dry ice. Both will freeze the amputated part.

Burns

Burns are caused by heat, chemicals, radiation, or electricity. They're classified according to depth (Figures 29-9 and 29-10):

Figure 29-9
Three categories of burns.

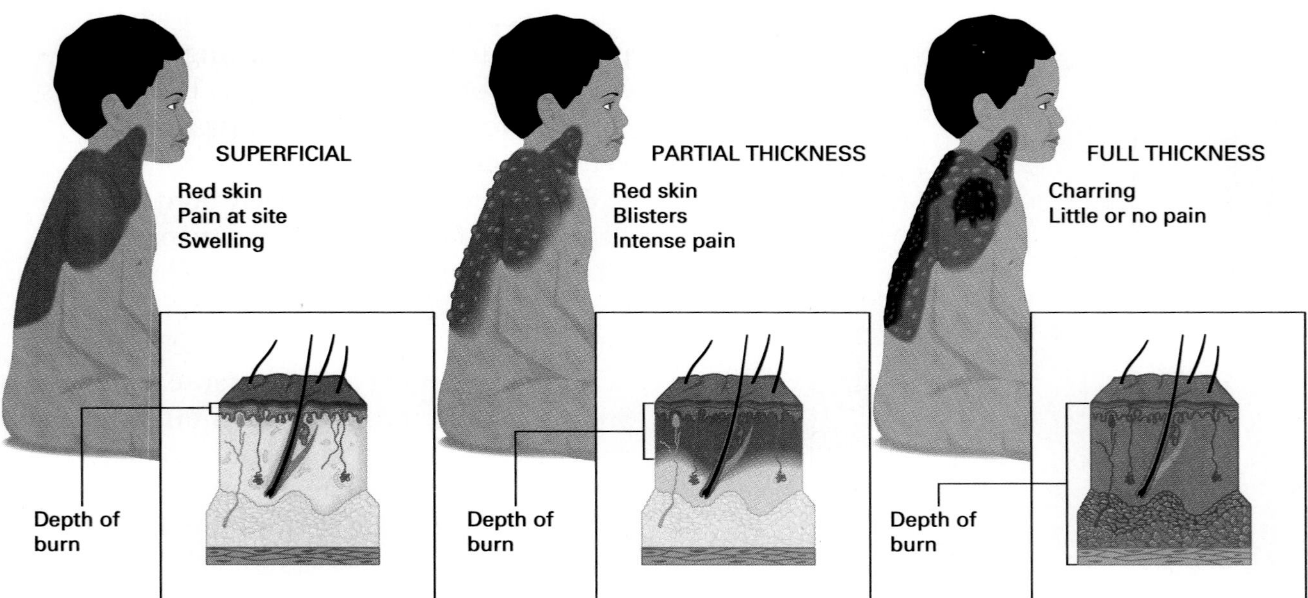

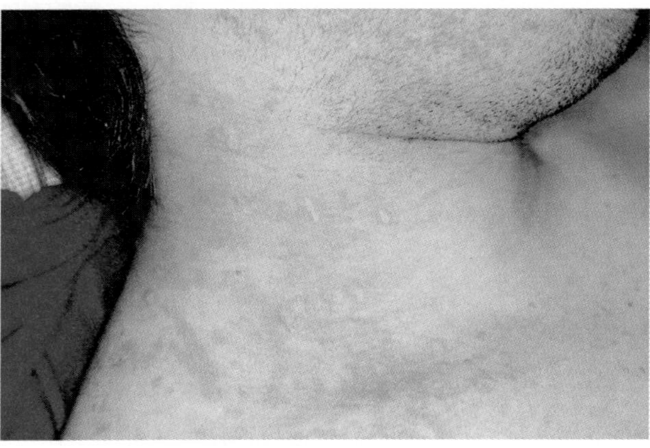

Figure 29-10a
Superficial burn.

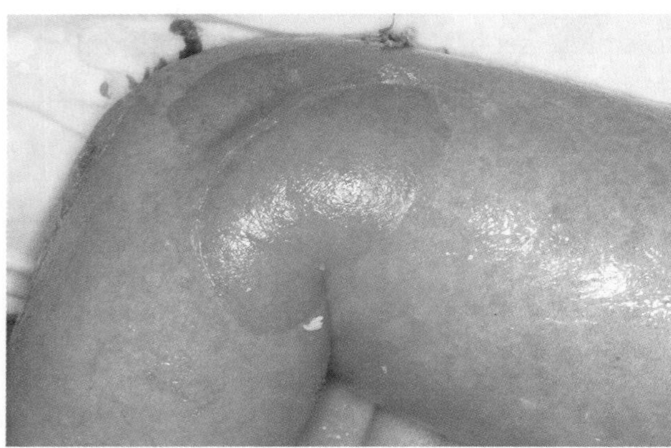

Figure 29-10b
Partial thickness burn.

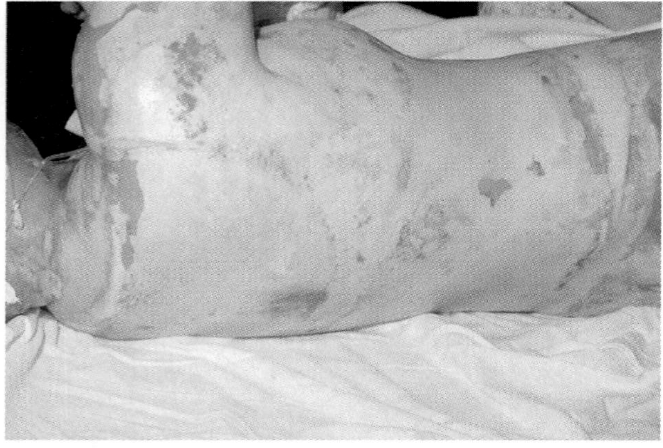

Figure 29-10c
Full thickness burn.

- A **superficial burn**, such as sunburn, involves only the epidermis. It's characterized by pain, reddening of the skin, and swelling.
- A **partial thickness burn** involves the epidermis and part of the dermis. It's characterized by deep intense pain, redness, and blistering. This type of burn usually is accompanied by superficial burns.
- A **full thickness burn** involves both layers of skin. It's characterized by charring and little or no pain. This type of burn usually is accompanied by both superficial and partial thickness burns.

Patient Management Stop the burning. This is your top priority. Flush the area with copious amounts of water until the burns feel cool to your touch. Remove all jewelry from the burned area. Remove all clothing from the burned area. However, if you feel resistance, leave the clothing in place. It may have melted to the skin. Cover the burns with dry, sterile dressings to prevent further contamination (Figure 29-11). Don't break blisters or use any type of ointment or antiseptic on the burns.

Once you've stopped the burning, monitor your patient for any breathing problems. Keep an eye on any patient who is pulled from an enclosed burning structure or burned on the face or chest. These burns can lead to swelling in the airway and severe respiratory distress.

Burns hurt a lot. The severely burned patient may in fact feel more pain than any other type of patient. Handle these patients very gently, taking care not to bump the burned area. Use a calm, empathetic approach.

Significant burns also can cause shock. Shock from burns occurs when fluids in the patient's body move to the burned area. However, this occurs slowly over several hours. One general rule of thumb is that if your burn patient appears to be shocky, look for another injury. Burn patients also

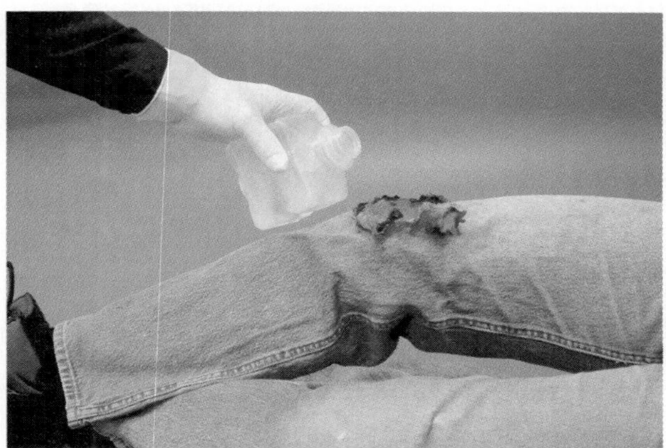

Figure 29-11a
Stop the burning process.

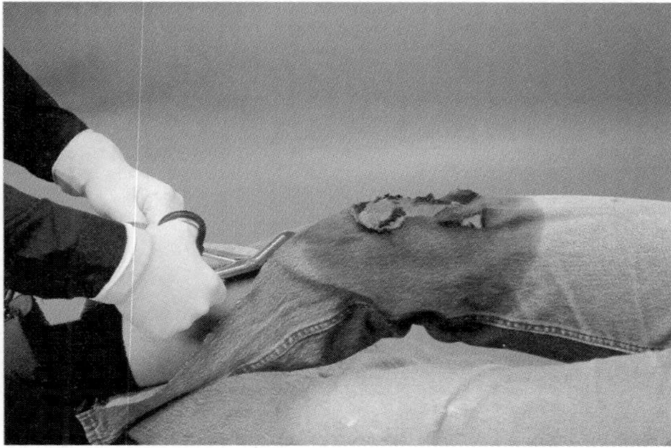

Figure 29-11b
Remove clothing and jewelry.

are at risk for hypothermia. Keep the patient as warm as possible.

Infants and children have a greater surface area relative to the size of their bodies. As a result, they tend to lose even more heat and fluids when burned than adults. This means that pediatric patients become more critical with less of their bodies burned.

Chemical Burns If the patient has been burned by chemicals, be sure to wear gloves and eye protection. Brush off any remaining dry powder from your patient (Figure 29-12). Flush the burns with copious amounts of water. Irrigate the eyes profusely if they've been exposed (Figure 29-13).

Electrical Burns When approaching a victim of electrical burns, make certain that the electricity has been turned off! Note that most of the damage of an electrical burn is hidden. The internal path of the electricity could be riddled with massive tissue and organ injuries. Also, when you examine your patient, look for two electrical burns—an entry wound and an exit wound. Monitor your patient closely. Significant electrical burns can lead to respiratory and cardiac arrest.

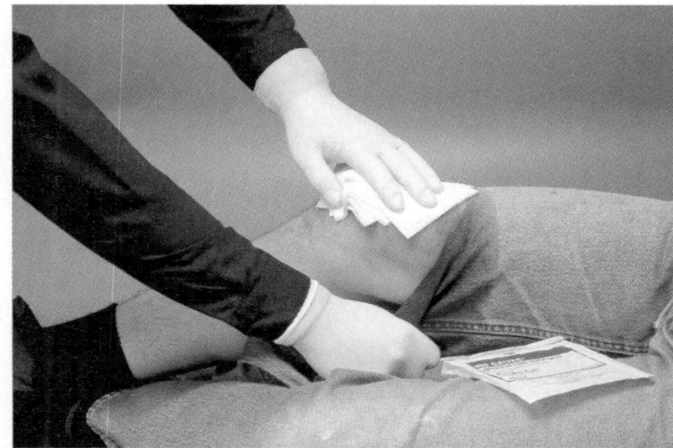

Figure 29-11c
Apply dry sterile dressings.

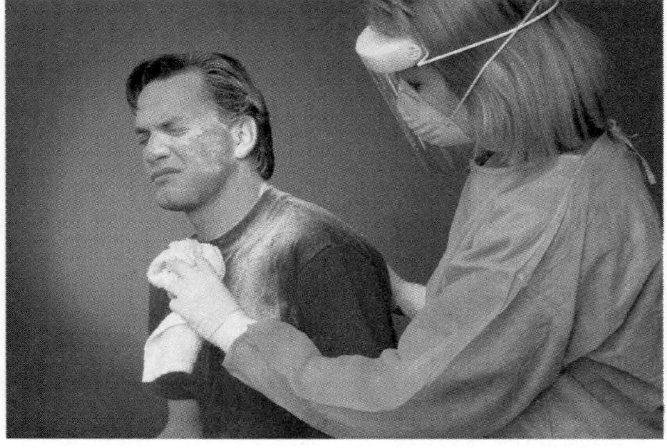

Figure 29-12
Brush off dry chemicals before flushing.

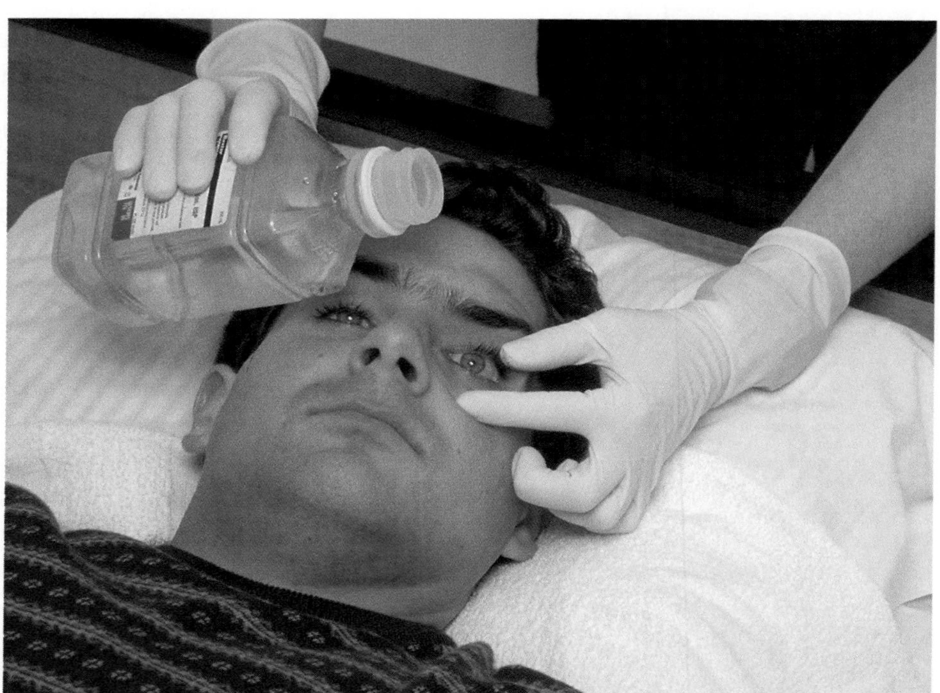

Figure 29-13a
Flush eyes with plenty of water. Method #1.

EMERGENCY CARE PLAN | PATIENTS WITH SOFT-TISSUE INJURIES

PRIORITIES

Your priorities for a patient with soft-tissue injuries are as follows:

- Always take BSI precautions.
- Support the patient's ABCs, paying careful attention to bleeding control and treating for shock.
- After bleeding is controlled, the burn cooled, and so on, gather an accurate physical exam and continue supportive treatment.
- Base emergency care on the patient's airway, breathing, and circulation status, not on how impressive the wounds appear to be. (Bullet holes are not nearly as impressive as large lacerations, but they sure demand close attention.)

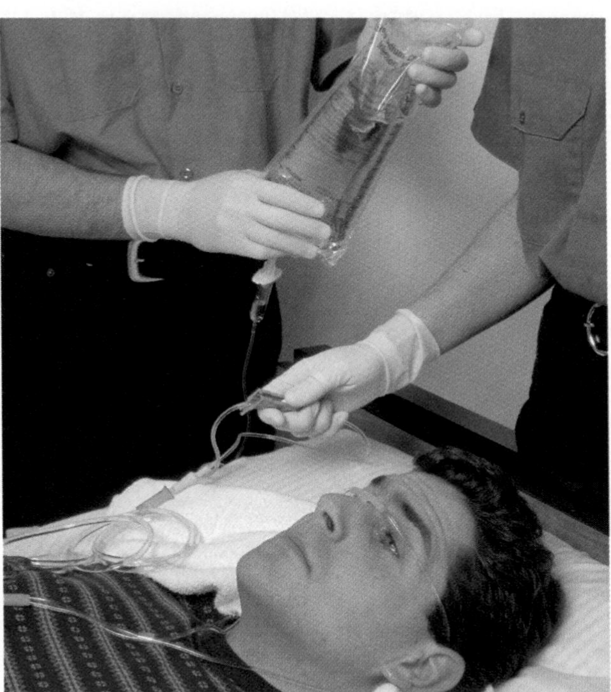

Figure 29-13b
Method #2

PATIENT CARE APPROACH

A soft-tissue injury can be very painful and ugly, without necessarily being a life threat. Be empathetic, no matter the severity of the injury. Don't minimize their pain.

DANGER SIGNS

Danger signs include:

- Burns to the face, throat, chest, genitals, or hands.
- Significant burns to an infant or child.
- Respiratory distress in a patient with burn injuries.
- Significant, uncontrolled external bleeding.
- Signs of shock.
- Puncture wounds to the neck, chest, or abdomen.

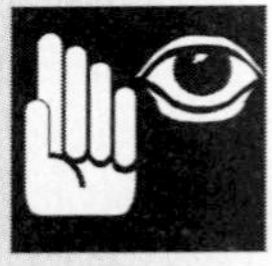

SCENE SIZE-UP

1. **ASSESS SCENE SAFETY.** Is the scene safe to enter? Is there any evidence that a shooting or stabbing has occurred? Are electrical wires down? Is there jagged metal close by? Take BSI precautions now.

2. **DETERMINE MECHANISM OF INJURY.** What caused the soft-tissue injury? Did heat, chemicals, radiation, or electricity cause the burns? What are the dimensions of the knife blade? What's the caliber of the bullet? Activate the EMS system if you haven't done so already.

3. **TRIAGE THE PATIENT.** How many patients are on scene? How serious are their injuries? Do you need to request more resources?

4. **DETERMINE ACCESS AND EXTRICATION NEEDS.** Does the patient need to be removed from a hazardous scene? Do you have enough room to assess and treat the patient?

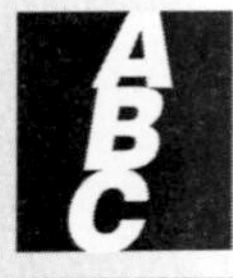

INITIAL ASSESSMENT AND TREATMENT

1. **FORM A GENERAL IMPRESSION.** What is your patient's sex and approximate age? What's your patient's level of distress? Posture? Chief complaint? Do soft-tissue injuries appear to be simple and isolated or are they life-threatening?

   Remember *If you're managing a burn patient whose wounds are still burning, begin flushing them with water immediately. Perform the initial assessment and treatment at the same time.*

2. **CHECK MENTAL STATUS.** Use AVPU (alert, verbal, painful, and unresponsive) to help estimate your patient's mental status. An altered mental status may indicate a head injury or shock. Also check for signs of alcohol intoxication as this can lead to altered mental status. If your patient has an altered mental status, place him or her on high flow oxygen if you're so equipped.

3. ASSESS THE ABCs.

- **Airway.** Is your patient's airway open? Is there any sign of an obstructed airway? If you have to open the airway of a suspected spine-injured patient, use a jaw-thrust maneuver. Watch for blood in the airway if your patient has suffered trauma to the face.

- **Breathing.** Is your patient breathing? If so, is it adequate? Are there signs of respiratory distress? Are there burns to the face or nasal hairs? Is there a sooty cough? Ventilate as necessary. If your patient is in respiratory distress, apply high flow oxygen if you're so equipped.

- **Circulation.** Does your patient have a pulse? Is it fast or slow? Strong or weak? What's the condition of your patient's skin? Is there any uncontrolled bleeding? Control bleeding and treat for shock as indicated.

Remember *An open neck or chest wound is life-threatening. Cover it with an occlusive dressing now.*

4. DETERMINE PRIORITY. Any patient with a soft-tissue injury who shows signs of airway, breathing, or circulation problems is a high priority. So is an infant or child with significant burns and any patient with burns to the face, throat, chest, genitals, or hands. Any patient suffering a significant blunt or penetrating injury to the head, neck, chest, abdomen, or pelvis also is a high priority.

PHYSICAL EXAM AND TREATMENT

1. GATHER A *SAMPLE* HISTORY.

(S)igns and symptoms? Is there obvious pain or bleeding? How much external blood loss? Is there any soot around the face or nasal hairs to indicate possible airway burns? Use DOTS (deformities, open injuries, tenderness, and swelling) to help you identify soft-tissue injuries.

(A)llergies to medications?

(M)edications? If the patient is taking a prescribed blood thinner such as Coumadin®, it may be more difficult to control bleeding.

(P)ertinent past history?

(L)ast oral intake?

(E)vents leading to the injury? How did the injury occur? Gather an accurate history of the event to better understand the mechanism of injury.

2. **PERFORM A HEAD-TO-TOE EXAM.**

- **Head.** Are there any injuries? Is there any bleeding? Is there evidence of burns to the airway? If there's an object impaled in the cheek, remove it.

- **Neck.** Are there any injuries? Is there any bleeding? Recheck the occlusive dressing if you've applied one.

- **Chest.** Are there any injuries? Is there any bleeding? Is there accessory muscle use with breathing? Are there any impaled objects? Recheck the occlusive dressing if you've applied one. Stabilize any impaled objects.

- **Abdomen.** Are there any injuries? Is there any bleeding? Is there an evisceration or an impaled object?

- **Pelvis.** Are there any injuries? Is there any bleeding? Are there signs of incontinence?

- **Extremities.** Are there any injuries? Is there any bleeding?

3. **TAKE VITAL SIGNS.** Pay close attention to signs of shock.

4. **PROVIDE TREATMENT AS NEEDED.** Continue to control bleeding. Dress and bandage any wounds. Cover an evisceration with moist dressings. Cover burns with dry sterile dressings after cooling. Continue to flush any chemical burns. Stabilize impaled objects. Check to make sure the occlusive dressings are properly sealing the wounds. Locate and preserve any amputated parts.

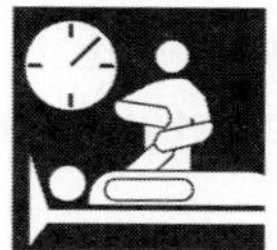

ONGOING ASSESSMENT AND TREATMENT

1. **REPEAT THE INITIAL ASSESSMENT.** All high priority patients should be reassessed every five minutes. Monitor closely for signs of shock.

2. **REPEAT THE PHYSICAL EXAM.** Focus on your patient's chief complaint, injuries, and vital signs. Check your interventions to make sure they're still effective.

3. **PROVIDE REASSURANCE.** Remember that patients with soft-tissue injuries may be experiencing extreme pain as well as the threat of disfigurements or permanent disability. Speak calmly. Maintain constant contact with your patient.

PATIENT HAND-OFF

1. **GIVE A PATIENT REPORT.** The following is an example of a patient report based on the scenario at the beginning of the chapter:

   This is Mitch, an 18-year-old male who was stabbed in the abdomen. The knife is still impaled there. Mitch is awake, but quiet. He initially was quite combative. His airway and breathing are intact. He's showing signs of shock. He appears to have no other injuries. His breath smells of alcohol. We're unable to complete a SAMPLE history on Mitch because he's been too combative. Other law enforcement officers told us that he ingested "speed" in addition to alcohol. Mitch has a rapid pulse and respirations of 28 per minute. We have Mitch restrained, and we're trying to place him on high flow oxygen. We've stabilized the knife with bulky dressings. Over the past few minutes, Mitch has gone from combative to quiet, and we're now unable to find a radial pulse although we do have a carotid pulse.

2. **CONDUCT THE TRANSFER OF CARE.**

3. **ASSIST IN EXTRICATION AND TRANSPORT.**

CONCLUSION

Soft-tissue injuries can range from simple cuts and scrapes to life-threatening eviscerations and amputations. Accurate assessment of your patient's ABCs is critical when determining your patient's priority. Management includes controlling bleeding, treating shock, and preventing further injury and contamination.

KEY TERMS

You may wish to use this list to review your understanding of key terms introduced in the chapter.

abrasions open injuries to the top layer of skin, usually occurring when the skin is scraped against a rough surface.

amputation the complete separation of tissue, usually involving the extremities.

bandage any material used to hold a dressing in place.

dermis layer of skin that lies beneath the epidermis; contains capillaries, nerves, and sweat glands.

dressing any cloth or paper material that is applied directly to a wound.

epidermis the outer, protective layer of skin.

evisceration open injuries that expose internal organs.

full thickness burn burn that extends through all layers of skin.

lacerations breaks or cuts in the skin; usually caused by the forceful impact of a sharp or sharp-edged object.

occlusive dressing an airtight dressing used to seal an open neck or chest wound.

partial thickness burn burn that involves the epidermis and some part of the dermis.

puncture wounds penetrating injuries; usually caused by a sharp, pointed object thrust through the skin.

soft tissue usually refers to the skin and underlying fatty layers.

subcutaneous fat layer of fat beneath the skin; insulates the body and anchors the skin to the muscle layer.

superficial burn burn that involves only the epidermis.

APPLICATION QUESTIONS

You may wish to use these questions to review your understanding of the chapter. For answers with page references, see Appendix 2.

1. You're managing a 27-year-old male who has been shot one time in the chest. Why is it important that you seal his open chest wound during your initial assessment and treatment of life threats, rather than after his head-to-toe exam?

2. You've arrived at the scene of an industrial accident where a worker has lacerated his upper arm. Bleeding is profuse. A coworker is applying direct pressure with little success. What other steps can be taken to help stop the bleeding?

CHAPTER 30 INFANTS AND CHILDREN

FIRST RESPONSE

Paul and Stacey, volunteer firefighters, are dispatched for a seizing child. Stacey is a new First Responder and hasn't had many EMS encounters with kids. "Don't worry," says Paul, "neither have I. We just don't see many sick kids in EMS."

They're met at the front door of the residence by the child's frantic father. They trot to keep up with him as he leads them to a bedroom. The three-year-old's name is Annie. The patient's mother is at her side, anxiously stroking the child's forehead. "We heard her groaning from the other room and found her shaking here on the bed," the distraught mother reports.

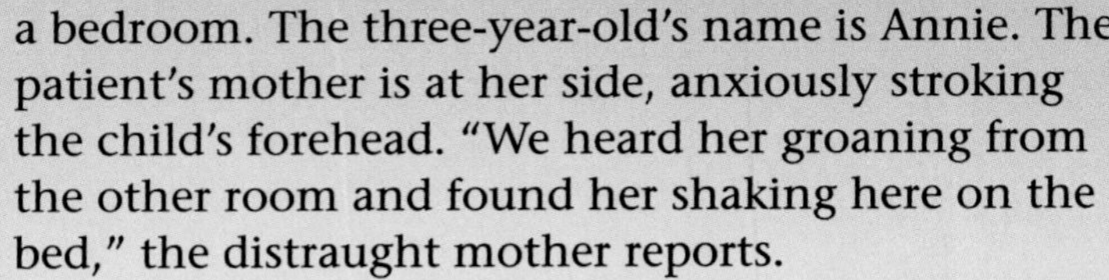

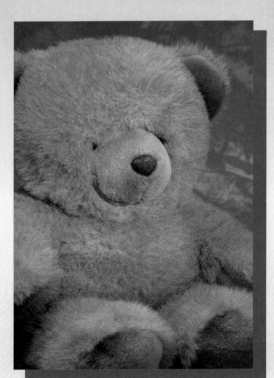

"Well, it looks like the shaking has stopped now. That's a good sign," Stacey tells them as she completes an initial assessment of the child. The patient's ABCs look good, but Annie clearly has an altered mental status. Her eyes are open but blank, and she doesn't respond to her parents. She's also hot to the touch. Stacey directs Paul to place the child on high flow oxygen.

"Has she ever had a seizure before?" Stacey asks.

"No. Is that what it is? A seizure?" asks the father.

"It's possible. Has she been running a fever?" asks Stacey.

"Yes, I was just about to give her some Tylenol," says Annie's mother. As Stacey continues with the physical exam, Paul reassures the parents and tries to keep them calm.

The Paramedics arrive as Annie begins to wake from her sleepy state. As the First Responders turn to leave, Annie's father catches them. "Thanks for helping us. We got pretty scared. I don't know what we'd do if something had happened to Annie. Thanks again."

As Paul and Stacey pull away from the residence, Paul looks at Stacey. "Not bad for a beginner, especially since we had three patients to take care of—the little girl and her mom and dad." Stacey nods. Not bad at all.

LEARNING OBJECTIVES

Caring for ill or injured **pediatric patients** (infants and children) presents a unique challenge for the First Responder. In some cases, assessment and treatment for infants and children aren't the same as for adults. This can make emergency care more complicated. As the First Responder in the scenario at the beginning of the chapter notes, infants and children make up a small percentage of calls in any EMS system. That means you have fewer chances to become comfortable with them. Infants and children also can evoke a very emotional response, one that can make it difficult for rescuers to keep a cool head.

The key to managing pediatric patients is to be prepared. This chapter will help you develop a plan that includes specific communication skills, as well as prioritized assessments and treatment.

***By the end of the chapter, you should be able to:*†**

- 6-2.1 Describe differences in anatomy and physiology of the infant, child, and adult patient. (pp. 394-395)
- 6-2.2 Describe assessment of the infant or child. (pp. 395-397)
- 6-2.3 Indicate various causes of respiratory emergencies in infants and children. (pp. 398-400)
- 6-2.4 Summarize emergency medical care strategies for respiratory distress and respiratory failure/arrest in infants and children. (pp. 398-400)
- 6-2.5 List common causes of seizures in the infant and child patient. (pp. 400-401)
- 6-2.6 Describe management of seizures in the infant and child patient. (pp. 400-401)
- 6-2.7 Discuss emergency medical care of the infant and child trauma patient. (p. 402)
- 6-2.8 Summarize the signs and symptoms of possible child abuse and neglect. (pp. 402-403)
- 6-2.9 Describe the medical-legal responsibilities in suspected child abuse. (p. 403)
- 6-2.10 Recognize need for First Responder debriefing following a difficult infant or child transport. (p. 403)

* Describe an emergency care plan for assessing and treating pediatric patients. (pp. 404-410)

†Numbered objectives are from the 1995 U.S. DOT "First Responder: National Standard Curriculum." Asterisks indicate supplemental material.

DIFFERENCES IN ANATOMY AND PHYSIOLOGY

There are some important differences between pediatric and adult patients. It's critical that you understand how those differences affect your field practice. They include the following (Figure 30-1):

- In infants and children the head is proportionately larger than the rest of the body. So they are much more likely to fall head first and the head is much more likely to be injured.
- In infants and children the body has a faster metabolic engine. Faster heart and breathing rates mean they have a greater need for a constant supply of oxygen. They also suffer more quickly when denied oxygen.
- In infants and children the airway is smaller and more easily blocked by secretions, swelling, and foreign bodies. Unresponsive or short-of-breath infants and children, particularly one- to three-year-olds, should always be checked for a blocked airway.

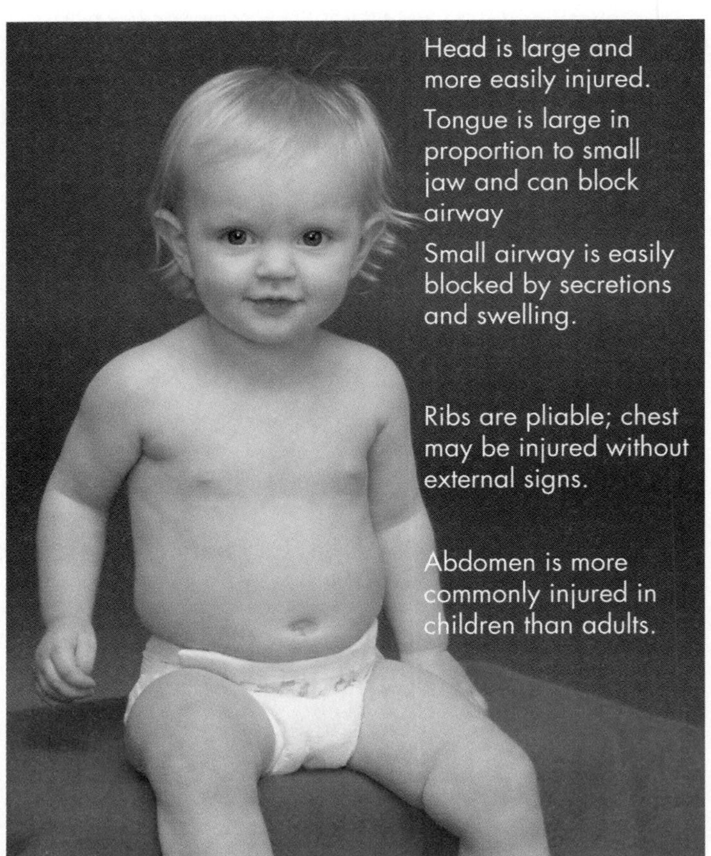
Head is large and more easily injured.
Tongue is large in proportion to small jaw and can block airway
Small airway is easily blocked by secretions and swelling.
Ribs are pliable; chest may be injured without external signs.
Abdomen is more commonly injured in children than adults.

Figure 30-1
Special areas of assessment in the infant and child.

- In infants and children the tongue is relatively large. Therefore, the tongue is more likely to block the airway when they are unresponsive.
- Infants and children have a soft, flexible windpipe (trachea). You can collapse it by hyperextending the head. So open the airway gently and take care to avoid hyperextension.
- The infant tends to breathe mainly through the nose. For this reason, it's important to keep the nose and upper airway clear of secretions.
- Infants and children can compensate for serious breathing and circulation problems for a short time. However, when they've compensated as much as they can, respiratory arrest, shock, and cardiac arrest may follow quickly.
- Infants and children can become cold much faster. This occurs because they have less mature temperature control mechanisms and because they have more surface area than adults relative to their size. Remember to protect them from heat loss.

PATIENT CARE APPROACH

Your approach to infants and children should vary according to the patient's age. At various stages of mental and emotional development, they will react differently to illness, injuries, and to strangers such as you. Consider the following developmental differences.

INFANTS

Age birth to one year, infants are physically dependent on their parents for all their needs. They usually begin to crawl at about six months of age and walk at about one year. They develop fear of strangers at about six months. Infants react mainly to physical cues in the environment, such as hot, cold, pressure, pain, and so on. They are pre-verbal (can't speak), but they do understand vocal tones.

A good approach is to allow a parent to hold the infant while you examine him or her. Avoid touching an infant with cold hands. Use a gentle, reassuring tone when talking to the infant.

TODDLERS

Age one to three years, toddlers are at the most dangerous stage of all. They're amazingly mobile with absolutely no common sense. Toddlers also make huge physical, language, and emotional leaps. They graduate from babbling to talking and have an opinion on almost everything. While they may act tough, they're quite fearful of separation from their parents. They may cry, scream, and push you away.

A good approach is to assess the toddler while he or she is on a parent's lap. Talk to the child using simple sentences. The two- or three-year-old may be able to tell you where he or she hurts. Be patient and flexible. Complete your assessments as opportunities arise, such as when the child is distracted by something. Try to provide a familiar object or toy that the child can take to the hospital. Be prepared to restrain this age group. They're very likely to try to squirm out of spinal immobilization.

PRESCHOOLERS

Age three to five years, preschoolers have excellent language skills. They're able to understand simple explanations, but often will take you quite literally. They're out of diapers and exploring their world with imaginative play. Children at this age often have unreasonable fears about their injury or illness. For example, a five-year-old with a broken arm may think the arm will be crooked or deformed forever.

A good approach is to provide the preschooler with simple explanations. Choose your words carefully, and keep your information and instructions short and simple. Be honest when you answer a question or address a concern. Keep the preschooler's parents nearby.

SCHOOL AGE

Age six to 12, school-age children are able to understand clear explanations of their illness or injury. They're quite concerned about being disfigured for life. This age group is beginning to develop strong ties to peer groups. When they're ill or injured in the presence of their peer group, they're often extremely embarrassed. School-age children are independent thinkers who want to feel in control of their bodies and their environment. However, when they're ill or injured, they may revert to baby talk and other immature behaviors.

A good approach is to include them in assessment and treatment. Explain every step of your care. Give them choices within limits, such as how they wish to be positioned and so on. Even though they appear to be listening attentively, confirm that they really understand what you're saying. Ignore immature behaviors. Encourage behavior that is age appropriate. If necessary, keep these patients safe from their peer group by sending onlookers away.

ADOLESCENTS

Age 13 to 18 years, adolescents have a heightened concern about their bodies and body image. They fear loss of control, and they may overreact to pain or injury. Though many are sexually active, they're still quite modest about their bodies. Older adolescents may appear to be adults physically. Emotionally they are not. They have wide mood swings, and they'll often revert to immature behaviors when ill or injured.

A good approach is to respect your patient's concerns about modesty. Allow him or her to make some decisions about the medical care you're providing. Explain your assessment and treatment. Ignore immature behaviors. Reassure your patient, and talk to him or her just as you would talk to an adult.

THE PATIENT'S PARENTS

When caring for the pediatric patient, you also must care for the patient's parents. If the patient is experiencing pain or discomfort, expect that the parents have an equal amount of anxiety. You'll find that parents display a wide range of emotions. The most common is fear. They also feel a loss of control because they have to turn over care of their infant or child to you.

There are several ways to effectively respond to parents in pediatric emergencies. Remain calm and appear in control of the situation. Parents want to know that you're competent and doing everything you can. Try to involve the parents in the care of the infant or child. Put them to work. It'll make them feel as if they're doing something, which will help to reduce their anxiety. Reassure parents, and honestly answer their questions. Don't lie to them or to the child. If parents are upset and agitated, your patient will respond by becoming more upset and agitated. So keep the parents calm. You'll have a much more cooperative patient by doing so.

COMMON INFANT AND CHILD EMERGENCIES

What follows are some notes and comments about specific childhood illness and injuries. Following this will be the "Emergency Care Plan" for all pediatric patients.

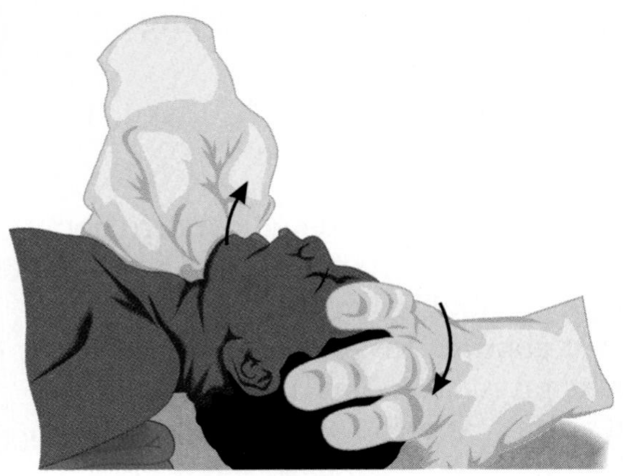

Figure 30-2a
Head-tilt/chin-lift maneuver.

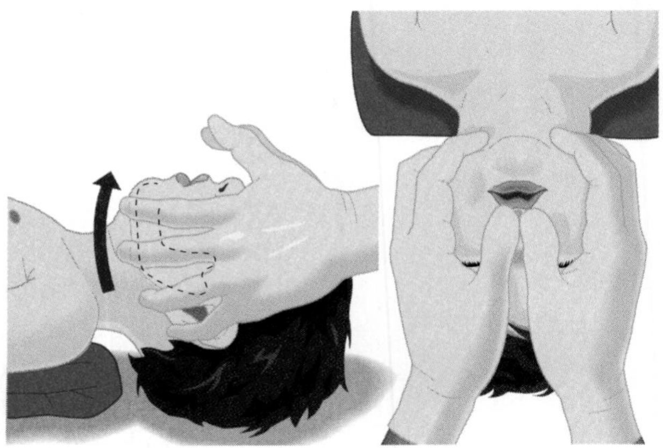

Figure 30-2b
Jaw-thrust maneuver.

AIRWAY OBSTRUCTION

As already stated, the tongue is the top cause of airway obstruction in infants and children. Use the head-tilt/chin-lift or jaw-thrust maneuver to open the airway of an unresponsive patient (Figure 30-2).

Suspect foreign body airway obstruction in all short-of-breath or unresponsive patients. Infants and children are particularly prone to swallow or choke on food, such as carrots, hot dogs, and hard candies. One- to three-year-olds in particular will place toys or small objects in their mouths.

Infants and children with a partial airway obstruction usually are alert and sitting up. They may have stridor or noisy breathing. They may use accessory muscles (retractions) to help them breathe. When they have a complete airway obstruction, they won't cry or make any other vocalizations. They'll be cyanotic, and they'll soon be unresponsive.

Refer back to Chapter 10 for a complete review of how to treat partial and complete airway obstructions.

OTHER RESPIRATORY EMERGENCIES

Illnesses involving the respiratory system are quite common in infants and children. Of the truly critical pediatric patients you'll see in your career, many will have a respiratory emergency. Signs and symptoms include (Figure 30-3):

- Rapid breathing. Respiratory rates may be higher than 60 per minute in infants, and over 30 or 40 per minute in children.

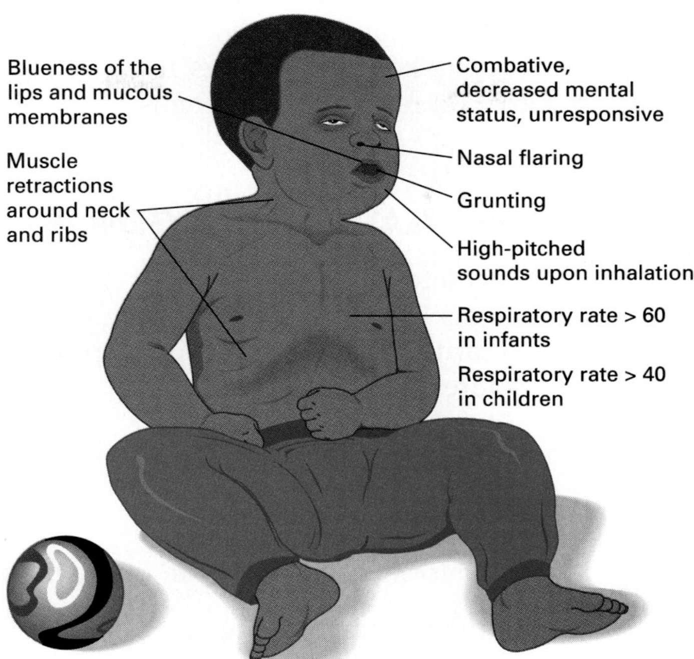

Figure 30-3
Signs and symptoms of respiratory distress.

- Nasal flaring. This helps infants and children inhale more air.
- Use of accessory muscles with breathing (retractions). You may see the patient use the muscles between the ribs, in the neck, and in the abdomen to assist with the work of breathing.
- Stridor.
- Seesaw breathing.
- Cyanosis.
- Altered mental status. The patient may be combative, lethargic, or even unresponsive.
- Grunting. (This helps to increase oxygenation of the patient's blood during exhalation.)

If untreated, respiratory distress can lead to respiratory failure. This usually occurs because the patient becomes too tired to continue the fight to breathe. Signs and symptoms of respiratory failure include an unusually slow respiratory rate (20 or less per minute in an infant and 10 or less per minute in a child). You'll also see limp muscle tone, altered mental status, a slow heart rate (below 100 in an infant and below 60 in a child), and cyanosis. Untreated breathing problems are the top cause of cardiac arrest in infants and children.

Refer back to Chapters 10 and 18 for a complete review of how to treat respiratory problems.

CIRCULATORY EMERGENCIES

Circulatory failure may result if a patient's respiratory or trauma emergency isn't treated or stabilized. Circulatory failure can lead to cardiac arrest. Signs and symptoms of the onset of circulatory failure include:

- Increased pulse rate.
- Poor skin condition.
- Abnormal capillary refill (more than two seconds).
- Mental status changes.

Manage the circulatory system by treating the patient for shock and, in the worst case, with CPR. Refer back to Chapters 11 and 12 for a complete review of how to treat cardiac arrest, shock, and bleeding.

ALTERED MENTAL STATUS

Rely on parents to help you identify normal vs. abnormal mental status in their infant or child. Those patients who are unusually quiet, sleepy, lethargic, or unresponsive need an immediate assessment.

A variety of conditions cause altered mental status. They include low blood sugar, poisoning, infection, head trauma, low oxygen levels, and seizures. Seizures in infants and children are most commonly caused by fever, specifically a rapid rise in temperature. These are called "febrile" seizures. Consider all seizures to be potentially life threatening.

By the time you arrive on scene, the seizure will probably be over. Assess the patient's ABCs, and check for injuries. If the patient has never had a seizure before, the parents will probably be very alarmed. Calm them. Then have them answer the following questions:

- Has the patient been running a fever?

- Has the patient had seizures in the past?
- If so, did today's episode appear to be like past seizures?
- Is the patient taking seizure medication?
- Is it possible that the patient may have ingested any other medications or substances?

Briefly, care of the pediatric patient with altered mental status is as follows. If the patient is seizing, protect him or her from further injury. Maintain an open airway, and ventilate if necessary. Provide oxygen if you're equipped to do so. If there are no signs of spinal injury, place the patient in the recovery position and keep suction equipment nearby. Have parents stay to help.

Refer back to Chapter 19 for a complete review of how to treat altered mental status.

SUDDEN INFANT DEATH SYNDROME (SIDS)

Sudden infant death syndrome, or **SIDS**, is defined as the sudden, unexplained death of an otherwise normal and healthy infant. It's a common cause of death in infants between the age of one week and one year. Though we know that more boys die of SIDS than girls and that the baby is most often discovered in the early morning, we know little else. There appears to be nothing yet that predicts SIDS or prevents it.

If you are called to a possible SIDS infant, assess the patient. Initiate CPR unless the baby is stiff (in *rigor mortis*). Trying to resuscitate an infant who is obviously dead offers false hope to the parents. They already feel overwhelming grief, remorse, and guilt. So in this situation, it's more important to support them. Follow all local protocols.

Be careful not to make any comments that might suggest blame to the parents. For example, don't tell the parents what they should or should not have done before you arrived. Acknowledge their feelings. Answer their questions truthfully. Be supportive as they experience their loss. Don't leave them alone. Request additional help from EMS as needed to manage the scene and to support the parents.

> **Remember** *In rare instances parents or family members experiencing the death of an infant may become violent. Make sure that the scene remains safe for all rescuers and family members.*

TRAUMA

Injuries due to trauma are the leading cause of death in infants and children in the U.S. today. Blunt injuries are a major cause of those deaths. As you're already aware, the anatomy of infants and children makes them prone to specific types of injuries. Their larger heads make them more prone to head injuries. Their soft flexible ribs translate to fewer rib fractures but more internal injuries. These patients also tend to have protruding abdomens. So abdominal injuries are more common and often a source of hidden internal injury.

Infants and children typically have different injury patterns than adults. Mechanisms of injury and injury patterns include the following:

- *Motor-vehicle crashes* — Infants and children who are not properly restrained typically suffer head and neck injuries. Children restrained with only a lap belt often suffer lower spine and abdominal injuries.
- *Bicycle or pedestrian crashes* — Children struck while on foot or riding a bicycle tend to suffer head, abdominal, and extremity injuries.
- *Falls*—Children commonly incur head injuries when they fall from a significant height.

Refer back to Chapters 26 through 29 for a complete review of how to treat trauma patients.

CHILD ABUSE AND NEGLECT

Child abuse and neglect are complex and disturbing problems seen in all areas of our society. **Abuse** may be defined as improper or excessive action that injures or causes harm. Child abuse includes emotional, physical, or sexual injury to an infant or child. **Neglect** may be defined as giving insufficient attention or respect to someone who has a claim to them. It refers to the failure of those responsible to provide for the nutritional, emotional, and physical needs of an infant or child. Physical child abuse and neglect are the two forms First Responders are most likely to see.

Signs and symptoms of child abuse may include:

- Multiple bruises in various stages of healing.
- Injury inconsistent with the mechanism described.
- Unusual injury patterns such as cigarette burns, scalding burns with glove or dip patterns, whip marks, or hand prints on the child's skin.

- Repeated calls to the same address.
- Parents who seem unconcerned about their child's injuries.
- Conflicting stories among caregivers.
- A child who appears to be fearful when asked how the injury occurred.
- **Shaken baby syndrome**. This condition occurs when a caregiver picks up an infant or child and shakes him or her violently. The altered mental status, seizure activity, and shock that can result may indicate internal organ or nervous system injury. (Note that some abusive behaviors leave no external evidence of trauma.)

Signs and symptoms of child neglect may include the following:

- No adult supervision.
- An unsafe living environment.
- Malnourishment in an infant or child.
- Untreated chronic illnesses such as asthma.
- Untreated cuts, bruises, and other injuries.

Child abuse and neglect may lead you to feel many emotions—sadness at the child's condition, rage at the abuser, and so on. However, remember that your top priority is to take care of the patient. Focus on the child's needs. The facts surrounding the injury can be sorted out after the patient is transported to an appropriate facility. Confronting the suspected abuser will only escalate the anxiety and tensions at the scene.

After providing medical care, your top priority is to make sure the child is removed from the abusive environment. *Never attempt to remove a child against a parent's will. This is a job for law enforcement only.*

It's important to follow your local protocols for reporting possible child abuse or neglect. Never hesitate to report your suspicions to the proper authorities. Report what you see and hear, and try to remain objective.

Remember *Calls involving serious injury or death of an infant or child have a way of affecting EMS rescuers very deeply. A critical incident stress debriefing (CISD) after the event can help. If your EMS system offers this service, make sure you take advantage of it.*

EMERGENCY CARE PLAN | INFANTS AND CHILDREN

■ PRIORITIES

The First Responder's priorities when managing infants and children are as follows:

- Calm and reassure both the patient and his or her parents.
- Recognize and treat life threats as early as possible in the call.
- Perform a physical exam that takes into account the patient's physical, emotional, and mental levels of development.

■ PATIENT CARE APPROACH

Your approach to an infant or child will vary depending on the patient's age. Generally, manage infants and children by taking a calm, gentle approach. Talk simply and honestly. Never lie about painful procedures. Focus the patient on positive, successful behaviors. Ease the child's fears with rewards or a favorite toy. Restrain the patient if he or she is too young or frightened to cooperate. Involve and inform the parents.

■ DANGER SIGNS

Don't let sick infants and children fool you. They have a remarkable ability to hide life-threatening breathing and circulation problems. Eventually the child will present with an altered mental status as well as severe problems with the ABCs. Watch for early signs of respiratory distress and shock.

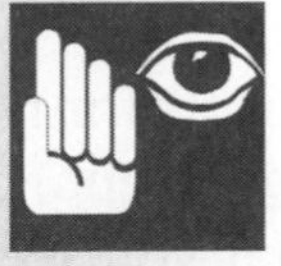

SCENE SIZE-UP

1. **ASSESS SCENE SAFETY.** Is the scene safe to enter? Are there any hazards? Take all BSI precautions now.

2. **DETERMINE MECHANISM OF INJURY OR NATURE OF ILLNESS.** Is this a sudden traumatic event? Is this a chronic or sudden illness? Pay close attention to whether or not the

child was restrained properly before the car crash, wearing a helmet during the bicycle fall, and so on. Activate the EMS system if you haven't already done so.

3. **TRIAGE THE PATIENT.** As you approach the infant or child, consider how ill or injured he or she appears to be. Do you need to call EMS for additional help?

4. **DETERMINE ACCESS AND EXTRICATION NEEDS.** Kids are quite portable. It's often easier to move the patient rather than rearrange furniture. Often the problem with managing a pediatric patient, particularly one who requires resuscitation, is not the small size of the work space but the small size of the child. Take a moment to organize other rescuers so that all tasks are completed in an efficient manner.

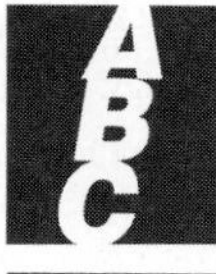

INITIAL ASSESSMENT AND TREATMENT

1. **FORM A GENERAL IMPRESSION.** What is your patient's sex and approximate age? What's your patient's chief complaint? Does your patient appear to be sick? What is the level of distress? The posture? Is the patient active, wiggling, crying? Does he or she appear to be healthy and acting in an age-appropriate way? Or does the patient appear to be listless, quiet, with poor muscle tone?

2. **CHECK MENTAL STATUS.** Is the infant or child interacting normally with the surrounding environment? Does your patient appear to recognize his or her parents? (That's an important indicator of level of responsiveness.) Is the patient awake and responding appropriately? Does the patient respond to your questions and verbal commands? Does your patient appear to be drowsy or lethargic?

   A general rule of thumb for pre-verbal patients is: "A distractible child is a perfusing child." In other words, if your patient reaches for a dangling penlight or set of keys, his or her brain is most likely getting enough oxygen. Depend on parents to give you an accurate assessment of the infant or child's mental status.

If your patient has an altered mental status, apply high flow oxygen by mask if you are so equipped. Position the patient as indicated by his or her level of responsiveness.

3. ASSESS THE ABCs.

- **Airway.** Is the airway open and clear? Is there any food, candy, or other foreign body in the patient's airway? Is there stridor? If necessary, open the airway and clear it of any foreign body obstructions. Be careful to avoid hyperextension. Use the jaw-thrust maneuver if there is any suspicion of spine injury. Avoid agitating a patient who is experiencing a partial obstruction of the airway.
- **Breathing**. Is the patient's rate and quality of breathing adequate? Are there any signs of respiratory distress such as nasal flaring, noisy breathing, grunting, use of accessory muscles, seesaw breathing? If the patient is having difficulty breathing, does he or she appear to be unusually tired? Administer high flow oxygen if you're so equipped. Ventilate if necessary.
- **Circulation**. Does your patient have a pulse? If so, is it normal? Is it weak and rapid? What's your patient's skin color and condition? Is capillary refill normal or delayed? Stop any major bleeding. If necessary, treat for shock or initiate CPR.

4. DETERMINE PRIORITY. If there is altered mental status or an airway, breathing, or circulation problem, consider your patient a high priority. Patients who appear to be uninjured but who have experienced a significant mechanism of injury are also high-priority patients.

PHYSICAL EXAM AND TREATMENT

1. GATHER A *SAMPLE* HISTORY.

(S)igns and symptoms? Remember that infants and children can hide signs of injury, and that they tend to suffer more internal injuries than broken bones. Rely on the parents to help gather the information you need.

(A)llergies to medications?

(M)edications?

(P)ertinent past history? Has the patient ever had this kind of episode in the past? When was the last time? What was done to treat the patient then?

(L)ast oral intake? Is there any possibility of poison ingestion?

(E)vents leading to the injury or illness?

2. **PERFORM A HEAD-TO-TOE EXAM**. Look and feel for any injuries to the head, neck, chest, abdomen, pelvis, and extremities. Use DOTS (deformities, open injuries, tenderness, and swelling) to help you locate any injuries. Observe patients under two years of age for signs of disability. That is, look to see if they are avoiding the use of a limb, for example, since they can't speak to tell you where they have pain. It also may help to perform a "toe-to-head" exam, starting at the patient's feet rather than the head (Figure 30-4). This will allow the patient to get used to your touch. Make sure you warm your hands. Always try to examine very young patients in their parent's arms. They are much more likely to stay still, and they'll be less frightened.

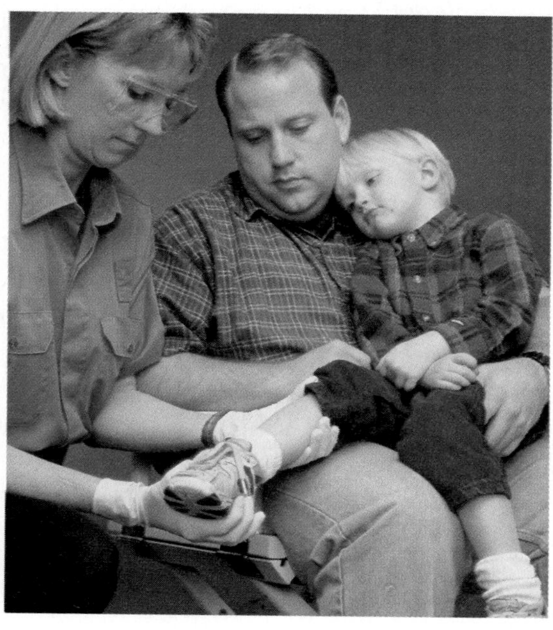

Figure 30-4
A toe-to-head exam may help the pediatric patient to be less afraid of you.

3. **TAKE VITAL SIGNS.** Refer to tables in Chapter 4 for normal rates in the infant and child. In general, pediatric respiratory and pulse rates are higher than adult rates. Blood pressure is lower. Capillary refill should be less than two seconds.

   Of all patient populations, infants and children benefit least from a blood pressure check. It's estimated that they would need to lose nearly half of their blood volume before there would be a significant drop in blood pressure. This makes blood pressure drops due to shock a very late sign, certainly not one you would wait to see before providing treatment. Depend on the other vital signs to help you assess your pediatric patient's circulation.

   Remember *To assess pulse in an infant or young child, use the brachial or femoral arterial pulse points.*

4. **PROVIDE TREATMENT AS NEEDED.** Treat for soft-tissue injuries, bandage and splint, and so on at this time.

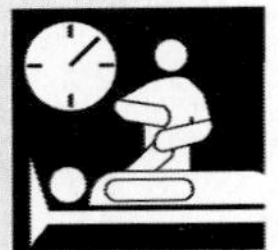

ONGOING ASSESSMENT AND TREATMENT

1. **REPEAT THE INITIAL ASSESSMENT.** Focus on changes in mental status, airway, breathing, and circulation. Find out if life threats and level of distress are getting better, staying the same, or getting worse.

2. **REPEAT THE PHYSICAL EXAM.** Reassess the patient's chief complaint, and check for changes in the signs and symptoms related to the chief complaint. Reassess vital signs. Recheck all interventions to make sure that they're still effective.

3. **PROVIDE REASSURANCE.** Remember that you'll usually have multiple patients to manage—the infant or child as well as the parents or other caregivers.

PATIENT HAND-OFF

1. **GIVE A PATIENT REPORT.** The following is an example of a patient report based on the scenario at the beginning of the chapter:

   This is Annie. She's three years old. About 30 minutes ago her parents heard her groaning on her bed and came in to find her shaking uncontrollably. They state that the shaking lasted about 45 seconds. They also state that during the event, Annie's eyes were rolled back in her head and she was incontinent of urine. They say that after the event, Annie was limp and unresponsive for a few minutes. We arrived to find Annie with her eyes open but unresponsive. Since then her mental status has improved to awake and appropriate, though sleepy. Her ABCs appear normal. She has no allergies, takes no medications, but has recently had a fever. She last ate this morning. Her head-to-toe is normal except for incontinence of urine. Vital signs include normal mental status, an open airway, respirations of 24 and unlabored, a pulse of 120 strong and regular. She has normal capillary refill and hot, dry, pink skin. We have had Mom remove her sleeper to cool her off. We've administered high flow oxygen via mask until a minute or so ago when she ripped off the mask. Her status has remained unchanged over the past several minutes.

2. **CONDUCT THE TRANSFER OF CARE.**

3. **ASSIST IN EXTRICATION AND TRANSPORT.** For the most part, the child's parents or other caregivers should be allowed to ride in the back of the ambulance to the hospital. This will keep both the patient and the caregiver calmer and feeling more secure. The only exceptions would be if rescuers are performing resuscitation of the infant or child or if a parent is so out of control as to hamper the rescuer's ability to provide care.

CONCLUSION

Caring for ill or injured kids can be difficult and intimidating for the First Responder. They have unique differences that we must take into account when assessing and treating them. They're by no means "little adults." However, if you approach each pediatric call in a systematic, prioritized fashion, you'll find managing pediatric patients extremely rewarding. As one First Responder put it, "I like taking care of kids. They have so much of their lives to lose. I like making a difference so that they'll have all of their lives to live."

KEY TERMS

You may wish to use this list to review your understanding of key terms introduced in the chapter.

abuse the improper or excessive action that injures or causes harm.

neglect giving insufficient attention or respect to someone who has a claim to that attention and respect.

pediatric patients patients who are infants or children.

shaken baby syndrome the injuries associated with this condition occur when a caregiver picks up an infant or child and shakes him or her violently.

sudden infant death syndrome (SIDS) the sudden death of an otherwise normal and healthy infant that remains unexplained by the patient's history and a thorough autopsy.

APPLICATION QUESTIONS

You may wish to use these questions to review your understanding of the chapter. For answers with page references, see Appendix 2.

1. You've been dispatched to care for a three-year-old child experiencing a seizure. Upon your arrival, the seizure has stopped but the child remains unresponsive. What kind of emergency care should you provide?
2. You've encountered a three-month-old infant who is a victim of SIDS. The patient is cyanotic and appears to be dead and stiff. The parents, who are extremely upset, ask you to do something. How will you proceed?

APPENDIX 1 DEFIBRILLATION

INTRODUCTION

This appendix is an introduction to the *automatic external defibrillator*, or *AED*. It's not intended to be used to train personnel on how to use an AED. Rely on your local, regional, or state guidelines for AED training when preparing to use an AED in the field.

***By the end of the chapter, you should be able to:*†**

* Define defibrillation. (p. 411)
* Discuss the importance of early defibrillation in a cardiac arrest patient's chain of survival. (p. 412)
* Describe the different types of AEDs. (pp. 412-413)
* List the indications for defibrillating a patient. (p. 413)
* List the contraindications for defibrillating a patient. (p. 413)
* Discuss when it is appropriate to interrupt CPR when using the AED. (p. 414)
* List the operational steps to using the AED. (p. 414)
* Describe key steps necessary to ensure that the AED is used safely. (pp. 414-416)
* Describe the correct procedure for reassessing the cardiac arrest patient following defibrillation. (pp. 414-416)

DEFIBRILLATION

Defibrillation is the application of an electrical shock to the patient's heart. It's probably the single most important intervention for a patient in cardiac arrest. In the past several years its importance has grown immensely. In fact, out of the American Heart Association's 1992 Emergency Cardiac Care Conference came the following endorsement:

†Asterisks indicate material supplemental to the 1995 U.S. DOT "First Responder: National Standard Curriculum."

All personnel whose jobs require that they perform basic CPR [should] be trained to operate and be permitted to use defibrillators, particularly automated external defibrillators.

Of all patients who experience sudden cardiac death, it's estimated that 90% could benefit from early defibrillation. Studies have shown that all four elements of the chain of survival matter: early access, early CPR, early defibrillation, and early advanced life support (ALS). However, studies also indicate that if a patient is still in cardiac arrest after the first 10 minutes of resuscitation, the chances of saving that patient from irreversible brain damage are slim to none. The true cardiac arrest "saves" are the ones the patient survives with adequate brain function to lead a relatively normal life. So a true "save" depends on the initial actions of citizens and First Responders like you. Early CPR and defibrillation are key.

AUTOMATIC EXTERNAL DEFIBRILLATORS

When the heart's normal electrical conduction system is disrupted by a heart attack, chaotic electrical activity can result. The heart literally quivers, or *fibrillates,* in the patient's chest. In this condition, it can't pump any blood. This electrical rhythm is called *ventricular fibrillation.* Another lethal rhythm that can be defibrillated is called *pulseless ventricular tachycardia* (Figure A-1). If these conditions remain uncorrected, the patient will die in a matter of minutes.

Automatic external defibrillators (AEDs) are machines designed to provide the heart with an electric shock. The shock allows the

ECG TRACINGS

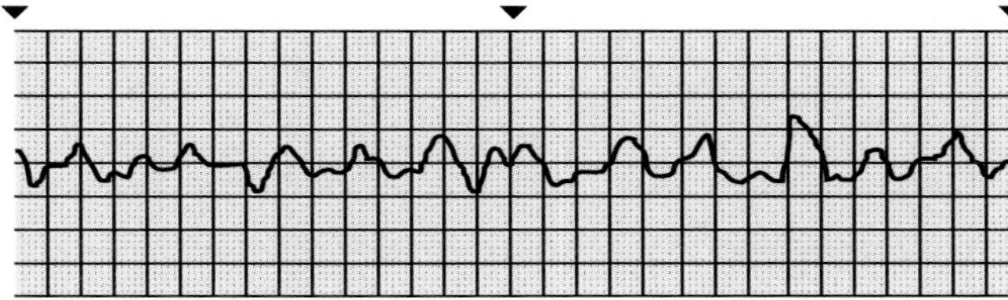

Ventricular Fibrillation

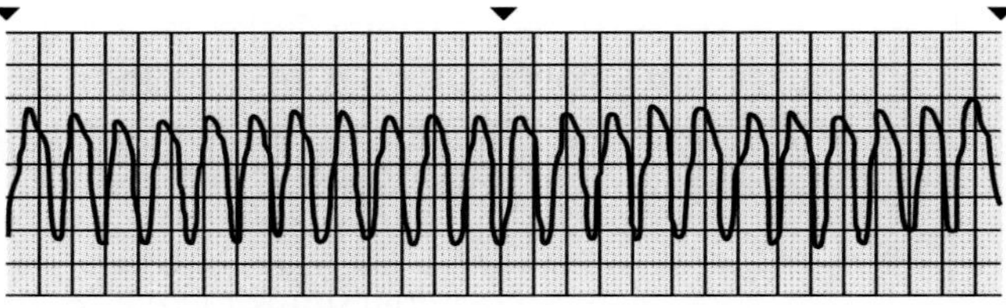

Ventricular Tachycardia

Figure A-1
Types of ECG tracings.

heart to reorganize its electrical activity so that it can again work effectively.

AEDs come in both fully automatic and semi-automatic models (Figure A-2). The fully automatic models analyze a patient's heart rhythm and shock the patient if needed, without the intervention of an operator. Semi-automated models analyze the patient's heart rhythms and suggest a shock if needed, but the shock itself must be administered by an operator.

INDICATIONS

The AED should be used only when a patient is breathless, pulseless, and doesn't show any obvious signs of death (rigor mortis, decapitation, and so on). The microprocessor in the AED is highly accurate. It will identify ventricular fibrillation and certain forms of ventricular tachycardia quickly. If the patient's heart has any other rhythm, the AED either won't shock the patient (the fully automated models) or it will advise not to shock (semi-automated models).

CONTRAINDICATIONS

A patient who has a pulse should not be defibrillated. Depending on the nature of the emergency, the AED may be applied but not turned on. Some local protocols allow rescuers to attach the AED to any unresponsive patient with signs of circulatory failure. This helps to reduce the time it'll take to shock the patient if the pulse is lost. Cardiac arrest "saves" are highest when defibrillation is provided immediately after cardiac arrest occurs. Follow your local AED protocols.

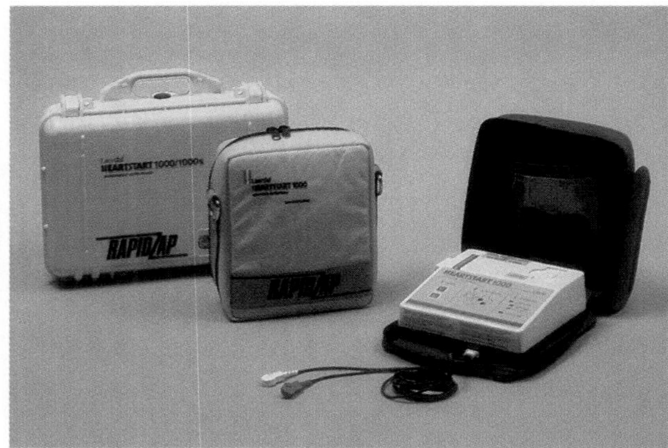

Figure A-2a
Fully automated AED.

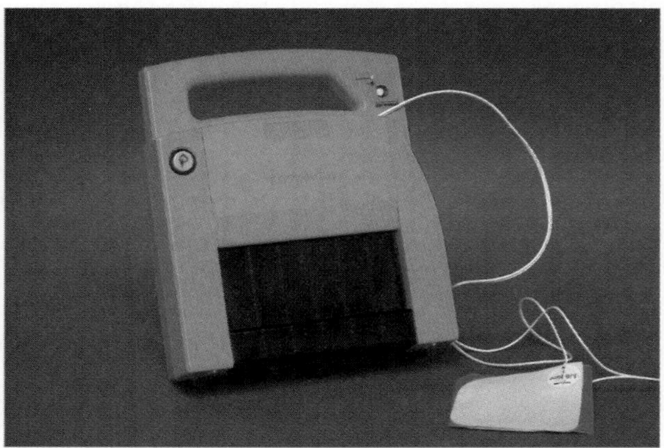

Figure A-2b
Semi-automated AED.

INTERRUPTIONS OF CPR

The AED is used in conjunction with CPR. It's necessary to interrupt CPR when the AED analyzes the patient's heart rhythm and delivers shocks. CPR may be stopped for up to 90 seconds if the AED advises that three consecutive shocks should be delivered. CPR buys you time while more effective therapies, such as defibrillation, are attempted. When it's appropriate, defibrillation is by far more effective than CPR in restoring a patient's pulse.

OPERATING AN AED

Your local, regional, or state EMS agency should have a specific protocol for applying and using the AED. Follow it. General guidelines for using an AED are (Figure A-3):

1. Ensure scene safety, and take BSI precautions.
2. Conduct an initial assessment. If CPR is in progress, stop it. Assure an open airway, breathlessness, and pulselessness. Prepare the AED. If you're part of a two-rescuer response, one rescuer should continue CPR while the other prepares the AED.
3. Attach the AED to the patient and turn on the power. Begin recording, if the AED has a recorder. If you're part of a two-rescuer response, stop CPR. Make sure no one is touching the patient. Push the "analyze" button to begin analysis of the patient's cardiac rhythm.

Warning *There must be no contact with the patient during analysis of the heart rhythm or during delivery of a shock. Before delivering a shock, say: "Clear the patient" or "I'm clear. You're clear. Everybody's clear." Always look to see that all rescuers have backed away from the patient before you deliver the shock.*

4. *If a shock is advised,* deliver a shock to the patient. Then reanalyze the heart rhythm. If the AED advises, deliver a second shock. If the AED advises, deliver a third shock. Then check for a pulse. If no pulse is found, perform one minute of CPR. Repeat the cycle of three shocks on scene, if indicated, and then transport.
5. *If no shock is advised,* check for a pulse.
   - *If a pulse is found,* see if the patient is breathing. If the patient is breathing, administer high flow oxygen by nonrebreather mask. If the patient is not breathing, ventilate with 100% oxygen if so equipped.

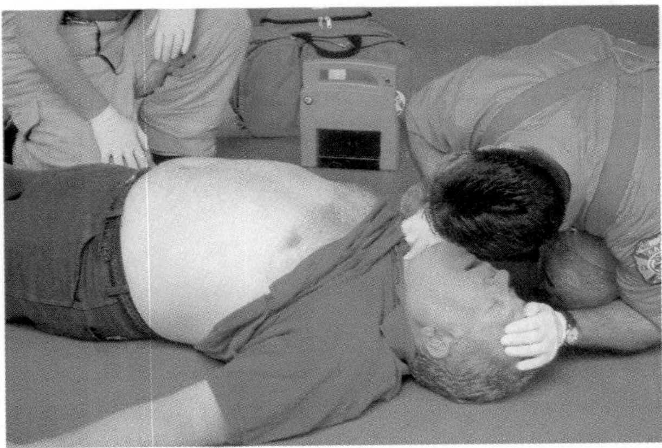

Figure A-3a
Verify breathlessness and pulselessness.

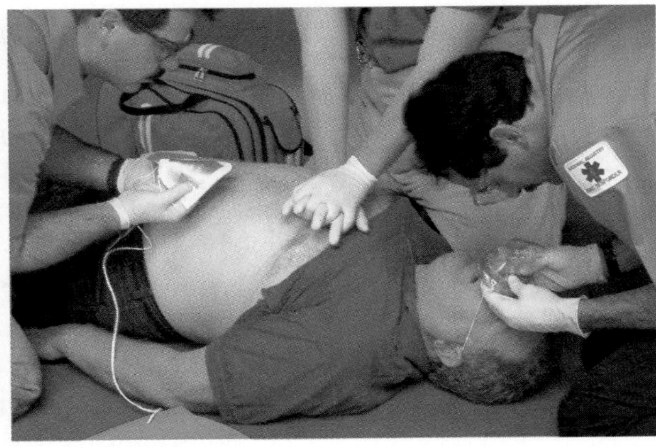

Figure A-3b
Prepare the AED while another rescuer continues CPR.

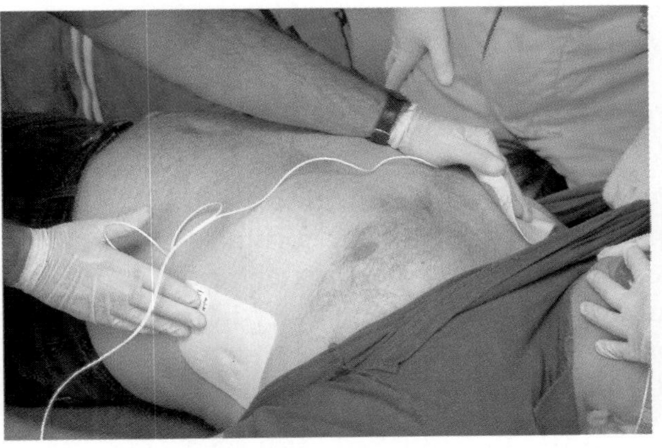

Figure A-3c
Position the electrodes properly.

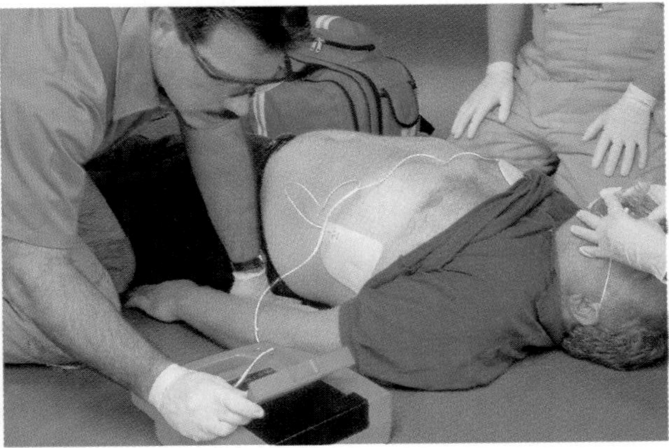

Figure A-3d
Turn on the AED. If CPR is being performed, stop it.

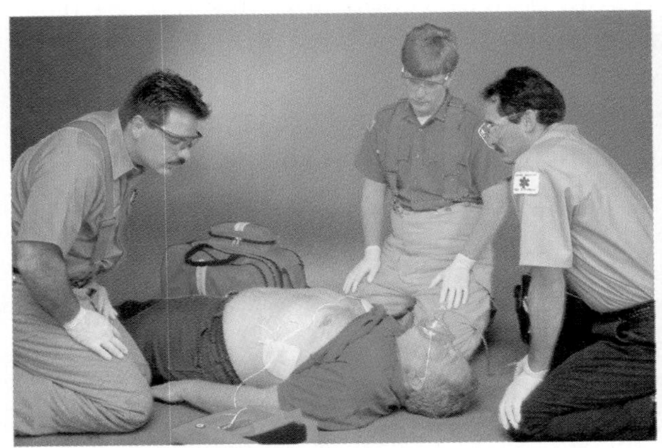

Figure A-3e
Back away from the patient while rhythm is analyzed.

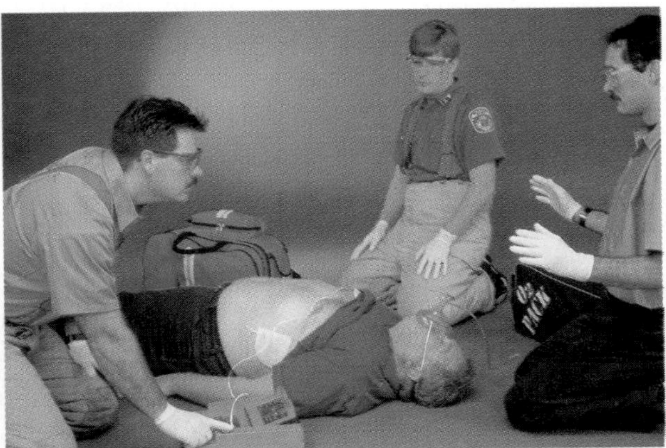

Figure A-3f
Stand clear and provide the shock.

- *If no pulse is found,* perform one minute of CPR. Analyze the patient's rhythm a second time. If the AED advises to shock the patient, do so using the three shock pattern listed above. If not, perform a third minute of CPR, check the rhythm, and shock if indicated. If a shock is not indicated, resume CPR and prepare for transport.

If you're a single rescuer (not part of a two-rescuer response) and equipped with an AED, the AED should be used prior to CPR. Activate EMS only after a "no shock" advisement, after the patient's pulse returns, after three shocks, or when help arrives.

When additional basic life support (BLS) or advanced life support (ALS) personnel arrive on scene, advise them of your assessment and treatment, including the number of shocks delivered and your patient's response.

Remember *Follow your local guidelines and the manufacturer's directions for use of the AED model you use in your EMS system.*

Additional points to remember when operating an AED:

- Reduce the chances of accidentally shocking another rescuer. Avoid defibrillating a wet patient. Water conducts electricity very well. Remove the patient from the water, and dry him or her as best you can. Metal also conducts electricity well. The AED operator should ensure that no one is touching metal and the patient at the same time.
- The AED should not be used on children under 12 years of age nor on patients weighing less than 90 pounds.
- Never forget the initial assessment.
- Remember to *assess* your patient's condition, *intervene* with CPR and defibrillation, and *reassess* to determine if your interventions were successful. Reassess frequently. If your patient regains a pulse, maintain the airway and breathing. Keep the AED attached to the patient in case he or she again becomes pulseless.

Practice AED operation on a regular basis. All EMS systems have guidelines. In addition, it's critical that you regularly maintain your AED. The most common cause of AED failure is improper battery maintenance and replacement. Follow the manufacturer's maintenance schedule. Complete a checklist (Figure A-4) every day to verify that the unit has been thoroughly checked and is ready for use.

AUTOMATED DEFIBRILLATORS: OPERATOR'S SHIFT CHECKLIST

Date: ____________ **Shift:** ______________________________ **Location:** ______________________________

Mfr/Model No.: ______________________ **Serial No. or Facility ID No.:** ______________________________

At the beginning of each shift, inspect the unit. Indicate whether all requirements have been met. Note any corrective actions taken. Sign the form.

	Okay as found	Corrective Action/Remarks
1. Defibrillator Unit		
Clean no spills, clear of objects on top, casing intact		
2. Cables/Connectors		
a. Inspect for cracks, broken wire, or damage b. Connectors engage securely		
3. Supplies		
a. Two sets of pads in sealed packages, within expiration date b. Hand towel c. Scissors d. Razor * e. Alcohol wipes * f. Monitoring electrodes *g. Spare charged battery *h. Adequate ECG paper *i. Manual override module, key or card *j. Cassette tape, memory module, and/or event card plus spares		
4. Power Supply		
a. Battery-powered units (1) Verify fully charged battery in place (2) Spare charged battery available (3) Follow appropriate battery rotation schedule per manufacturer's recommendations b. AC/Battery backup units (1) Plugged into live outlet to maintain battery charge (2) Test on battery power and reconnect to line power		
5. Indicators/*ECG Display		
* a. Remove cassette tape, memory module, and/or event card b. Power on display c. Self-test ok * d. Monitor display functional *e. "Service" message display off *f. Battery charging; low battery light off g. Correct time displayed — set with dispatch center		
6. ECG Recorder		
a. Adequate ECG paper b. Recorder prints		
7. Charge/Display Cycle		
* a. Disconnect AC plug — battery backup units b. Attach to simulator c. Detects, charges and delivers shock for "VF" d. Responds correctly to non-shockable rhythms *e. Manual override functional f. Detach from simulator *g. Replace cassette tape, module, and/or memory card		
8. *Pacemaker		
a. Pacer output cable intact b. Pacer pads present (set of two) c. Inspect per manufacturer's operational guidelines		
☐ **Major problem(s) identified** **(OUT OF SERVICE)**		

****Applicable only if the unit has this supply or capability**

Signature: ______________________________

Figure A-4

An example of an operator's checklist.

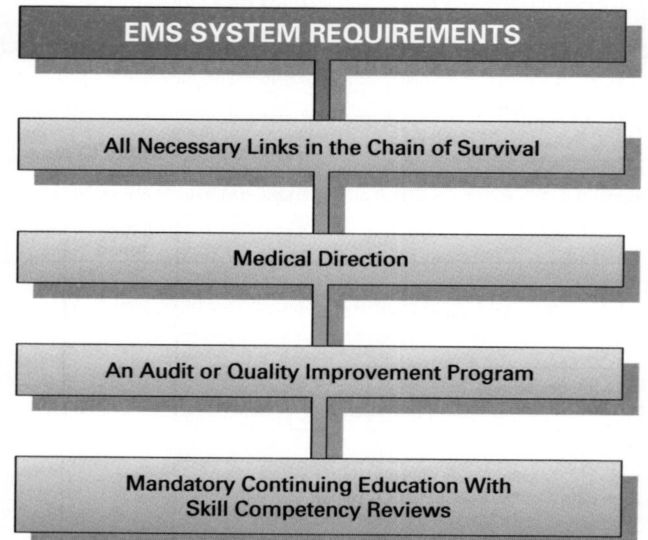

Figure A-5
EMS system requirements for AED use.

Note that your EMS system's medical director or an appointed designee must review every event in which the AED is used (Figure A-5). Usually, this is accomplished through written reports, a review of voice and EKG recordings, and/or solid-state memory modules and magnetic tape recordings stored in the device.

CONCLUSION

The American Heart Association statement quoted at the beginning of this appendix states that you should be using an AED if you're performing CPR as part of your job. Early defibrillation is the single most important factor in whether or not a patient's pulse is restored following cardiac arrest. The key to successful defibrillation is:

- *Assess* your patient to quickly determine if defibrillation is indicated.
- *Intervene* with sets of three shocks followed by a minute of CPR.
- *Reassess* your patient for any changes.

Work to bring this life-saving piece of equipment to your service if you're not currently using it. The introduction of the AED has saved many lives that otherwise would have been lost. EMS experts nationally believe that the adoption of an AED program is time and money well spent.

APPENDIX 2 ANSWERS TO APPLICATION QUESTIONS

Answers below are followed by page numbers, which refer to text where relevant concepts are taught.

CHAPTER 1

1. Your first task in any emergency is to *assure scene safety*. If you can't, you must notify EMS dispatch immediately and ask for help. Don't enter the scene until trained personnel have made it safe. (p. 6)

2. As a First Responder, you will assure scene safety, gain access to the patient, assess and treat the patient for life-threatening problems, and assist more highly trained EMS personnel—such as the EMT-Paramedic. The EMT-Paramedic will provide much more advanced medical care. (pp. 5, 7)

CHAPTER 2

1. To convince another EMS worker to attend a CISD meeting, you might point out the following: critical incident stress is a normal stress response to extremely abnormal circumstances. To help avoid "burnout," she could talk about the call with the same people who were there working with her. Remind her that everyone will be openly discussing their feelings, fears, and reactions. And that everything said is absolutely confidential. (pp. 13-15)

2. Ways to stay fit for handling stress include: eating right, as well as reducing intake of sugar, fat, caffeine, and alcohol; getting enough sleep; exercising regularly; encouraging family support by methods such as shutting off the EMS beeper when with the family; reducing stress at work by methods such as reassignment to a low-volume area or to another shift; participating in critical incident stress services offered by your EMS system. (pp. 13-15)

CHAPTER 3

1. It's not enough for the caregiver to tell you the patient should not be resuscitated. It's necessary for you to see the actual written document. In this case you should start life-saving emergency care. However, you might also consider contacting on-line medical direction to get their help. (pp. 22-25)

2. Anything the patient tells you about his medical history is confidential. The only other people who should get that information at the scene are the EMS workers who take over care of the patient. (pp. 19-20)

3. It's your job to make sure the patient understands the risks of refusing care. If you have done all you can and the patient still refuses care, call medical direction for instructions. (p. 21)

CHAPTER 4

1. In general a child's bones are more flexible than an adult's. Though they are less likely to break, they provide less protection to the organs that lie beneath. Therefore, the adult will be more likely to have broken bones in the chest and less injury to the organs underneath. The child may have fewer broken bones, but more internal injuries to the organs. (p. 39)

2. Immobilize the cervical spine first. Remember that the cervical spine is the most poorly supported part of the spinal column. Together with the additional weight of the head, this can lead to a higher incidence of injury. (p. 39)

3. Choose to assess her mental status. Remember that the brain is very sensitive to drops in the oxygen supply. So mental status makes an excellent indicator of how well the respiratory and circulatory systems are working. (p. 37)

CHAPTER 5

1. First thing's first. Protect yourself by putting on the appropriate personal protective equipment. Then assist your coworker so that he can glove up. After the call, you also might want to find out why he didn't choose to wear gloves. Emphasize that he has jeopardized his own health. Help him to figure out how he'll handle future calls so that he doesn't risk an exposure like that again. (pp. 46-48)

2. Since childbirth can involve exposure to large amounts of bodily fluids, you will want to be fully covered. Wear protective gloves, goggles, a surgical mask, and gown. (pp. 46-48)

CHAPTER 6

1. An emergency move may be made when the rescuers are unable to provide life-saving care to a patient because of his or her location or position. So, this patient qualifies for an emergency move. (pp. 54-55)

2. Don't move the patient. She has no life threats, there are no scene hazards, and she has neck pain, which could indicate a injury to the spine. More advanced EMS workers need to be called to extricate and evaluate her. (pp. 54-55)

3. You need to come to agreement on the following: What type of move will you use? Who will do what and in what order will it be done? In what direction and to what location will you move the patient? Who will lead the move; that is, who will signal and count-off? (pp. 52-53)

CHAPTER 7

1. Gentle honesty is the best policy. You might try, "I'm so sorry, but your baby has passed away. The baby's signs indicate that it would do no good to try to resuscitate him. I've so very sorry." The next step is to let the parents express their feelings. Give them the information they ask for, if you can do so confidently. Ask if there's anything you can do to help, if there are family or friends you can call. Don't be afraid to just be with them as they grieve. Above all else, stay alert for potential violence. (pp. 66-68)

2. You may want to try a gentle approach, reassuring the patient from a distance that you are concerned about him and just want to check to be sure he is safe and uninjured. Use slow movements. Speak quietly. Be alert. Call the police for help at your first suspicion of violence. (p. 70)

CHAPTER 8

1. You must stay safe if you mean to help this patient. So stay put! The scene has not yet been secured by law enforcement, and you absolutely must wait for their "all clear" before entering the scene. (pp. 86-87)

2. Flares, barricades, even rescue vehicles can be effective deterrents. (p. 86)

3. The priority level for each patient is (pp. 90-91):

   a. Second priority is given to major painful, swollen, deformed extremities.

   b. Third (lowest) priority is given to dead patients.

   c. First (highest) priority is given to airway and breathing difficulties.

   d. Third (lowest) priority is given to minor soft-tissue injuries.

CHAPTER 9

1. This patient is alert, but he doesn't remember the accident, is repeating himself, and seems confused. (pp. 000-000)

2. This is a low priority patient. She doesn't appear to be in distress. Her skin appears to be normal, and she is well enough to socialize. She can be examined further at the scene. (p. 106)

CHAPTER 10

1. Conduct a scene size-up. Take all proper BSI precautions. Form a general impression, assess responsiveness, and then assess airway and breathing as outlined in Chapter 10. (Chapters 8 and 9 plus pp. 112-113)

2. Conduct a scene size-up. Take all proper BSI precautions. Form a general impression, assess responsiveness, and assess airway and breathing as outlined in Chapter 10. Since this is a trauma patient, be sure to immobilize the spine and use a jaw-thrust maneuver to open the airway. (Chapters 8 and 9 plus pp. 112-115)

3. The child may have a partial airway obstruction with adequate air exchange. Don't do anything except keep the child calm and activate the EMS system. (pp. 135-136)

CHAPTER 11

1. Your first action should be to reassess the child to confirm that she isn't breathing and has no pulse. It's not uncommon for CPR to be started on patients that aren't in cardiac arrest. (pp. 154-155)

2. Blue is bad! Reassess, reassess, reassess! If this patient does have a pulse, it's possible that the other First Responder hadn't opened the airway or isn't providing adequate ventilations. Reposition the airway, assess breathing, and ventilate. Look for the chest to rise and fall. Then assess the patient's pulse to see if chest compressions also are required. (Chapters 8 and 9 plus p. 152)

CHAPTER 12

1. Disagree! This patient is in shock and can use all the oxygen he or she can get. If you have oxygen and are trained to use it, always apply high flow oxygen to all of your patients who show signs and symptoms of shock. (pp. 164-166)

2. The "time rule" says that time is a shock patient's most precious commodity and that the longer the patient is in shock, the more likely it is that he or she will die. This rules serves to focus on identifying and treating life threats, and then rapid transport to an appropriate medical facility. (p. 166)

CHAPTER 13

1. While it's true that the physical exam and treatment step is important, it clearly has a lower priority than the treatment of life threats. This First Responder has an inflexible approach that could lead him to making a mistake when he determines priorities for his patient. (p. 169)

2. Stop everything and reassess your patient's level of responsiveness, airway, breathing, and circulation. Remember to recheck a patient's ABCs every time you observe a significant status change. (p. 177)

3. No! You have enough information about this patient's status. Your time would be much better spent reassessing his ABCs and treating him for shock. (pp. 180-181)

CHAPTER 14

1. While reassessing all of the patient's vital signs is important, level of responsiveness would be the top vital sign to monitor. Remember that reassessment should in large part be based on your patient's chief complaint. This patient's level of responsiveness was your top finding. It's also the best gauge of the

severity of a head injury. The other vital signs listed are important but not nearly as important as level of responsiveness. (pp. 189-190)

2. Repeat your initial assessment immediately! Remember that any time your patient has a significant status change you must "go back to home base" and assess the patient all over again, starting with level of responsiveness, airway, breathing, and circulation. (pp. 189-190)

CHAPTER 15

1. Henry is an 87-year-old male who is complaining of head and chest pain. He is a low priority patient and appears to be awake and alert. He has a patent airway; normal, unlabored breathing; a strong radial pulse; normal skin color, temperature, and moisture. Henry was stepping up onto the curb when he fell forward, striking his head and chest on the sidewalk. He has a large bruise to his forehead and scrapes and bruises to his chest and hands. He has no allergies to medications. Henry takes medication for high blood pressure, arthritis, and Parkinson's disease. He has had a stroke and a heart attack in the past year. Henry last ate this morning. We are holding manual stabilization of his spine and have bandaged his abrasions. (p. 194)

2. This patient has a compromised airway. Nothing else matters if we can't get it cleared! I have been assessing and managing this patient's airway, breathing, and circulation and consider this to be a much higher priority than a physical exam. (pp. 195-196)

CHAPTER 16

1. - Check the scene to see if it's safe.
   - Take BSI precautions.
   - Form a general impression of the patient.
   - Assess her mental status.
   - Check her airway, breathing, and circulation status, and apply oxygen at this time.
   - Gather a SAMPLE history.

- Complete a head-to-toe exam.
- Take vital signs.
- Repeat the initial assessment.
- Complete a patient hand-off. (Chapters 8-15)

2. Because of the change in status, you should immediately complete an initial assessment. (p. 205)

CHAPTER 17

1. a. Make sure the patient's airway is open.
   b. Assure the adequacy of the patient's breathing. If possible, administer high-flow oxygen.
   c. If the patient has low blood pressure, place him or her in the shock position.
   d. Comfort and reassure the patient.
   e. Do not allow the patient to move unnecessarily.
   f. Assist in packaging and transporting the patient as requested. (pp. 216-221)

2. Patients who have been prescribed medications should follow their physician's directions, which are written on the prescription label. If the doctor has instructed the patient to take the medication in the event of chest pain, then the patient may take it according to the doctor's orders. You are not allowed to administer this medication to the patient. Follow all local protocols! (p. 219)

CHAPTER 18

1. Lucille required immediate intervention. She needed to sit up, and she needed high-flow oxygen. Ed should have focused on the initial assessment and treatment of her shortness of breath, not on her physical exam. (pp. 224-225)

2. This is Lucille. She is 72 years old. Lucille's complaining of severe shortness of breath. She says that she also feels some chest tightness. Lucille is a high priority patient. She's awake, but tired. Her airway is open. Lucille has labored, rapid breathing at 32 breaths per minutes and marked accessory muscle use. Her pulse is rapid and strong at 120 beats per

minute. We have Lucille sitting up, and we're administering oxygen at 15 liters per minute by mask. There has been no change in her status over the past 10 minutes or so. (Chapter 15 and pp. 223, 224-225, 233)

CHAPTER 19

1. Under no circumstances should you give anything by mouth to a patient who can't administer it himself. Giving the patient orange juice might be a good idea if the patient could hold the glass and drink it himself. Your priorities for this patient should be early activation of the EMS system; aggressive treatment for airway, breathing, and circulation problems; continuous reassessment; and an accurate patient history and physical exam. Focus on the patient's ABCs and protecting him from injury. (pp. 242, 244)

2. Activate the EMS system. Protect the patient from injury by moving objects away from the patient. Assess the adequacy of the airway. Don't force anything into the patient's mouth during the seizure. Provide high flow oxygen, if you're so equipped. Ventilate if necessary. (p. 239)

CHAPTER 20

1. Patients who describe a history of vomiting should be considered infectious. Always wear gloves with these patients. You may want to consider wearing protective eye wear and a gown if you suspect that patient may vomit again. (Chapter 5)

2. a. Activate the EMS system.

   b. Treat any airway, breathing, or circulation problem.

   c. Position the patient in the shock position. Keep the patient warm, and provide nothing by mouth.

   d. Administer oxygen to the patient if you are trained and equipped to do so. (Chapter 12 and pp. 248-253)

CHAPTER 21

1. What kind of medication is in the bottle? How many pills were in the bottle? How long has the child been playing with the bottle? Is it possible that the child got into other medications or poisons as well? Is the child behaving normally? (pp. 257-258, 262)

2. Immediately complete an initial assessment and treat the patient's airway, breathing, and circulation as necessary. Attempt to gather as much history as possible regarding the patient's drug use. (p. 258)

CHAPTER 22

1. This patient may be showing a rapid progression of airway and breathing problems. Since he is already showing signs of an airway obstruction, place the patient on high flow oxygen if you can and be prepared to manage his airway with ventilations if necessary. (Chapter 10 and pp. 272-276)

2. If the patient is having respiratory distress, she'll probably be most comfortable sitting upright. It's unlikely that she'll allow you to place her in a shock position. However, be prepared to reposition her if she beings to feel dizzy or is unable to manage her upright position. (Chapter 10 and pp. 272-276)

CHAPTER 23

1. Disagree! This patient will require internal warming at a hospital. There's no way that you'll be able to warm this patient in the field. Your top priority is to ventilate this patient and to keep him from losing any more body heat. (Chapter 10 and pp. 280-282, 290)

2. The first thing to do for a seizing patient is to protect him from injury. As soon as his seizure stops, roll this patient onto his side to help maintain his airway. Suction if necessary and repeat your entire initial assessment. (Chapter 19 and pp. 284-285)

CHAPTER 24

1. Transport. Given the frequency and interval of contractions, it appears that this patient has some time before delivery. Since there are no signs of crowning, you need not consider this an imminent delivery. However, depending on how many children the patient has had in the past, things can still progress rapidly. So assess the contractions frequently and be prepared to deliver if necessary. (pp. 295-296)

2. The patient may be having a miscarriage, or spontaneous abortion. Watch for signs of tissue discharge from the vagina and continually assess the amount of blood loss. Provide

emotional support for the patient as she will likely be upset over the problem. Send any tissue that passes or evidence of blood loss to the hospital with the patient. Treat for shock as needed. (p. 302)

CHAPTER 25

1. Yes. The patient hasn't only made statements about suicide, he's also made a physical attempt at suicide. Talk to the patient and try to gain his cooperation. If you're not successful and the patient still refuses transport, you'll need to request assistance from law enforcement. Make contact with medical control to confirm that you can transport the patient against his will. (p. 315)
2. No! You should wait for law enforcement to arrive and secure the scene. Many EMS rescuers are injured because they enter scenes that are unsafe. You'll not be able to render aid to the patient if you become a victim yourself. (p. 315)

CHAPTER 26

1. The rescuer needs to get his priorities straight. The patient is a high priority trauma patient who needs support for his airway, breathing, and circulation. Splinting can wait. (Chapter 9 and pp. 324-326)
2. Complete the physical exam and treatment and then the ongoing assessment and treatment. (pp. 329-331)
3. The greater the time that elapses from the moment of injury to definitive care, which is often surgery, the greater the likelihood of permanent disability and death. Time is the big killer of critical trauma patients. (p. 323)

CHAPTER 27

1. This patient's spine must take a back seat to his airway in this instance. Spinal protection is critical, to be sure, but it doesn't rate higher than maintaining a patient's airway. (p. 350)
2. You may want to start by saying that you're pleased he can feel all of his fingers and toes, but even so, he still could have an injury to his spine. Tell him that the fact that he rolled his

car, has a bruise to his head, and a stiff neck are reasons enough to suspect a spine injury. The signs and symptom of this injury may be masked by the alcohol. He risks permanent injury, even death, by refusing to allow you to stabilize his spine. If he still refuses, carefully document the call. Make sure other rescuers witness the refusal, and call your medical director. (Chapter 3 and pp. 337-338, 348)

CHAPTER 28

1. This patient's extremity fractures should be stabilized by strapping them to a backboard. This patient is in critical condition, and there's no time to splint each leg. (p. 361)
2. Have the patient cradle the injured arm with his good arm. Often the simplest splinting method is the best. (p. 364)

CHAPTER 29

1. An open wound to the chest can cause a severe compromise of his breathing. Life threats are managed as they are recognized. Treat this injury during your initial assessment. (pp. 379, 387)
2. In addition to direct pressure, you can elevate the arm and apply pressure to the brachial artery. These three methods—direct pressure, elevation, and pressure points—are highly effective in controlling even the most severe external bleeding. (Chapter 12 and pp. 376-377)

CHAPTER 30

1. In your care of the patient, it's important to calm and reassure both the patient and the parents. While you're waiting for the arrival of an ambulance: protect the patient from further injury, maintain an open airway, provide oxygen if you are equipped to do so, and ventilate if necessary. If there's no possibility of spine injury, place the patient in the recovery position. Be prepared to suction. (Chapter 19 and pp. 400-401)
2. If the patient is obviously dead, attempting resuscitation may be offering the false hope to the parents that the infant will recover. It's more important that you provide care to the parents under these circumstances. Provide grief support, as the

parents will obviously be experiencing severe emotional distress, remorse, and guilt.

Be careful not to make any comments that might suggest blame to the parents. For example, don't tell the parents what they should or should not have done prior to your arrival. Don't leave the parents alone. Call for the most appropriate EMS resources for managing the scene and supporting the parent's grief. Also be aware that people who are experiencing extreme grief may occasionally become violent. Assess the parents or other caregivers for safety. (p. 401)

INDEX